Advanced Clinical Practice
at a Glance

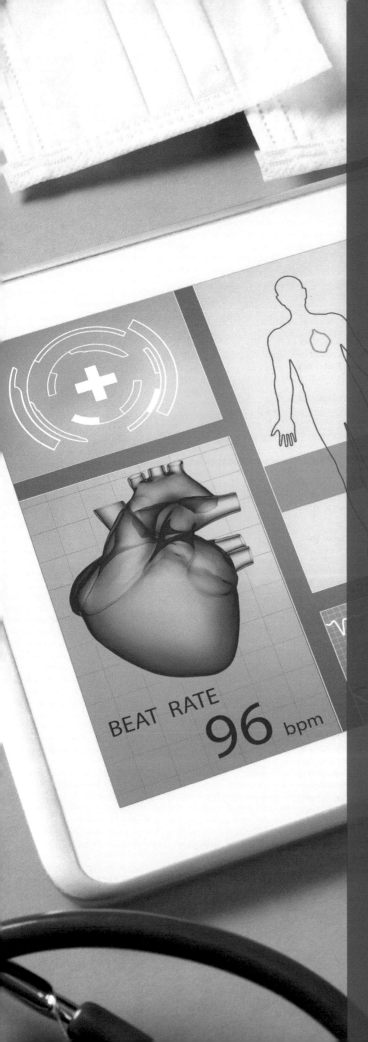

Advanced Clinical Practice

at a Glance

Edited by

Barry Hill,
MSc AP, PGCAP, BSc (Hons), DipHE/OA Dip,
SFHEA, TEFL, NMC RN, RNT/TCH, V300.
Assistant Professor and Lead for Nursing
Midwifery and Health Employability,
Northumbria University

Sadie Diamond Fox,
MCP ACCP, BSc(Hons) RN, PGC AHP, NMP
(V300), FHEA
Advanced Critical Care Practitioner (FICM
member) and Assistant Professor in Advanced
Critical Care Practice, ACP and ACCP Lead,
Northumbria University

Series Editor: Ian Peate

WILEY Blackwell

Registered Offices
John Wiley & Sons, Inc., 111 River Street, Hoboken, NJ 07030, USA
John Wiley & Sons Ltd, The Atrium, Southern Gate, Chichester, West Sussex, PO19 8SQ, UK

Editorial Office
9600 Garsington Road, Oxford, OX4 2DQ, UK

For details of our global editorial offices, customer services, and more information about Wiley products visit us at www.wiley.com.

Wiley also publishes its books in a variety of electronic formats and by print-on-demand. Some content that appears in standard print versions of this book may not be available in other formats.

Library of Congress Cataloging-in-Publication Data applied for
Paperback ISBN 9781119833284

Cover Design: Wiley
Cover Image: © Khakimullin Aleksandr/Shutterstock

Set in MinionPro 9.5/11.5 by Straive, Pondicherry, India

Printed and bound by CPI Group (UK) Ltd, Croydon, CR0 4YY

C9781119833284_220524

Dedication

This book is dedicated to my friends and family, in particular my dad Ray Hill and friend Helen Jackson who passed away in 2021. I will love you for eternity. Thanks to my co-editor Sadie Diamond-Fox and the Wiley team for your support, and all the book contributors for sharing your knowledge

BH

To my 'cheerleaders'; my friends and family, in particular my husband, Alexandra Gatehouse and my co-editor Barry Hill

SDF

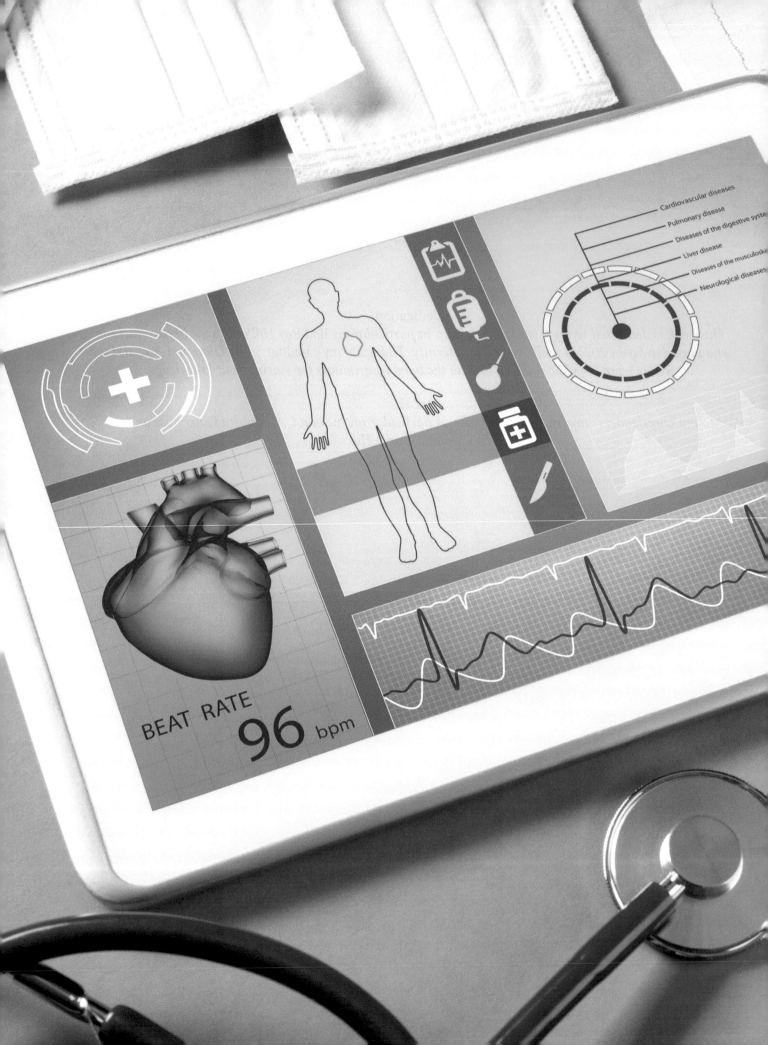

Contents

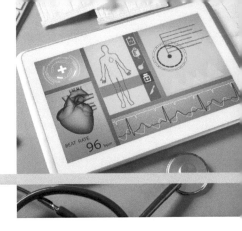

Contributors

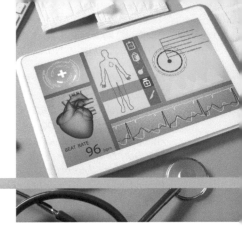

Clare Allabyrne *Chapter 11*
Associate Professor and Programme Lead for Advanced Clinical Practice Mental Health, London Southbank University

Jill Bentley *Chapters 37, 38*
Lecturer in Advanced Clinical Practice, Non-Medical Prescribing and Adult Nursing, and Advanced Critical Care Practitioner (FICM member), Salford Royal Foundation Trust

Lee Berry *Chapter 25*
Advanced Critical Care Practitioner (FICM member), Southampton General Hospital

Helen Bone *Chapter 17*
Advanced Critical Care Practitioner (FICM member), James Cook University Hospital

Roberta Borg *Chapter 8*
Advanced Critical Care Practitioner (FICM member)

Natalie Brady *Chapter 51*
Occupational Therapist and Advanced Clinical Practitioner in Frailty, Warrington and Halton Teaching Hospitals NHS Trust

Phil Broadhurst *Chapters 47, 50*
Advanced Critical Care Practitioner (FICM member), Stockport NHS Foundation Trust

Emma Bryant *Chapter 9*
Advanced Critical Care Practitioner (FICM member), Oxford University Hospitals NHS Foundation Trust

Ashton Burden Selvaraj *Chapter 19*
Trainee Advanced Critical Care Practitioner University Hospital Coventry & Warwickshire and Intensive Care Society equality, diversity and inclusion group collaborator

Steph Burrows *Chapter 35*
Advanced Critical Care Practitioner (FICM member), Nottingham University Hospitals NHS Trust

Mark Cannan *Chapter 34*
Advanced Critical Care Practitioner, North Cumbria Integrated Care NHS Foundation Trust

Enrique Castro-Sanchez *Chapter 43*
Associate Professor in Infection Prevention and Improvement, University of West London

Eddie Chaplin *Chapter 11*
Director of Research and Enterprise at London South Bank University and Head of the Scientific Committee of the European Association of Mental Health in Intellectual Disability

Karen Chivers *Chapter 14*
Consultant Nurse and Advanced Clinical Practitioner, Frimley Health NHS Foundation Trust

Esther Clift *Chapter 32*
Consultant at Southern Health NHS Foundation Trust, visiting lecturer at University of Winchester, clinical advisor for Wessex Academic Health Science Network, and Professional Adviser for NHSE&I

Rebecca Connolly *Chapter 10*
Advanced Clinical Practitioner at United Lincolnshire Hospitals NHS Trust and Nottingham University Hospitals NHS Trust, and Senior Lecturer at University of Lincoln

Hannah Conway *Chapters 23, 26*
Advanced Critical Care Practitioner, Assistant Professor of Advanced Clinical Practice, University of Nottingham, Intensive Care Society (ICS) FUSIC and Education Committee Member, Deputy Chair Advanced Practitioners in Critical Care Professional Advisory Group (APCC), Co-Chair Advanced Clinical Practitioners Academic Network (ACPAN) and PRORVnet

Stuart Cox *Chapter 34*
Advanced Critical Care Practitioner (FICM member), University Hospital Southampton NHS Foundation Trust and Dorset & Somerset Air Ambulance

Sarah Curr *Chapter 42*
Lecturer in Nursing Education, King's College London

Jo Delrée *Chapter 11*
Associate Professor and Head of Division Mental Health and Learning Disability Nursing, London South Bank University

Joanna De Souza *Chapters 42, 52*
Senior Lecturer in Nursing, King's College London

Sadie Diamond Fox *Chapters 1, 5, 7, 8, 12, 16, 17, 20, 42, 49, 52, 55*
Advanced Critical Care Practitioner (FICM member) at Newcastle upon Tyne Hospitals NHS Foundation Trust, Assistant Professor in Advanced Critical Care Practice at Northumbria University, Council Member, Education Committee Member and Chair of the Advanced Practitioners in Critical Care Professional Advisory Group (APCC PAG) at the Intensive Care Society (ICS) and Co-Chair at Advanced Clinical Practitioners Academic Network (ACPAN)

Leanne Dolman *Chapter 52*
Lecturer in Nursing, King's College London

Brigitta Fazzini *Chapter 44*
Advanced Critical Care Practitioner, Royal London Hospital, Deputy Chair of Intensive Care Society (ICS), Advanced Practitioner in Critical Care (APCC) Professional Advisory Group (PAG), and Co-Chair of Advanced Clinical Practitioners Academic Network (ACPAN)

Jill Featherstone *Chapter 30*
National Professional Development Specialist in Medical Education for Organ and Tissue Donation and Transplant, NHS Blood and Transplant

Helen Francis-Wegner *Chapter 2*
Lecturer in Advanced Clinical Practice (FHEA), University of Plymouth, and Advanced Clinical Practitioner in Emergency Medicine (RCEM Member), Royal Cornwall Hospitals Trust.

Alexandra Gatehouse *Chapters 16, 20, 31, 55*
Advanced Critical Care Practitioner (FICM member), Newcastle upon Tyne Hospitals NHS Foundation Trust

Kirstin Geer *Chapter 34*
Advanced Critical Care Practitioner (FICM Member), North Cumbria Integrated Care NHS Foundation Trust

Daniel Gill *Chapter 30*
Advanced Critical Care Practitioner, Northern Care Alliance

Jo-Anne Gilroy *Chapter 41*
Advanced Critical Care Practitioner (FICM member) and Director of HEE London Advanced Critical Care Programme

Fiona Greenfield *Chapter 28*
Speciality Lead of Pleural Services (BTS & UK Pleural Society member, Northwest Anglia NHS Foundation Trust

Lucy Halpin *Chapters 4, 5*
Advanced Critical Care Practice and Program Director in Thames Valley, Advanced Critical Care Practitioner (mFICM)

Jo Hardy *Chapter 29*
Advanced Physiotherapy Practitioner in Critical Care, Leeds Teaching Hospitals NHS Trust.

Matt Harris *Chapter 25*
Senior Advanced Critical Care Practitioner (FICM member), University Hospital Southampton NHS Foundation Trust

Alex Hemsley *Chapter 24*
Trainee Advanced Clinical Practitioner and Emergency Care (RCEM member), Royal Victoria Infirmary at Newcastle upon Tyne Hospitals NHS Foundation Trust

Barry Hill *Chapters 5, 13, 15, 20, 21, 22*
Director of Education (Employability), Programme Leader and Assistant Professor, Northumbria University

Rebecca Hoskins *Chapter 40*
Consultant Nurse in Advanced Practice and NMP lead, University Hospitals Bristol and Weston NHS Foundation Trust, Senior Lecturer and Faculty Strategic Lead Advanced Practice, University of the West of England Bristol

Rachael Hosznyak *Chapter 54*
Supervision and Assessment Lead for Frailty, Rehabilitation and Social Work and Advanced Practitioner in Urgent Care specialising in Frailty at Health Education England, and Registered Paramedic

Robin Hyde *Chapter 46*
Assistant Professor (Children's Nursing) and Advanced Paediatric Nurse Practitioner and Programme Lead in Children's Nursing, University of Northumbria, Newcastle

Jo Jennings *Chapter 33*
Advanced Clinical Practitioner Simulation and Clinical Skills Lead, South Warwickshire NHS Foundation Trust, Assistant Professor in Advancing Practice, Coventry University, and Advanced Practice Development Lead for Older Adults, Health Education England

Maureen Jersby *Chapter 53*
Programme Leader in Advance Clinical Practice and Assistant Professor in Adult Nursing, Northumbria University

Timothy Kuhn *Chapter 27*
Advanced Critical Care Practitioner (FICM member) and Senior Lead Nurse in Critical Care and Critical Care Outreach Team, Croydon Health Services NHS Trust

Laura Elliott *Chapter 12*
Programme Lead Advanced Clinical Practice Apprenticeship and Senior lecturer (FHEA) Advanced Practice, University of Northampton

Janine Mair *Chapter 39*
Acute Care Nurse Consultant, East Kent Hospital University NHS Foundation Trust, and Visiting Senior

Lecturer in Advanced Practice, Canterbury Christ Church University

Tracey Maxfield Chapter 29
Trainee Advanced Clinical Practitioner in Acute Medicine, Airedale NHS Foundation Trust

Caroline McCrea Chapter 18
Advanced Critical Care Practitioner (FICM Member), Portsmouth Hospitals NHS Trust

Elizabeth Midwinter Chapters 48, 49
Matron for Resuscitation and Simulation Services and Advanced Clinical Practitioner in Emergency Medicine, Lancashire Teaching Hospitals NHS Foundation Trust

Gerri Mortimore Chapter 5
Senior Lecturer Advanced Practice and NICE Nurse Expert Advisor, University of Derby

Stevie Park Chapter 30
Trainee Jo Advanced Critical Care Practitioner, University Hospitals Coventry & Warwickshire

Ollie Phipps Chapters 2, 3
Senior Lecturer & Course Director for MSc Advanced Clinical Practice and Non Medical Prescribing, Canterbury Christ Church University, Hon. Associate Professor, University of East Anglia, & Advanced Clinical Practitioner, Maidstone & Tunbridge Wells NHS Trust

Jaclyn Proctor Chapter 51
Senior Lecturer Advanced Clinical Practice, Edge Hill University

Julie Reynolds Chapter 5
Lecturer in Adult Nursing, Keele University

Vikki-Jo Scott Chapter 44
Senior Lecturer, University of Essex, Senior Fellow of Higher Education Academy, and Registered General Nurse in Critical Care Nursing

Ian Setchfield Chapters 3, 4, 6, 39
Acute Care Consultant Nurse and Advanced Practice Lead, East Kent Hospitals University Foundation NHS Trust, Visiting Senior Lecturer, Canterbury Christ Church University

Sonya Stone Chapters 1, 19
Assistant Professor and Programme Director of Advanced Clinical Practice, University of Nottingham, Advanced Critical Care Practitioner (FICM member), Nottingham University Hospitals NHS Trust

Vanessa Taylor Chapters 45, 46
Deputy Head of School (Nursing) (Students and Teaching) and Professor of Learning, Teaching and Professional Practice (Cancer and Palliative Care), University of Central Lancashire

Dave Thom Chapters 35, 36
Anaesthesia Associate, Dorset County Hospital

John Wilkinson Chapter 7
Anaesthetic Registrar, Health Education England North East

Joe Wood Chapter 24
Advanced Critical Care Practitioner, Physiotherapist and Point of Care Ultrasound Educator, Medway NHS Foundation Trust

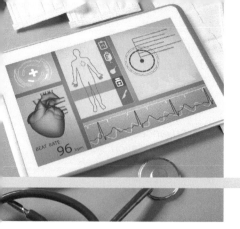

Preface

Advanced clinical practice is a defined level of expertise within health and care professions such as nursing, pharmacy, paramedics, and occupational therapy. Practice at this level is designed to transform and modernise pathways of care, enabling the safe and effective sharing of skills across traditional professional boundaries. Advanced clinical practitioners (ACPs) are equipped with the skills and knowledge to allow them to expand their scope of practice to better meet the needs of the people they care for.

Advanced level practitioners are deployed across all healthcare settings and work at a level of clinical practice that pulls together the four pillars of clinical practice, leadership and management, education, and research. ACPs are educated to master's level or equivalent, although not all advanced level practitioners in England hold a master's; they have achieved this level of practice through experience and expertise. The need for master's level education is advised, but it is not set by law, nor is 'ACP' a qualification that can be registered with a professional body; it has yet to be made a legally protected title that requires professional registration.

The increasing demand on health services and continued financial constraints mean that it has never been more important to have educated and competent staff delivering the best care possible. It has therefore been recognised that the changing landscapes of both the NHS and the private sector require an advancing level of practice extending beyond initial registration.

Advanced clinical practice is delivered by experienced, registered health and care practitioners. it is 'a level of practice characterised by a high degree of autonomy and complex decision making' and includes the analysis and synthesis of complex problems across a range of settings, enabling innovative solutions to enhance people's experience and improve outcomes. In addition, advanced clinical practice embodies the ability to manage clinical care in partnership with individuals, families, and carers.

This definition of advanced clinical practice has been developed to provide clarity for service users, employers, service leads, education providers and health professionals, as well as potential ACPs already practising at an advanced level. This is the first time that there has been a common multiprofessional definition that can be applied across professional boundaries and clinical settings. The definition serves to support a consistent title and recognises the increasing use of such roles across the UK.

HEE (2017), in partnership with NHS Improvement and NHS England, developed a multiprofessional framework for advanced clinical practice, which includes a national definition and standards to underpin the multiprofessional advanced level of practice.

The RCN's (2018) definition of advanced clinical practice is in line with that of HEE, in that it acknowledges 'advanced practice is a level of practice, rather than a type of practice'.

HEE's (2017) multiprofessional ACP framework, which built on a preceding NHS England document outlining an advanced practice model (NHS England, 2010), set out a new, bold vision in developing this critical workforce role in a consistent way to ensure safety, quality, and effectiveness. It has been developed for use across all settings, including primary care, community care, acute, mental health and learning disabilities.

The framework recognises that, as the health and care system rapidly evolve to deliver new models of care, health and care professionals have adapted to meet the increasing health needs of individuals, families and communities. For the first time in England, the HEE (2017) framework sets out an agreed definition for advanced clinical practice for all health and care professionals and articulates what it means for individual practitioners to practise at a higher level from that achieved on initial registration.

The multiprofessional framework offers opportunities for mid-career development of new skills, such as prevention, shared decision-making, and self-care. It aims to ensure a common understanding of advanced clinical practice and supports individuals, employers, commissioners, planners, and educators in the transformation of services to improve the patient experience and outcomes.

Written by academics and clinicians, this book provides an essential practical and theoretical resource for healthcare students related to advanced clinical practice. The book utilizes a framework of advanced level practice and is multi-professional and inclusive. This book is the most contemporary at a glance style book of its kind in the UK aimed at all health and social care professionals aiming to work, or working within advanced level practice. This book is the only book to address advanced clinical practice at a glance focusing on NMC and HCPC regulatory body requirements and also aligned to nationally recognised advanced practitioner training curricula such as Faculty Intensive Care Medicine (FICM), Royal College of Emergency Medicine (RCEM), and the Royal College of Nursing (RCN).

This book has been created specifically for the at a glance series, and it is made for the practicing clinician, being only 150 pages, it is the perfect size for busy healthcare professionals. The snapshot figures and key points make this book accessible, appealing to a variety of learning styles, and focused for busy healthcare professional. Each chapter is written in a format that enables the reader to review the chapter as a complete unit, and therefore the reader can choose in which order they wish to read this book.

A multitude of professional bodies have updated guidance on undergraduate and post graduate education programmes preparing students to prepare for more advanced level roles. The Nursing and Midwifery Council (NMC) updated future nurse pre-registration programme standards, standards for nurses, standards for midwives, standards for nursing associates and standards for post registration Programmes. Additionally, the HCPC and FICM identify and advocate the importance of advanced level practice and this book facilitates the key points at a glance.

This book adheres to the current at a glance series and provide information in a concise and comprehensive manner, which will engage readers by including full-colour images and graphics as well as accurate and useful information and a user-friendly overview of key advanced practice topics utilising nationally recognised competency frameworks set by bodies such as Health Education England (HEE), FICM and RCEM. The book will also be available in a range of formats, including eBook, to increase accessibility. In summary, we hope this book acts as a good source of reference for our readers. We hope that this book creates a desire for our readers to learn more about advanced clinical practice and use key knowledge to teach and support others who are providing care for patients, with the fundamental principles being the provision of safe and effective care for all patients.

Barry Hill and Sadie Diamond Fox

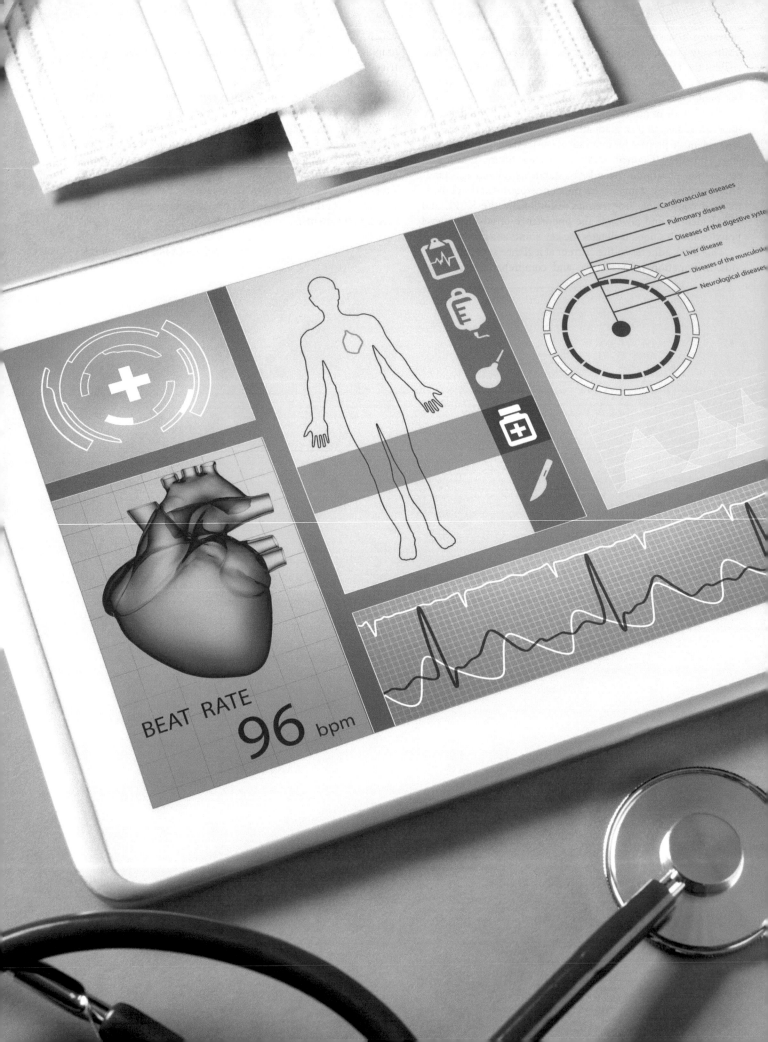

Advanced clinical practice

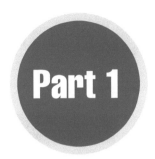

Part 1

Chapters

1 Introducing advanced clinical practice

Figure 1.1   The four pillars of advanced clinical practice based on the Health Education England Multiprofessional Framework.

ADVANCED CLINICAL PRACTICE

CLINICAL

- Practice in compliance within their code of conduct and within their scope of practice
- Demonstrate critical understanding of their broadened level of responsibility and autonomy
- Act on professional judgement about when to seek help, demonstrating critical reflection on own practice, self-awareness, emotional intelligence, and openness to change.
- Work in partnership with individuals, families and carers, using a range of assessment methods as appropriate
- Demonstrate effective communication skills, supporting people in making decisions, planning care or seeking to make positive changes a person-centered approach
- Use expertise and decision-making skills to inform clinical reasoning approaches Initiate, evaluate and modify a range of interventions
- Exercise professional judgement to manage risk
- Work collaboratively
- Act as a clinical role model/advocate for developing and delivering care that is responsive to changing requirements
- Evidence the underpinning subject-specific competencies i.e. knowledge, skills and behaviours relevant to the role setting and scope

LEADERSHIP & MANAGEMENT

- Develop effective relationships, fostering clarity of roles within teams, to encourage productive working.
- Role model the values of their organisation/place of work, demonstrating a person-centred approach to service delivery and development.
- Evaluate own practice, and participate in multi-disciplinary service and team evaluation, demonstrating the impact of advanced clinical practice on service function and effectiveness, and quality
- Engage in peer review to inform own and other's practice, formulating and implementing strategies to act on learning and make improvements.
- Lead practice and service redesign solutions
- Actively seek feedback and involvement from individuals, families, carers, communities and colleagues in the co-production of service improvements.
- Critically apply advanced clinical expertise to provide consultancy across professional and service boundaries, to enhance quality, reduce unwarranted variation and promote the sharing and adoption of best practice.
- Demonstrate team leadership, resilience and determination, managing situations that are unfamiliar, complex or unpredictable and seeking to build confidence in others.
- Continually develop practice in response to changing population health need, engaging in horizon scanning for future developments
- Demonstrate receptiveness to challenge and preparedness to constructively challenge others, escalating concerns that affect individuals', families', carers', communities' and colleagues' safety and well-being when necessary.
- Negotiate an individual scope of practice within legal, ethical, professional and organisational policies, governance and procedures, with a focus on managing risk and upholding safety.

EDUCATION

- Critically assess and address own learning needs by negotiating a personal development plan that reflects the breadth of ongoing professional development across the four pillars of advanced clinical practice.
- Engage in self-directed learning, critically reflecting to maximise clinical skills and knowledge, as well as own potential to lead and develop both care and services.
- Engage with, appraise and respond to individuals' motivation, development stage and capacity, working collaboratively to support health literacy and empower individuals to participate in decisions about their care and to maximise their health and well -being.
- Advocate for and contribute to a culture of organisational learning to inspire future and existing staff.
- Facilitate collaboration of the wider team and support peer review processes to identify individual and team learning.
- Identify further developmental needs for the individual and the wider team and supporting them to address these.
- Supporting the wider team to build capacity and capability through work-based and inter-professional learning, and the application of learning to practice
- Act as a role model, educator, supervisor, coach and mentor, seeking to instill and develop the confidence of others

RESEARCH

- Critically engag e in research activity, adhering to good research practice guidance, so that evidence based strategies are developed and applied to enhance quality, safety, productivity and value for money.
- Evaluate and audit own and others' clinical practice, selecting and applying valid, reliable methods, then acting on the findings.
- Critically appraise and synthesise the outcome of relevant research, evaluation and audit, using the results to underpin own practice and to inform that of others.
- Take a critical approach to identify gaps in the evidence base and its application to practice, alerting appropriate individuals and organisations to these and how they might be addressed in a safe and pragmatic way.
- Actively identify potential need for further research to strengthen evidence for best practice. This may involve acting as an educator, leader, innovator and contributor to research activityix and/or seeking out and applying for research funding.
- Develop and implement robust governance systems and systematic documentation processes, keeping the need for modifications under critical review.
- Disseminate best practice research findings and quality improvement projects through appropriate media and fora (e.g. presentations and peer review research publications).
- Facilitate collaborative links between clinical practice and research through proactive engagement, networking with academic, clinical and other active researchers

Table 1.1   Key advanced practice resources

Resource	Website
Advanced Clinical & Critical Care Practitioner Academic Network (ACCPAN)	www.accpan.net
Council of Deans for Health	www.councilofdeans.org.uk/
HEE Advanced Practice Credentials	https://advanced-practice.hee.nhs.uk/credentials/ https://advanced-practice.hee.nhs.uk/hee-commissioned-advanced-practice-learning-and-development-resources/ https://advanced-practice.hee.nhs.uk/centre-credential-approval-and-assurance-process-faqs/
HEE Advanced Practice Toolkit	www.hee.nhs.uk/our-work/advanced-clinical-practice/advanced-clinical-practice-toolkit
HEE Advanced Practice reports and publications	https://advanced-practice.hee.nhs.uk/resources/reports-and-publications/
HEE Centre for Advancing Practice	https://advanced-practice.hee.nhs.uk/
Institute for Apprenticeships and Technical Education Apprenticeship standards	www.instituteforapprenticeships.org/apprenticeship-standards/?
NHS Leadership Academy	www.leadershipacademy.nhs.uk/
Royal College of Paediatric and Child Health – Advanced Clinical Practitioner (ACP) paediatric curricular framework	www.rcpch.ac.uk/education-careers/supporting-training/acp-curriculum
Faculty of Intensive Care Medicine Curriculum for Training for Advanced Critical Care Practitioners	www.ficm.ac.uk/careersworkforceaccps/accp-curriculum
Royal College of Emergency Medicine Emergency Care Advanced Clinical Practitioner Curriculum	https://rcem.ac.uk/emergency-care-advanced-clinical-practitioners/
Respiratory ACP Network	www.respiratoryacpnetwork.co.uk/

Advanced Clinical Practice at a Glance, First Edition. Edited by Barry Hill and Sadie Diamond Fox.
© 2023 John Wiley & Sons Ltd. Published 2023 by John Wiley & Sons Ltd.

The evolution of advanced clinical practice roles within the UK began in the 1980s[1] and has continued to develop in various forms internationally since.

The *NHS Long-Term Plan*[2] together with Health Education England's (HEE) Multiprofessional Framework (MPF)[3] have been the most recent key drivers for advanced clinical practice within England. The MPF outlines the capabilities expected of practitioners working at advanced level across the four key pillars of advanced practice: clinical practice, leadership and management, education and research[3] (Figure 1.1).

'Advanced clinical practice is delivered by experienced, registered health and care practitioners. It is a level of practice characterised by a high degree of autonomy and complex decision making. This is underpinned by a master's level award or equivalent that encompasses the four pillars of clinical practice, leadership and management, education and research, with demonstration of core capabilities and area specific clinical competence.'[3]

Both the MPF and the *NHS Long-Term Plan* acknowledge that advanced practitioners (APs) are central to transforming service delivery to meet dynamic local healthcare needs, and as such there has been a large investment in the training and development of these roles. Increasing life expectancy, complexity and disease burden, the European Working Time Directive and a subsequent shortage of medical personnel have often been cited as drivers for the implementation of AP roles. However, caution is advised when rationalising their introduction and development to that of the medical substitution paradigm. Advanced practice roles complement existing medical models and are not designed to replace them.

Since their inception, there has been great diversity in AP roles along with some controversy surrounding them. Nevertheless, a colossal effort from professional bodies such as the Council of Deans of Health (CoDoH), the Association of Advanced Practice Educators (AAPE UK) and the royal colleges as well as HEE has led to a huge investment in workforce development in this area of service delivery, to meet patients' needs in the future. Development in this area has also included the introduction of a multiprofessional definition of advanced clinical practice, the first of its kind, to provide clarity for employers, service leads, education providers, health professionals and APs themselves.

Before the release of the *NHS Long-Term Plan*, the CoDoH was commissioned by HEE, as part of the development and implementation of the multiprofessional framework for advanced clinical practice in England,[3] to revolutionise the interface between HEE and universities. Since the seminal CoDoH report[4] and in line with the *Five Year Forward View*,[5,6] there have been several important developments for the advanced clinical practice arena. As a result of significant investment and infrastructure, multiple initiatives are either well established or under way, including the following.

- Advanced Clinical Practitioner Level 7 Apprenticeship standard – the standard, published by the Institute for Apprenticeships and Technical Education[7] and created in consultation with key stakeholders including healthcare providers and higher education institutes (HEIs), incorporates skills development, technical knowledge and practical experience through a work-based training programme. This integrated training model allows for achievement of both a Master's degree in advanced clinical practice and an apprenticeship, whilst providing an important alternative funding stream for NHS and private sector healthcare providers.
- HEE accreditation of ACP university training programmes.
- Guidance for the supervision of advanced practitioners.[8]
- Launch of the Centre for Advancing Practice to support education and training for advanced practitioners.
- Centre for Advancing Practice directory of practitioners to recognise those working at an advanced level of practice across specialties.
- Development and adoption of national specialist standards into university training programmes.
- Development of core capability and credentialling frameworks for ACP roles – several credentialing schemes already exist, such as the Faculty of Intensive Care Medicine (FICM)[9] for advanced critical care practitioners (ACCPs) and the Royal College of Emergency Medicine (RCEM)[10] for emergency care ACPs (ECACPs).

There remains variation in the adoption of AP roles across the UK. However, much work is ongoing to develop standardised governance processes, training expectations and supervision for this group to bring parity and ensure quality. This work will be central to promoting recognition of the level of practice, and ensuring patient safety across all sectors.

Advanced Practice Toolkit (APT)

The APT is an online, interactive repository for 'consistent, credible and helpful resources relating to Advanced Practice'. There are specific areas for practitioners, apprentices, employers, workforce and commissioners and those involved in higher education, training and accreditation. The toolkit is hosted by HEE e-learning for healthcare: https://cs1.e-learningforhealthcare.org.uk/public/ACP/ACP_01_001/index.html#/

Centre for Advancing Practice

A central resource commissioned by HEE to help with delivery of workforce transformation for advanced clinical practice via five key functions.
1 Programme accreditation
2 Recognition of education and training equivalence
3 Advanced Practice Directory
4 HEE credentials
5 Workforce solutions

The website also hosts details of the multiprofessional AP faculties which are present in seven regions across England (https://tinyurl.com/y3a4eyju).

Conclusion

Exciting times lie ahead for the development of new AP roles and the expansion of existing AP posts within the NHS. We still have a way to go when considering the long-term workforce development support for this group of clinicians, who, by nature of the career path they have chosen, are inherently driven to progress. The HEE Centre for Advancing Practice will no doubt prove to be the hub for such activity. Medical colleges and professional groups such as the RCEM, FICM and the Intensive Care Society (ICS) have representation from advanced practitioners on central committees, and in clinical lead roles for key workstreams, giving this workforce an important opportunity to shape the development of these specialties for the future. Other networks created to provide education, support and research opportunities are now developing, building an important infrastructure to support this growing workforce (Table 1.1).

2 Scope of practice

Table 2.1 A timeline of political drivers for advancing and advanced level practice

Date	Policy/document name and organisation
1994	United Kingdom Central Council for Nursing, Midwifery & Health Visiting *The Future of Professional Practice Following Registration*
2004	NMC *Consultation on a Framework for the Standard for Post-registration Nursing*
2007	Health Professions Council (now HCPC) *Standards of Proficiency: Generic Statement*
2008	Council for Healthcare Regulatory Excellence (CHRE) *Advanced Practice: Report to the Four UK Health Departments*
2009	NHS Wales *Framework for Advanced Nursing, Midwifery and Allied Health Professional Practice in Wales*
2010	Department of Health *Advanced Level Nursing: A Position Statement*
2012	NHS Education for Scotland *Scottish toolkit* (updated); first released in 2008 www.advancedpractice.scot.nhs.uk/
2014	NHS England *Five Year Forward View*
2015	Department for Health and Social Care *NHS Constitution*
2017	NHS Health Education England *Multiprofessional Framework for England*
2018	NMC *Future Nurse: Standards of Proficiency for Registered Nurses*
2019	NHSE *NHS Long-Term Plan*
2020	International Council of Nurses *Guidelines on Advanced Practice Nursing*
2020	NHS *We are the NHS: People Plan for 2020/2021 – Action for Us All*
2021	Health and Care Professions Council *Advanced Practice: Research Report*

Advanced Clinical Practice at a Glance, First Edition. Edited by Barry Hill and Sadie Diamond Fox.
© 2023 John Wiley & Sons Ltd. Published 2023 by John Wiley & Sons Ltd.

There have been many drivers for the evolution, growth and governance of advanced practice and all have shaped and sculpted the landscape. These changes have all attempted to realign alternative solutions to the provision of healthcare services in the UK based on several different factors. The European Working Time Directive (for junior doctors' working hours) has expedited this evolution and needs to be considered; however, it is not the only influencing factor.

Table 2.1 details the main policy drivers and key documents that have shaped the trajectory of advanced practice. These need to be considered, fully recognised and understood before we can truly determine where the level of advanced practice sits within UK healthcare.

Defining scope of practice

For healthcare professionals, acknowledging one's scope of professional practice is important, as it defines the limit of knowledge, skills and experience. This scope is supported by professional activities undertaken in the working role and essential boundaries must be identified, acknowledged and maintained. It is acknowledged that a professional's scope will change over time as their knowledge, skills and experience develop.

With the evolution of advanced practice and the expansion of entrustable professional activities, traditional professional boundaries, for example of the nurse, paramedic and physiotherapist, have significantly changed, and this is demonstrated as the multiprofessional workforce comes together at an advanced level.

The provision of healthcare has evolved and is incorporated into many settings, from primary care to secondary care, from a generalist stance or within specialties. This variability and breadth have meant that advanced practice has become immersed in attempts to define and provide structure. Competency frameworks are developed based on interpretation of the clinical environment but two main factors remain ever present: advanced practice must include elements of clinical work, and it is a level of practice, not a job role or title. This level of practice will be different depending on the work environment but involves work in direct care and is complemented by generic competencies that inform the individual's ability to challenge professional boundaries and pioneer innovations.

As this level of practice is unique to the work setting, it is acknowledged that no one profession can encompass all the expertise needed to treat and care for patients. For all, it must include the four fundamental strands of advanced practice: clinical element, research element, educational element and management/leadership element. Technological and clinical advances across all sectors have brought about changes to practice and have contributed to the level and quantity of postqualification education required to advance.

Often contentious is the definition of what advanced practice is. No one definition will fit perfectly to all advanced practitioners or indeed all work environments. Advanced practice is occasionally described as a blurring of the boundaries of traditional roles of registered healthcare professionals. Yet this blurring of boundaries implies assuming aspects of a variety of roles which is needed to provide better, more holistic care to all, which can be seen as a positive evolution of healthcare.

Expanding scope of practice

Those training and working at an advanced level must be aware of their competence and capability. With various curriculums and capability frameworks being developed and implemented, advanced practitioners have guidance on where their knowledge, skills and professional behaviour must sit. However, someone beginning their advanced practitioner journey must acknowledge that it will take years to acquire the knowledge, skills and experience to work at an advanced level.

For some, advanced practice touches upon the knowledge and skills which were traditionally associated with medicine. However, with the development of the multiprofessional workforce, bringing a different set of knowledge and skills, the advanced practitioner is seen as being 'value added' rather than a role substitute. After all, the word *substitution* has no place in advanced practice.

Dunning–Kruger effect

The Dunning–Kruger effect is pertinent in advanced practice. Here, incompetence and metacognitive defects can lead to an overestimation of an individual's abilities and performance. People in this group find it a challenge to recognise genuine levels of competence when applied to themselves or (objectively) in more competent peers. Gaining insight into one's own limitations and inadequacies is also a challenge by social comparison demonstrating an inability to 'see' their own deficits in relation to their peers' performance. The presence and prevalence of this effect in advanced practice must be recognised and challenged to counterbalance the effect of imposter syndrome, thus creating a balanced, objective practitioner.

Imposter syndrome

Imposter syndrome is a common phenomenon amongst advanced practitioners and can be interpreted both positively and negatively. Here, the practitioner doubts their credentials and their ability to function, and is often plagued by a fear of being exposed as inadequate. This phenomenon is driven by anxiety and self-doubt, or because of attempted perfection. Often, it is associated with high-pressure environments, especially in healthcare, and with comparing oneself to another colleague. Imposter syndrome is the sense that someone else is better than you.

Regulation

As this evolution of an alternative 'arm' to provide healthcare in the UK continues, mechanisms of governance have been difficult to hone due to the variability in roles and environments where advanced practice can be found. In 2008, calls to have a new part added to the NMC and HCPC registers were not acted upon as the Council for Healthcare Regulatory Excellence (CHRE) deemed that regulators should ensure that their codes of conduct adequately reflect the requirement for health professionals to stay up to date and operate safely within their areas of competence.

In addition, organisations are encouraged to develop local governance frameworks, policies and procedures to support and regulate advanced practice, taking support and guidance from relevant advisory groups for the disciplines involved.

All these factors play a pivotal role in the continued expansion and prevalence of advanced practice roles and all professionals involved in these roles. Encompassing the four fundamental strands of advanced practice is essential but interpersonal skills and insight are equally important, ensuring that advanced practice is a sustainable development in the future workforce planning and longevity of the NHS.

3 Professional, legal and ethical considerations of advanced practice

---

Box 3.1 Ethical principles

Autonomy
Health professionals must respect a patient's decision to accept or refuse care. Advanced practitioners should be the patient's advocate, to ensure that patients receive all the necessary information to make a well-informed decision. This information must include potential risks, benefits and complications. Care should be discussed and planned with the patient, putting their wishes at the centre of what is done. Many influences will affect a patient's decision, including culture, age, social system, previous experience, general health and awareness of other patients' experiences.

Non-maleficence
The main principle of 'non-maleficence' within medical ethics is – 'do no harm'. The advanced practitioner should select interventions that will cause the least amount of harm to achieve a beneficial outcome (benefit versus risk). The patient is at the centre of the decision. Non-maleficence has many implications for advanced practitioners. An example of this is when treating the terminally ill and withdrawing treatment.

Beneficence
The principle of beneficence ensures that the advanced practitioner takes positive actions to help others. This can be as simple as consoling an upset patient, through to administering analgesia to someone in pain. Beneficence is at the centre of all professional actions while engaging with patients. On occasion, beneficence may clash with a patient's autonomy.

Justice
Care is provided on a fair and equal basis, no matter what the patient's financial or social status.

The development of advanced practice within the UK has seen changes in traditional professional boundaries. Due to this, professionals working in this sphere must be aware of the professional, legal and ethical considerations that they may face.

Professional issues

Advanced practitioners are pioneers of a new style of practice which challenges the traditions associated with professional roles. With the development of the advanced practitioner role, which is undertaken by members of the multiprofessional workforce, working within professional silos has significantly changed. Within areas such as acute and emergency care, nurses, physiotherapists and paramedics, for example, despite keeping their own professional identity, will work together undertaking the same role, undertaking the same procedures and working alongside one another. Each profession brings its own dimension of expertise to the patient, while embracing its own scope of practice. This is seen as being 'value added' for both the patient and the healthcare team. However, each professional group has its restrictions, often associated with legislation or its professional regulator, i.e. independent prescribing.

Competence

Each advanced practitioner must possess the correct knowledge, skills and behaviour to undertake their role and to demonstrate competence, professionally and educationally. Although embracing the four pillars of advanced practice, as experts, advanced practitioners must be professionally mature and have significant experience of practice. They must always work within their scope of professional practice and acknowledge their professional limitations and restrictions.

Responsibility

All healthcare practitioners working either at their base registration or at an advanced level must understand that they are both responsible and accountable for the decisions they make. Expanding one's scope of practice should be done following the correct preparation, education and experience. The concepts of accountability and responsibility are closely linked and are at the centre of the codes of conduct for those professionally regulated by the Nursing and Midwifery Council (NMC) and the Health and Care Professions Council (HCPC). Advanced practitioners have an obligation to undertake their role, and associated tasks, using sound professional judgement. As their level of practice expands, they should realise that this will increase the level of responsibility.

Accountability

Regulated healthcare professionals are responsible for maintaining their competence in practice. They are answerable for decisions made within professional practice, and the consequences of those decisions. Advanced practitioners should be able to justify their decision making and understand the associated legislation, ethical principles, professional standards and guidelines, including evidence-based practice.

Indemnity

Legal accountability involves advanced practitioners ensuring that they have professional indemnity insurance in case there is a substantiated claim of professional negligence. Regulators need to ensure that registrants have this indemnity arrangement in place, and it is now a condition of their registration. The indemnity insurance must be appropriate for the level of practice undertaken.

If you are employed, your employer has vicarious liability for your actions and omissions while in its employment and is responsible for your actions. However, the practitioner must have been working within their level of competence and following their organisation's policies, procedures and guidelines.

Regulation

Despite not regulating advanced practice within separate registers, primarily due to the variability in roles, the NMC and HCPC were tasked with ensuring that their codes of conducts adequately reflected not only those at the base of professions but also those working at an advanced level, ensuring that professionals stay up to date and work within their scope of practice.

Governance

With the development of advanced practice across the UK, the four nations have taken a different approach to its implementation. However, clear local governance structures must exist to support the development, implementation and ongoing strategy for both the employer and advanced practice employee. There should be policies clearly highlighting the differences between base registration, enhanced practice and advanced practice which explore the agreed scope of practice and freedom to act. Appropriate governance meetings of an advanced practice assurance group, or similar, should exist with a reporting route to the trust board or similar. An executive should be identified to hold the portfolio of advanced practice and an advanced practice lead should be appointed, where possible, to steer the development of advanced practice within an organisation.

Legal issues

Advanced practice will often involve exploring new ways of working and touching upon roles that were traditionally performed by other professional groups, for example medical staff. Therefore, it is essential that any legal implications are fully explored to ensure that new areas of practice are appropriate for the obligations of current legislation and statutes. It must be noted that ignorance of the law is not an appropriate or sufficient defence.

The law relates to rules that govern and oversee our society, with the purpose of maintaining justice, upholding social order and preventing harm to both individuals and property. The UK Parliament can implement laws across the four countries (England, Wales, Scotland, Northern Ireland). However, the devolved nations all have powers and judicial systems to implement laws that affect an individual country on devolved issues, and health is one.

Ethics

Advanced practitioners should be prepared to make appropriate ethically informed judgements to support their practice. However, this is not easy, as professionals have struggled with understanding ethics and ethical dilemmas for centuries. Ethics is supported by ethical principles which consist of rules, standards and guidelines which come from theoretical positions regarding what is good for humans. For advanced practitioners to practise in an ethically sound way, they must balance ethical considerations with professional values and relevant legislation.

An individual, usually a patient, will sit at the heart of ethical decision making. The advanced practitioner should seek advice in complex situations where legal, ethical and professional issues need to be considered. Sometimes, the advanced practitioner will be expected to discuss the ethical problem with the individual/patient, to see how their needs can be compassionately met while addressing the challenges of clinical practice for the individual/patient involved. On other occasions, if the individual is unable to discuss their needs, the advanced practitioner will need to weigh up the ethical considerations and, if necessary, consider the individual's/patient's best interests. Four key principles must be considered: autonomy, non-maleficence, beneficence and justice (Box 3.1).

Consent

The principle of consent is associated with international human rights law and is a key aspect of the principle of autonomy. It allows an individual, where capacity exists, to make their own decision. Consent is essential, and failure to obtain it could be interpreted as 'trespass against the person'; if a patient is touched without consent, this may constitute a crime of battery in English law or assault in Scottish law. All practitioners have a responsibility to ensure that they gain consent before proceeding with care or treatment.

4 Advancing to consultant-level practice

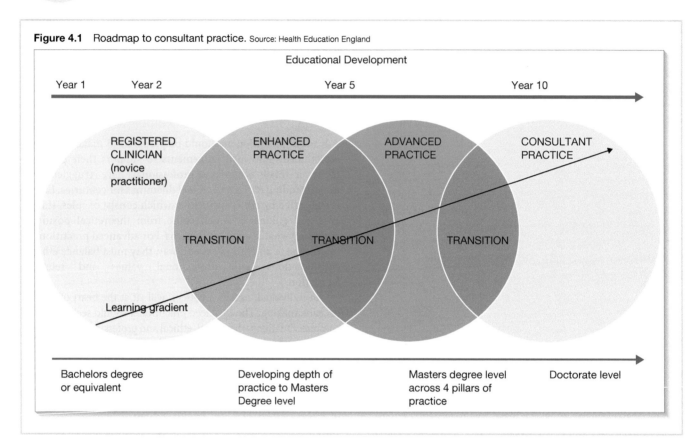

Figure 4.1 Roadmap to consultant practice. Source: Health Education England

Consultant practitioners, like advanced practitioners, are not a new phenomenon within healthcare practice. Over the years, there has been a consistent lack of role clarity for autonomous practitioners working in consultant and advanced practice roles. This has resulted in the potential for this multiprofessional workforce to provide innovative models of person-centred safe and effective care to be underutilised. Consequently, both the NHS *Interim NHS People Plan*[1] and the *NHS Long-Term Plan*[2] underpin the need to invest and develop the advanced and ultimately consultant practitioner workforce as a strategic priority for the NHS. Therefore, Health Education England (HEE) is developing clear deliverables through the Centre for Advancing Practice (CAP) to maximise the potential of advanced and consultant practice.

It is imperative that current and future healthcare practices learn lessons from the past regarding the lack of understanding of the advanced/consultant practitioner role. To ensure this is effective, employers require support to ensure that opportunities for robust career development pathways are put in place from advanced to consultant practitioner.

Consultant-level practice

In 1998, the UK government introduced the role of the consultant nurse[3] as a way of expanding the clinical career pathway and also improving patient care and experience by enhancing clinical leadership. Today, consultant-level practice requires significant clinical expertise and experience along with working towards a level 8 academic qualification.

There are numerous benefits of the consultant practitioner role.
- System leadership
- Expert clinical practice
- Role modelling and supporting a positive work-based culture
- Facilitation
- Quality improvement
- Forging strong links with higher education institutes
- Clinical and academic supervision

However, there are also challenges.
- Lack of clarity regarding the scope of the role, which should not include people management responsibilities
- Unrealistic expectations as to what the consultant practitioner can achieve
- Job plans that enable the benefits of the consultant practitioner to be realised, as the consultant practitioner job plan is recommended to be 50% clinical with the other 50% devoted to utilising the other three pillars in order to influence whole-system working, ensuring person-centred patient care

Therefore, the role of the consultant practitioner can be seen as the pinnacle of the clinical career ladder and provides expertise, clinical and strategic leadership in clinical practice, practice-based research, inquiry, development and improvement approaches that change practice sustainably through individual, team and organisational learning, cultural change and improving effectiveness.[4]

A recent HEE multiprofessional capability and impact framework for consultant-level practice[5] shows how the role of the consultant practitioner is structured around the following four pillars of practice (Figure 4.1).
1 Expert practice
2 Strategic and enabling leadership
3 Learning, developing and improving across the system
4 Research and innovation

Whilst the above four pillars are like those described in the HEE advanced clinical practice framework,[6] by introducing an overarching fifth pillar, 'consultancy',[5] the consultant-level practice framework provides a navigable platform within which the journey from advanced to consultant level practice can be achieved.

The journey from advanced to consultant practice

The HEE consultant-level practice framework[5] clearly identifies the capabilities required for each pillar and provides evidence-based examples of how the impact of the consultant practitioner can be demonstrated. How the practitioner can demonstrate impact is central if the potential of consultant practitioners to influence whole-system working is to be realised due to the complexity of the role. Whilst the framework is of benefit to an advanced practitioner starting their journey towards consultant practice and the employer supporting them, there is no prescriptive formula as to how that journey is achieved.

How this journey is travelled is integral to its success and can only be achieved if the advanced practitioner has a robust job plan, appraisals undertaken by a line manager who understands the role, clinical supervision that provides high support and high challenge, targeted continuing professional development (CPD) and, most importantly, has a personal desire to push boundaries and take opportunities to develop their practice across all pillars.

The Venus model[7] consists of five interdependent stems which articulate the behaviours required to elicit workforce transformation and change across complex systems. The five stems require an individual to be able to:
1 facilitate an integrated approach to learning, using the workspace as a valuable resource
2 act as a transformational and collective leader
3 act as a skilled practice developer
4 utilise improvement skills to measure and evaluate what is valued
5 understand the system enablers and use them to facilitate culture change at a microsystem level.

It could be suggested that the Venus model can be used as a navigable blueprint with which to guide professional development on the journey to consultant practice.

Development of facilitation skills is also key if the journey towards consultant practice is to be successful. Being able to act as a facilitator not only promotes a positive work-based culture, improves resilience and safety cultures, recognises the value of the workplace as a learning environment and provides effective clinical leadership but also operationalises the ability to traverse the different levels of the organisation.[8] This enables person-centred practice and the ability to influence and meet organisational priorities.

Leadership within the NHS has over recent years evolved from a 'top-down approach' to recognising the need to grow transformational, collective and compassionate leaders who are able to articulate a clear vision and inspire others to promote sustainable change. The NHS Leadership Academy healthcare leadership model uses nine leadership dimensions,[9] identifying effective leadership behaviours. Using a model such as this allows individuals to identify strengths and areas for improvement, thus providing a foundation upon which to develop a 'leadership toolkit'. This is essential as a consultant practitioner must be able to work as a system leader, navigate complexity and develop expertise in all four pillars so having the ability to catalyse collective action in others.

Conclusion

To develop the necessary expertise across all pillars, the practitioner is required to develop a synergistic approach to both professional and CPD development. Adopting a model such as the Venus model can aid in their journey towards consultant practice.

5 Transitioning to advanced practice

Figure 5.1 Seven fundamental considerations which underpin supervision in advanced clinical practice. Source: Health Education England[1]

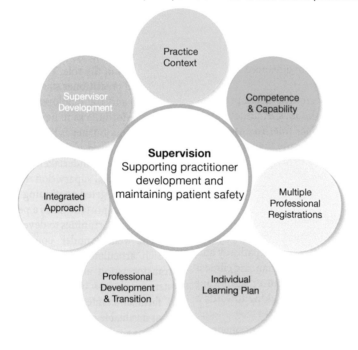

Box 5.1 Some of the investments in advanced level practice

- ACP level 7 apprenticeships, incorporating skills development, technical knowledge and practical experience through a work-based training programme
- HEE accreditation of ACP university training programmes
- Guidance for the supervision of ACPs
- Launch of the Centre for Advancing Practice to support education and training for advanced practitioners
- Development and adoption of national specialist standards into university training programmes
- Development of core capability and credentialling frameworks for ACP roles – several credentialling schemes already exist such as the Faculty of Intensive Care Medicine (FICM) for advanced critical care practitioners (ACCPs) and the Royal College of Emergency Medicine (RCEM) for emergency care ACPs (ECACPs)

Becoming an advanced clinical practitioner

Trainee advanced clinical practitioners (ACPs) arise from a variety of backgrounds, such as nurses, operating department practitioners (ODPs), paramedics, pharmacists, physiotherapists and speech and language therapists. Many were senior clinicians within their original fields of practice. Because of this fact, becoming an ACP often represents a significant change in role and many will underestimate how difficult this transition can be. From being an expert in their previous role to becoming a novice in their new ACP role is challenging. This is compounded by the fact that trainee ACPs can be on rotation, for example through different medical or surgical wards, with each rotation requiring a period of adjustment. There is often a temporary loss of confidence until they not only become familiar with their new environment but feel valued and able to contribute.

Acceptance

An additional challenge, often not considered, is that, frequently, newly appointed trainee ACPs will take up their role in the trust where they previously worked. Tension can occur between long-time colleagues, which can be attributed to personal jealousy, feeling threatened or simply because there is an expectation that the ACP should contribute like they did before in their previous role.

Prescribing

Legislation sets out which professions may act as prescribers. A range of non-medical healthcare professionals can prescribe medicines for patients as either independent or supplementary prescribers. However, disparity currently exists between APs due to the base profession in which they trained. For example, ODPs are exempt by law from completing a relevant qualification to enable them to use the title of independent or supplementary prescriber.

Advanced Clinical Practice at a Glance, First Edition. Edited by Barry Hill and Sadie Diamond Fox.
© 2023 John Wiley & Sons Ltd. Published 2023 by John Wiley & Sons Ltd.

The nature of AP roles often calls upon the individual to be accountable for the assessment of patients with previously undiagnosed or diagnosed conditions and for decisions about the clinical management required, including prescribing. A lack of prescribing rights for ODPs directly impedes their career prospects of progressing to ACP roles, particularly in emergency and critical care, as they are exempt from gaining professional credentials/membership with their respective royal college/faculty (Royal College of Emergency Medicine and the Faculty of Intensive Care Medicine), a prerequisite that is now an essential criterion for many employers.

Uniforms

In some trusts, the ACP is denoted by a particular uniform. However, it may not be obvious whether they are a trainee ACP or a senior ACP. This can cause undue anxiety for a trainee who may feel they are not meeting the expected standard of a senior ACP, and this can have serious consequences for self-esteem and confidence.

Academic study

As well as coping with new role transition, another difficulty encountered is undertaking academic study. To attain ACP status requires the completion of a Master of Science degree in advanced clinical practice. Masters-level academic study can be an intimidating experience if trainees have not undertaken study for some years. However, there are positive outcomes from being in senior roles before ACP training. Many ACPs will have transferable skills such as excellent communication skills and positive behaviour characteristics, as well as knowledge and experience in their field of expertise, which can be employed to educate other trainee ACPs and health professionals.

Mentorship and supervision

Mentorship and supervision are of paramount importance to support transition but, unfortunately, this can be limited due to time constraints and availability of mentors/supervisors. Good mentorship has been shown to increase the attainment of clinical skills and to reduce any feelings of isolation a new trainee may feel. Interestingly, since 2018 the Nursing and Midwifery Council (NMC) no longer uses the term 'mentor' but instead uses the terms *practice supervisors* and *assessors*.

A seminal document concerning this area has been produced by Health Education England (HEE)/Centre for Advancing Practice.[1] It provides guidance for workplace supervision of ACP development which will be useful for supervisors, employers, those driving workforce development and educators, and sets out seven fundamental considerations which underpin supervision in advanced clinical practice (Figure 5.1).

Supervisors of both trained and trainee ACPs are highly encouraged to complete the HEE Educational and Clinical Supervisors programme (www.e-lfh.org.uk/programmes/educational-and-clinical-supervisors/) and attend further online or face-to-face training with HEE. A number of regions have developed their own minimum standards for supervising ACP professionals, which will probably become a nationwide initiative co-ordinated centrally by HEE.

Transitioning to advanced clinical practice

According to HEE, ACPs enhance and supplement service provision by supporting continuity of care and offering a holistic approach to patient management and outcomes. There is also evidence that patients are comfortable with ACP consultations.

The road to becoming an ACP is fraught with challenges and tribulations, as mentioned within this discussion, all of which can affect confidence and self-assurance. Becoming an ACP offers great rewards in the form of job satisfaction and autonomy, and the ability to provide timely care to patients makes the journey worthwhile. Careful consideration is required by any healthcare professional looking to transition into the world of advanced practice. The individual should establish the requirements of both the clinical and academic pathway to fully understand the scope of practice within the proposed role. Being able to function with a high degree of autonomy and make complex decisions are foundation features of advanced practitioners. The pathways are evolving to meet the demands of a strained healthcare system. As a direct result of this, advanced practitioners are often functioning at the very fringes of their professional licences.

Whilst advanced nurse practitioners have been in place since the early 1990s, some of the key outward concerns surrounding the continued evolution of these advanced roles remain. The need for role clarity, training standards and ongoing professional growth within the roles are not always well defined and standardised. When transitioning into any advanced practice role, it is important to feel professionally safe within your practice. ACPs not only enhance patient safety, but also could potentially compromise it if their training standards and scope of practice are not clearly defined.

Scope of practice

Many advanced practice roles are underpinned by a professional registration such as the NMC or the Health and Care Professions Council (HCPC). Roles such as physician associate are not at present regulated, and this is currently under review in conjunction with the General Medical Council (GMC). It is felt that often these regulatory bodies do not meet or indeed understand the increasing scope of advanced practice, nor do they set a standard for the use of the title 'advanced practitioner'. This is a common argument made against advanced practice roles. The true role of an advanced practitioner is far more than a title. Ensuring you are entering into a pathway which is underpinned by all four pillars of advanced practice in conjunction with a defined scope of practice, clear lines of clinical responsibility and supervision are key when choosing an advanced practice pathway to follow.

Advancing the advanced clinical practitioner

The provision of ACP-led care is safe and effective and has a positive impact on patient care and experience, service efficiency and capacity. However, it is recognised that there is a lack of continuing professional development (CPD) opportunities and unclear career pathways exist. A recent national evaluation of both the ACP and advanced critical care practitioner (ACCP) role has also highlighted these issues and as such, a number of support networks have been established, particularly on the social platform Twitter.

Conclusion

Exciting times lie ahead for the development of new ACP roles (Box 5.1) and the expansion of existing ACP posts within the NHS. We still have a way to go when considering the long-term workforce development support for this group of clinicians who, by the nature of the career path they have chosen, are inherently driven to progress. The HEE Centre for Advancing Practice (https://tinyurl.com/y3a4eyju) has already proven to be a hub for such activity, but there are also smaller networks that can provide support for both clinicians and educators.

6 Continuing professional development and lifelong learning

Box 6.1 CPD activities

- Mandatory training
- E-learning
- Attendance at organised learning events
- Simulation training
- Reflection
- Structured learning events such as intermediate and advanced life support
- Participating in small group practice-based learning
- Evidence of audit, research or publications
- Work-based assessments such as case-based discussions
- Reading and reflecting on peer-reviewed articles in professional publications
- Webinars

Box 6.2 Theoretical CPD framework theories

- Transformation of the individual's professional practice
- Transformation of skills to meet society's changing healthcare needs
- Transformation of knowledge to enable knowledge translation
- Transformation of workplace culture to implement workplace and organisational values and purpose

---

Advanced Clinical Practice at a Glance, First Edition. Edited by Barry Hill and Sadie Diamond Fox.
© 2023 John Wiley & Sons Ltd. Published 2023 by John Wiley & Sons Ltd.

Continuing professional development (CPD) is a requirement of both regulatory and professional bodies, so enabling employers and employees to provide safe and effective patient-centred care. However, CPD can no longer be viewed by the individual as the attainment of isolated blocks of learning but rather as a 'lifelong learning' journey forging links between professional practice and organisational objectives.

There is little research on advanced practitioners and their CPD needs. Therefore, if the benefits of the advanced practitioner are to be realised then CPD needs to be targeted, enabling a multiprofessional workforce that ensures that patients are seen by the right person, at the right place at the right time.[1]

Continuing professional development

The onus for undertaking CPD rests with the individual to meet their professional body's revalidation requirements. However, employers also have a responsibility to support individuals to undertake CPD. One of the challenges facing the attainment of CPD for the multiprofessional advanced practitioner workforce is the varying numbers of mandated hours and CPD cycles set by the professional regulatory bodies. This provides employers with a challenge to make sure that robust governance and supervision standards are in place to protect both the patient and the advanced practitioner.

Rather than being reactive or passive, CPD allows learning to become a proactive and conscious undertaking. There is a synergistic relationship between improved patient safety and a workforce that participates in high-quality CPD. The provision of high-quality CPD not only allows for the delivery of high-quality patient care but plays a pivotal role in the retention of experienced staff and allows for robust succession planning. There are numerous recognised CPD activities noted in Box 6.1.

The complexity of delivering CPD to a diverse healthcare workforce has resulted in many organisations having less than effective learning strategies. However, a recent theoretical framework comprising four theories can be seen in Box 6.2. This is underpinned by context, mechanism and outcome relationships and has the potential to provide employers with a platform with which to develop robust, effective CPD delivery[2] strategies.

Continuing professional development and the four pillars of advanced practice

As the advanced practitioner workforce grows, so will the need to view CPD not as updating knowledge in isolation or a means of obtaining a specialist skill but as a platform within which to demonstrate the value and impact of this innovative workforce model. The four pillars of advanced practice provide a navigable framework for the advanced practitioner to not only demonstrate impact and value but to also start their journey towards consultant-level practice.

It is understandable that the 'clinical' pillar receives particular attention from both the advanced practitioner and the employer as it enables both service delivery and safe patient-focused care. However, the other three pillars are of equal importance if their value and impact are to be measured and realised. Therefore, it is essential that advanced practitioners do not deconstruct the four pillars when undertaking CPD but view them as an interlinked framework which allows them to work at an advanced level of practice.

Enablers for effective continuing professional development and lifelong learning

One of the most pressing challenges facing effective CPD attainment is funding. Therefore, it is vital that advanced practice leads within organisations work collaboratively with corporate leads to ensure that advanced practice strategies exist which allow for advanced practitioner CPD requirements to be articulated clearly in education and training plans. Appraisals should also be undertaken by individuals who understand the role of the advanced practitioner, so enabling effective personal development plans to be agreed.

Whilst adequate funding is important for CPD, there is a wealth of free CPD activities, such as Health Education England (HEE) e-learning for healthcare (e-LfH) which has over 200 programmes covering all aspects of healthcare. Fellowships and scholarships are available providing advanced practitioners with unique CPD experiences across all four pillars. The NHS Leadership Academy provides a host of resources and tools, many of which at a regional level are free.

Access to appropriate educational and clinical supervisors is also essential if targeted CPD is to be effective. This will promote the workplace as a valuable place of learning and facilitate an effective workplace culture.[2]

Another key enabler for effective CPD is robust job planning which gives the individual protected non-clinical time allowing all four pillars of advanced practice to be attained. This empowers the advanced practitioner to develop into a facilitator and change agent. One result of this is effective clinical leadership, enabling an improvement-focused culture and utilising their tacit experience and knowledge to enable effective workplace learning.

The future of continuing professional development and lifelong learning

To deliver CPD against the backdrop of fiscal and operational challenges facing the NHS will require the adoption of technology to augment traditional face-to-face CPD activities, something that has been brought into stark reality by the COVID-19 pandemic.[3]

The pandemic has resulted in the use of synchronous and asynchronous learning, both of which have advantages and limitations for the learner. For example, technology has enabled individuals to participate in synchronous and asynchronous learning events that may not have been accessible due to funding or practical reasons such as attendance at international conferences or webinars.

Aside from providing a platform for innovative CPD activities for advanced practitioners, such as podcasts or educational blogs, technology provides a means for connecting individuals. Across the country, there are already well-established advanced practitioner networks and with the advent of the new HEE regional advanced practice faculty leads, there is an opportunity to grow communities of practice. Communities of practice not only enable collective learning but also provide support to advanced practitioners who are in highly specialist roles.

One thing is for certain – the pandemic has acted as a catalyst for the evolution of CPD attainment, which is something that advanced practitioners should embrace, embedding CPD within everyday practice.

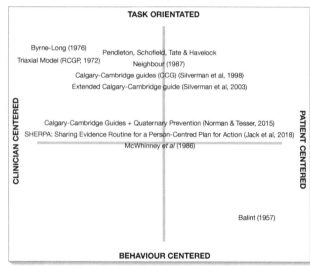

7 Consultation models

Figure 7.1 Consultation models and their differing emphasis on four common domains. Source: Mehay *et al.* (2012)[4]/Taylor & Francis

TASK ORIENTATED

Byrne-Long (1976)
Triaxial Model (RCGP, 1972)
Pendleton, Schofield, Tate & Havelock
Neighbour (1987)
Calgary-Cambridge guides (CCG) (Silverman et al, 1998)
Extended Calgary-Cambridge guide (Silverman et al, 2003)

Calgary-Cambridge Guides + Quaternary Prevention (Norman & Tesser, 2015)
SHERPA: Sharing Evidence Routine for a Person-Centred Plan for Action (Jack et al, 2018)
McWhinney *et al* (1986)

CLINICIAN CENTERED — **PATIENT CENTERED**

Balint (1957)

BEHAVIOUR CENTERED

Box 7.1 Enhanced Calgary-Cambridge consultation model

Initiating the session
- Preparation
- Establishing rapport
- Identifying the reason(s) for consultation

Gathering information
Exploration of the patient's problems to discover the:
- *Biomedical perspective:*
- *Patient's perspective:*
- *Background information – context:*
  - Past medical history
  - Drug and allergy history
  - Family history
  - Personal and social history
  - Review of systems

Physical examination

Explanation and planning

Closing the session

Figure 7.2 A pictorial representation of the Open to Closed Cone described in the three-function model of the medical interview. Source: Based on Bird & Cohen-Cole 1990.[6]

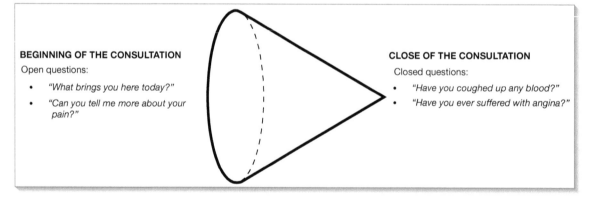

BEGINNING OF THE CONSULTATION
Open questions:
- *"What brings you here today?"*
- *"Can you tell me more about your pain?"*

CLOSE OF THE CONSULTATION
Closed questions:
- *"Have you coughed up any blood?"*
- *"Have you ever suffered with angina?"*

Box 7.2 Alternative agendas and suggested communication tools Modified from [4][4]

Breaking bad news
A	Anxiety – acknowledge
K	Knowledge – what do they already know?
I	Information – how much information do they want? Keep it simple, avoid overload
S	Sympathy + emotional management
S	Support – ask what would help
S	Support + ask what would help
S	Summarise strategy and key points

Conflict situations
D	Disagree
A	Agree
N	Negotiate a compromise
C	Counsel
E	Educate
R	Refer to third party

Dealing with an angry patient
A	Avoid confrontation
F	Facilitate discussion
V	Ventilate feelings
E	Explore reasons
R	Refer/investigate

Ethical considerations
A	Autonomy (patient) – be fair (justice)
B	Beneficence
C+C	Consent + confidentiality
D	Do not lie
E	Everybody else (society vs individual) – virtue, duty, utility and rights

The process of conducting a patient consultation and performing a subsequent clinical assessment has historically been termed 'the most powerful and sensitive and most versatile instrument available to the physician'.[1] Despite the rapid growth of healthcare technology, this remains the case today. A skilled ACP has the potential to make a significant contribution to several fundamental outcomes, including patient satisfaction, patient concordance with prescribed therapies and interventions, overall diagnostic accuracy, and overall measurable changes in health or quality of life that result from safe patient care. Evidence suggests that, by conducting a high-quality medical history alone, 60–80% of the information needed to form a diagnosis can be ascertained.[2,3] The overall aim is to identify symptoms and physical manifestations that represent a final common pathway of a wide range of pathologies, which may be highly suggestive or even pathognomonic of one such pathology, or multiple concurrent pathologies.

Various established consultation models exist to give structure to the consultation, aiming to effectively, efficiently and accurately collect the required information from the patient while continuing to build rapport with them.

Classification of consultation models

To maximise the efficiency and efficacy of the consultation, several models and frameworks have been proposed. These can be task oriented, clinician centred, behaviour centred and patient centred. Although most models have been developed for use within the primary care/GP setting, they are applicable to secondary care and tertiary care settings, with adaptation as necessary.

Mehay[4] classifies consultation models as differing in three ways.

- *Concept versus implementation*: conceptual frameworks have clear aims but lack integration of the process of implementation into practice. The more recent frameworks (2003 and onwards) include both aspects.
- *Clinician versus patient centredness*: frameworks vary in their degree of focus on the consultation's agenda, process and outcome in respect of the practitioner's perspective (biomedical/disease framework) versus the patient's perspective (illness framework). Although disease and illness usually coexist, the same disease can lead to markedly different experiences of illness in different patient populations.
- *Task-oriented versus behavioural focus*: the degree to which frameworks focus on the tasks to be achieved in the consultation versus the range of behaviours required in the consultation.

Mehay[4] proposes a simple diagram which details the degree to which existing frameworks differ, in terms of their focus on the three classifications. Figure 7.1 has been adapted from this original work to include more recent consultation frameworks.

Calgary-Cambridge Guide to the Medical Interview

The Calgary-Cambridge guides (CCG), which have evolved to become the enhanced Calgary-Cambridge guides,[5] serve to give structure to the whole patient–practitioner interaction (Box 7.1).

Cone technique

This established aid, described in the three-function model of the medical interview,[6] guides the practitioner using open to gradually more closed questions (Figure 7.2). This aims to collect information:

- thoroughly, reducing the risk of missing pertinent information using open questions
- efficiently, using closed questions

- whilst allowing the patient time to express the elements of their presentation which are significant to them.

When moving to closed questions, there are a variety of mnemonics available to act as a mental aid to ensure completeness of information. Examples of commonly used mnemonics are given in Chapter 8.

Ideas, concerns and expectations (ICE)

Whilst the consultation's primary aim is to collect information to formulate a differential diagnosis and management plan, additional objectives are to build rapport, explore concerns, improve patient satisfaction, review the patient's agenda and promote shared decision making. Bearing in mind the acronym ICE throughout the consultation helps to achieve these objectives.

Communication

Communication with patients is key to all aspects of clinical practice. Seminal NHS frameworks and policy drivers place effective communication at the core of providing a person-centred approach in health and care. Communication skills are consequently core strands of ACP training and ongoing professional development. Effective communication with patients can lead to improvement in both treatment quality and safety metrics; conversely, poor communication has been highlighted as one of the main concerns leading to complaints to the Parliamentary and Health Service Ombudsman. In order to develop effective ACP–patient relationships, we must consider some of the fundamental principles of effective/therapeutic communication within the healthcare setting, such as patient health literacy, cultural understanding and language barriers.

Triggers to consultation

Considering the trigger to consultation can be a powerful tool in setting up and directing the consultation appropriately.

Triggers may include:
- interpersonal crisis
- interference with social or personal relations
- sanctioning or pressure from family or friends
- interference with work or physical activity
- reaching the limit of tolerance with symptoms.

Consultations with an alternative agenda

A typical agenda for a medical consultation is to gain information to assist with creating a differential diagnosis. However, not all interactions between patient and practitioner are attempting to achieve this agenda. It is undeniable that therapeutic communication is complex, and several constructs have been proposed to aid the clinician/practitioner in working with patients as partners. Examples of these alternative agendas and communication tools to approach them are detailed in Box 7.2.

Assessing the quality of consultations

Burt *et al.*[7] developed the Global Consultation Rating Scale as a tool to assess the quality of a consultation and identify areas for improvement. It is based on the Calgary-Cambridge models and assesses the subject on 12 different areas from 'Initiating the session' to 'Closure'. Each area is scored as:
- not done or poor
- adequate
- good.

A total consultation score between 0 and 24 is obtained by summing the scores from the 12 domains.

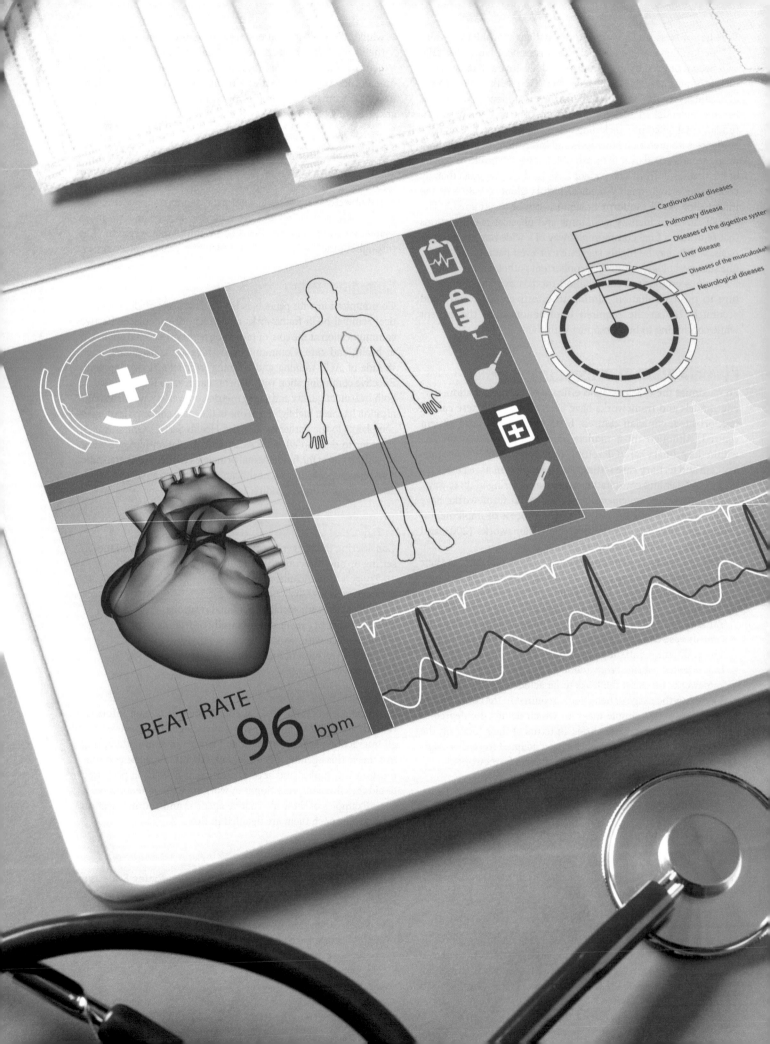

Advanced history taking and physical examination

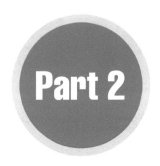

Part 2

Chapters

8 Principles of history taking and physical examination skills

Figure 8.1 Concept map as a history-taking template. Source: Irfan M (2019) *The Hands-on Guide to Clinical Reasoning in Medicine*, Figure 2.3, p.16. Wiley-Blackwell, Chichester

Symptom + Semantic Qualifiers + Severity of illness

Well → Provisional Diagnoses / Explore all causes in order of relevance

ill / Very ill → Rule out life-threatening causes first

Dying → Search for quickly reversible causes / Weigh risk v/s benefit ratio of intervention / Consider palliation if more appropriate

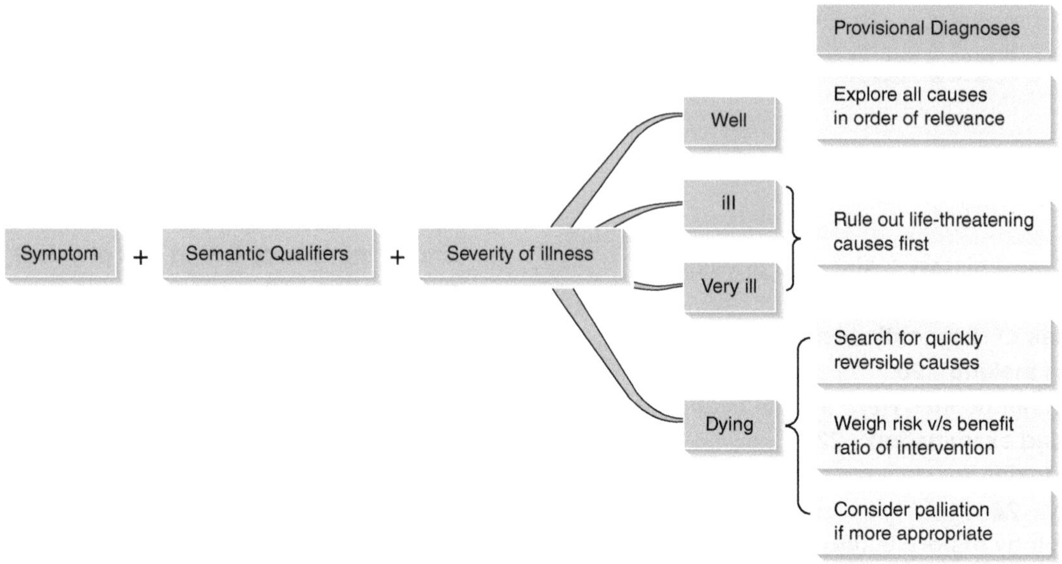

Figure 8.2 Concept map as a history-taking template for chest pain. Source: Irfan M (2019) *The Hands-on Guide to Clinical Reasoning in Medicine*, Figure 2.4, p.16. Wiley-Blackwell, Chichester

History taking
Chest pain
54 year old male. Chest pain-2 hours. History of hypertension and diabetes mellitus. In extremis. Low BP and saturations, high HR and RR, normal temperature and blood sugar.

Aetiology of chest pain

Chest pain + Semantic Qualifiers: Middle aged man / Acute chest pain / Vascular risk factors + Severity of illness Very ill = Life threatening causes: Acute myocardial infarction / PE / Aortic dissection (h/o hypertension)

Questions to ask: Exertional, pleuritic, tearing?

Exertional (worse on exertion):
Character - squeezing, heavy
Duration - minutes rather than seconds or hours
Site - centre of chest
Radiation - to arm, jaw, neck
Associated symptoms - autonomic features of sweating, sickness, palpitations, lightheadedness
Risk factors - vascular risk factors, recreational drugs

Pleuritic (worse on inspiration, coughing):
Character - stabbing, a catch when breathing in
Duration - can be hours to days
Site - unilateral or central
Radiation - if diaphragmatic pleura involved radiates to shoulder tip
Associated symptoms - breathlessness, lightheadedness
Risk factors for venous thrombo-embolism

Tearing:
Character - tearing ripping
Duration - minutes to hours
Site - centre of chest
Radiation - to back
Associated symptoms - breathlessness, lightheadedness, neurological deficits etc
Risk factors - hypertension, connective tissue diseases

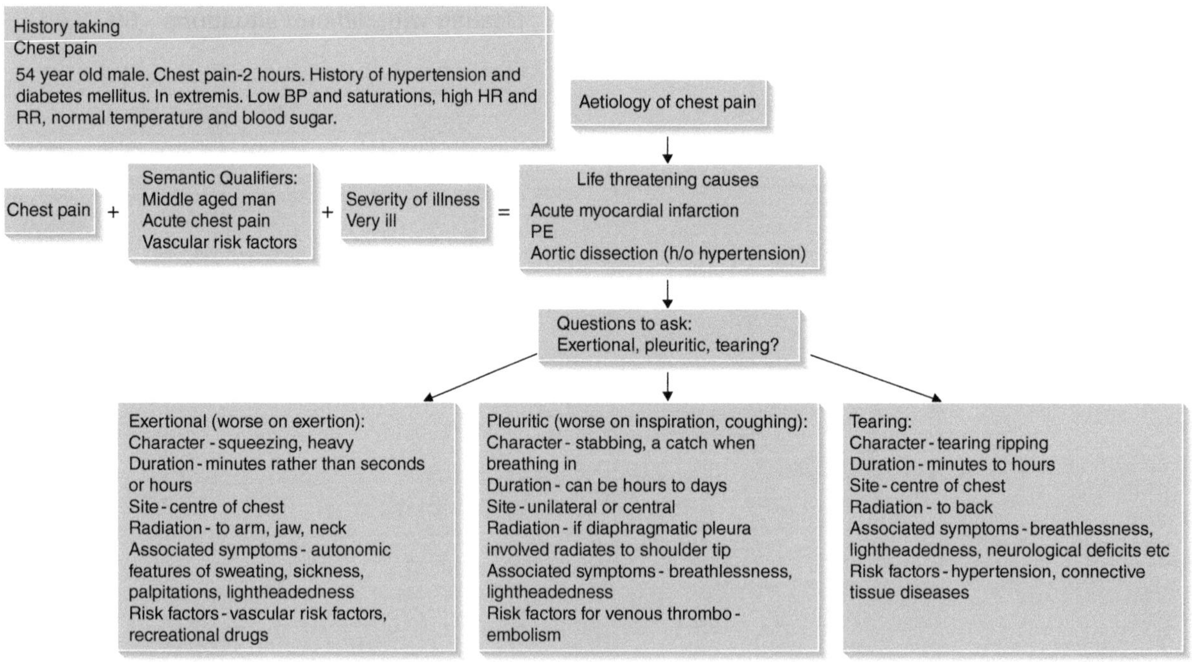

The knowledge obtained about the patient through a comprehensive history and physical examination informs the diagnostic reasoning and in turn the treatment options and clinical decisions.

History taking

Obtaining a medical history is a crucial part of any consultation, both to gather the information required to treat the patient, and to open communication and establish a rapport, which enables the

Advanced Clinical Practice at a Glance, First Edition. Edited by Barry Hill and Sadie Diamond Fox.
© 2023 John Wiley & Sons Ltd. Published 2023 by John Wiley & Sons Ltd.

patient to become a partner in managing their health. The value of a health interview is often underestimated, particularly in an era with high-end technology and point-of-care diagnostic tools, but evidence over the years has shown that a thorough medical history remains the major contributor to making an accurate diagnosis, despite the significant medical advances.[1-3] To achieve this, the medical history must be robust and accurate; we need to be asking the right questions, and more importantly, listening to the answers!

> *'Listen to your patient, he is telling you the diagnosis'*
> (Sir William Osler[4])

A comprehensive history commonly consists of several components and data pertaining to these components.

Skills needed to elicit information

Communication skills

The practitioner's verbal and non-verbal communication can instill trust, build rapport, and ensure understanding. Without this, the patient is unlikely to speak openly and honestly, preferring instead to withhold vital information.

The ability to listen and observe

Good communication begins with listening and observing to know how to respond and pitch the consultation. This includes the ability to be flexible and adapt the style of communication to the patient's cultural, education and socioeconomic backgrounds. A lot of information can be elicited from observing patients and their environment, whether it's a home visit, a first responder on the site of incident, in a clinic or hospital bed.

Clinical knowledge

Knowledge and experience of conditions and their presentation are vital. This enables the practitioner to ask the right questions to include or exclude differential diagnoses.

Appropriate use of questions

Open, closed and probing questions all have their uses. Generally, open questions are used at the start of a consultation. Practitioners often talk about 'a golden minute' when the patient is given the opportunity to explain their situation without interruption.[5] Probing questions help direct the conversation while closed questions elicit straightforward answers, useful to explore a problem in more detail and drill down to conclusive information. Negative questions should be avoided as these may be confusing and leading.

Time management

Once the problem becomes clear, it may become necessary and entirely appropriate to control the flow of the conversation. A note of caution when doing this however, as sometimes the patient's main concerns may differ from those of the practitioner. In general, one should aim to be quick and efficient at obtaining ancillary information (PMH, DH, allergies, SH, FH), to spend more time where it matters (PC/PS). Some practitioners prefer to quickly go through the ancillary questions first before then asking, 'What brings you to see us today?' whereas others start with the presenting complaint. Find a pattern that works best for you and then rehearse it until it becomes second nature.

Ability to summarise information succinctly

The information gathered from the health interview must be documented. In certain situations, it may be useful to quote patients directly. Using a systematic list like the one found in.

History taking for special situations

The traditional history-taking format meets many challenges in scenarios where time-critical interventions are required and a quick, focused history is more appropriate. The mnemonic 'AMPLE', originally developed for use in the context of trauma,[5] may be applied to quickly glean pertinent information.

- A = Allergies
- M = Medications
- P = Past medical history
- L = Last meal (timing)
- E = Events related to presentation

General aspects of physical examination

Physical examination is the process of obtaining information using the following techniques.

- *Inspection* – a visual examination of the patient and their surroundings.
- *Palpation* – the process of using different parts of one's hand under varying degrees of pressure to evaluate underlying tissue tension, structure size, temperature, swelling, static position, presence of crepitus and provocation of pain.
- *Auscultation* – listening over an area of the body using a stethoscope and noting things like the quality, duration and frequency of the noise heard.

Physical examination for special situations

A full examination of each body system may not always be necessary. Having taken a full history, formulate a handful of key questions and then focus your examination towards answering them or at least excluding one or two differentials. In time-critical scenarios, it is wise to apply the familiar ABCDE approach (see: www.resus.org.uk/library/abcde-approach); at other times you may tailor your examination technique to the question at hand.

Evidence-based physical diagnosis

The information yielded from the history taking and physical examination exercises cannot be taken at face value; the practitioner is required to undertake a clinical reasoning process. This involves hypothesis generation, refinement, summary of findings and the formulation of a management plan. Throughout this process, the practitioner is required to undertake critical appraisal of the evidence, acceptability and clinical relevance of findings from the HTPE activity. The SNAPPS tool and concept mapping are two key resources that can help immensely.

SNAPPS and concept mapping

The SNAPPS tool is designed to aid the more junior practitioner in structuring their patient presentations, but it is a useful tool for all involved in conducting HTPEs. Concept maps are diagrams that start from generalised ideas and progress to more specific ideas represented in circles or boxes called 'nodes'.[6] The nodes are connected to each other with 'linking words' that show relationships between the concepts. They are unique to the individual and are meaningful representations of a person's thought process in the complex world of clinical reasoning. Figure 8.1 details how a concept map may be used as a history-taking template and Figure 8.2 details how this may be used for the presenting complaint of chest pain.

9 Principles of diagnostic testing and clinical decision making

Table 9.1 Clinical situation

Consultation and assessment of an immobile postoperative gynaecology patient with pleuritic chest pain includes pulmonary embolism (PE) as a differential diagnosis. A hypothetical diagnostic test (Test A) for pulmonary embolism has a sensitivity of 75% and specificity of 90%. Is this an accurate test? Is there an alternative test with higher accuracy?

Table 9.2 Sensitivity and specificity Based on [2]

Sensitivity True positives (75) True positives (75) + False negatives (25)		The ability of a test to correctly identify patients **with** disease
True positive	The patient has disease and is correctly identified by a positive test	75% of patients with pulmonary embolism will be detected, but 25% of patients with pulmonary embolism will not be identified by the test. They may go untreated and suffer associated complications
False negative	A patient has disease but is not identified due to a negative test	
Specificity True negatives (90) True negatives (90) + False positives (10)		The ability of a test to correctly identify patients **without** disease
True negative	A patient without disease is correctly identified by a negative test	90% of patients without pulmonary embolism will be identified by a negative test result, but 10% of patients without pulmonary embolism will have a positive test and may receive unnecessary treatment
False positive	A patient without disease has a positive test	

Figure 9.1 A receiver operator curve (ROC) to compare hypothetical diagnostic tests for pulmonary embolism

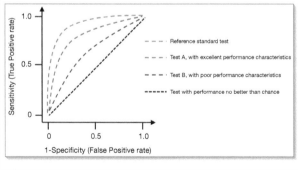

Table 9.3 True positives and true negatives Based on [2]

Positive predictive value (PPV)	True positives (75) True positives (75) + False positives (10)	A positive test has 88% probability of accurately identifying PE
Negative predictive value (NPV)	True negatives (90) True negatives (90) + False negatives (25)	A negative test has 78% probability of accurately identifying patients without PE

Table 9.4 Statistical terms pertaining to evidence-based diagnosis/diagnostic accuracy

Term	Description
Likelihood ratio (LR)	Finding/sign/test results sensitivity divided by the false-positive rate. A test of no value has a LR of 1. Therefore, the test would have no impact upon the patient's odds of disease
Positive likelihood ratio	Proportion of patients with disease who have a positive finding/sign/test, divided by proportion of patients without disease who have a positive finding/sign/test. The more positive a LR (the further above 1), the more the finding/sign/test result raises a patient's probability of disease. Thresholds of ≥4 are often considered to be significant when focusing a clinician's interest on the most pertinent positive findings, clinical signs or tests
Negative likelihood ratio	Proportion of patients with disease who have a negative finding/sign/test result, divided by the proportion of patients without disease who have a positive finding/sign/test. The more negative a LR (the closer to 0), the more the finding/sign/test result lowers a patient's probability of disease. Thresholds <0.4 are often considered to be significant when focusing a clinician's interest on the most pertinent negative findings, clinical signs or tests
Prevalence	Equal to the pretest probability
Post-test probability	The probability of the presence of a condition after a diagnostic test is performed
Pretest probability	The probability of the presence of a condition prior to a diagnostic test being performed
Pretest odds	Pretest odds = pretest probability/(1 – pretest probability)

Advanced Clinical Practice at a Glance, First Edition. Edited by Barry Hill and Sadie Diamond Fox.
© 2023 John Wiley & Sons Ltd. Published 2023 by John Wiley & Sons Ltd.

The advanced practitioner assimilates information gathered through patient consultation, history taking and physical examination, to establish a list of differential diagnoses. The number of differentials may be refined through use of a range of diagnostic tests where necessary, to confirm or refute a diagnosis. An understanding of the principles, advantages and limitations of diagnostic testing enables the practitioner to use sound professional judgement regarding which test to request for any given patient, depending upon the clinical context. In turn, this allows appropriate use of healthcare resources, and may avoid potential harms from the test itself or harms that may arise as an indirect result of the test data. The ability to understand and critically review the accuracy of a diagnostic test is paramount for clinical decision making. This chapter provides an overview of the principles of using diagnostic tests for clinical decision making, using the clinical example in Table 9.1 to demonstrate clinical applicability.

Key principles

The key principle of a diagnostic test is its accuracy. New diagnostic tests should always be evaluated by comparing them with the most accurate available source of disease status, such as post-mortem findings, or the current 'gold standard' test for diagnosis of the relevant disease.[1] This may also be referred to as the 'reference standard'. Accuracy is usually reported using the characteristics of sensitivity and specificity, with an accurate test being both highly sensitive and highly specific.

Sensitivity (Table 9.2) is the ability of a test to correctly identify patients *with* the disease.[2] 100% sensitivity means that a positive result would correctly identify all those *with* the disease in question (true positives). However, most diagnostic tests are not perfect, and some patients *with* the disease may still have a negative test (false negative), and this is reflected by a decreased sensitivity value. The risk of tests with low sensitivity is that they can allow patients who have the disease to remain undiagnosed.

Specificity (Table 9.2) is the ability of a test to correctly identify patients *without* the disease.[2] 100% specificity means a negative result would correctly identify all those *without* the disease in question (true negatives). However, some patients *without* the disease may still have a positive test (false positive), which is reflected by a decreased specificity value. False positives resulting from tests with low specificity can cause distress to patients and subject them to further unnecessary investigations and treatment.

Predictive value is another way of reviewing the accuracy of a diagnostic test, by calculating the proportion of patients with a positive test having the disease, or the proportion of patients with a negative test not having the disease.[3] Table 9.3 highlights the factors used to calculate predictive value. Unlike sensitivity and specificity, predictive values are influenced by disease prevalence in the population.[2] In a clinical setting where prevalence of the disease is high, it is more likely that a patient with a positive test does indeed have the disease; therefore, the positive predictive value of a test will increase. Conversely, in a population with low levels of the disease, it is more likely that a patient with a negative test does not have the disease, leading to an increase in negative predictive value. In the hypothetical example, the prevalence of pulmonary embolism in this context is probably higher than may be found in the outpatient setting, and therefore the test may have a higher positive predictive value in this population.

When critiquing diagnostic tests, the impact of prevalence needs to be considered, as the population tested within the study influences the predictive value.[3] Further scrutiny of the cohort would be needed before assuming generalisability of the test across different populations.

Receiver operator curves (ROC) graphically plot sensitivity and specificity characteristics for tests, thereby helping to define the optimum cut-off point for a negative or positive test result where the data is non-binary.[3] The inverse relationship between sensitivity and specificity is such that as one value increases, the other decreases. A cut-off seeking to maximise both characteristics would be ideal if equal value was placed on both. However, there may be situations where greater value is placed upon one characteristic over the other.

Area under the receiver operator curve (AUROC) summarises test accuracy, with values of 1.0 representing perfect accuracy. Tests with AUROC of 0.5 have a discriminatory value no better than chance alone.[1] The AUROC can be used for comparison of different diagnostic tests for a specified disease.

The ROC curve in Figure 9.1 demonstrates the performance of several hypothetical tests to detect pulmonary embolism. The green line is the reference standard, with high sensitivity and specificity, and an AUROC value close to 1.0. Test A (red line) has an AUROC less than the reference standard but is more closely aligned with it than test B (blue line). Test A is more accurate than test B, but not as accurate as the reference standard. The black line has an AUROC of less than 0.5, indicating a poor test. The reference standard has the best diagnostic accuracy, but is it the right test for the patient? Are there other risks to consider, such as exposure to radiation? Is the patient too unwell to have this test? What are the risks compared to the benefits?

Diagnostic accuracy and clinical decision making

Appraisal of diagnostic accuracy studies supports clinical decision making. Further statistical terms pertaining to appraising diagnostic accuracy are detailed in Table 9.4. Toolkits to guide the appraisal process, such as the Critical Appraisal Skills Programme (CASP),[4] are available, and meta-analyses of diagnostic test studies are also reported within the Cochrane Library.[5] In time-limited situations, evidence-based decision-making tools and artificial intelligence software are increasingly used.

The number of diagnostic tests performed tends to decline with increasing clinical experience, reflecting an intuitive component to clinical decision making that develops through pattern recognition.[6,7] Shared decision making with the patient, their family and the wider multidisciplinary team should be considered in complex situations, in order to discuss the appropriateness and choice of diagnostic testing within the clinical context, taking into account factors such as test availability, the ease and accuracy of performance, associated risks and benefits, the wishes of the patient, and how the test result may ultimately influence management.

10 The psychiatric interview: mental health history taking and examination

Table 10.1 The Mental State Exam (MSE)

Component	Clinical significance/important clues	Specific considerations
Appearance	• Patients with severe depression may present with weight loss or appear dishevelled • Patients with histrionic personality disorders may wear what is considered contextually or culturally inappropriate clothing (e.g., inappropriately seductive outfit in contrast to how they previously dressed)	• Estimated age by appearance vs stated age • Body habitus • Posture • Hygiene (level of grooming)
Behaviour	• Psychomotor agitation is common in patients with mania, whereas psychomotor retardation can be seen in depression • Glancing repeatedly at different parts of the room can be seen in patients experiencing visual or auditory hallucinations (e.g., in schizophrenia) • Abnormal motor activity can be a sign of an underlying neurological disorder or a side-effect of psychotropic medication	• Eye contact (level and type) • Attitude toward the ACP • Level of distress • Ability to gain rapport • Apathy/abulia/akinetic mutism
Sensorium and cognition	• Level of consciousness – are they orientated to person, place and time? • Awareness to time is lost first, followed by orientation to place, and lastly to self • Consider common causes of a reduced GCS: AEIOU-TIPS • Consider hypo- and hyperactive delirium which is usually the result of an underlying medical condition (e.g. acute kidney injury)	• Describe level of consciousness: *Alertness* (state of awareness – a normal finding) *Somnolence* (state of drowsiness in which patient responds normally except for slight delay) *Lethargy* (impaired consciousness from which can be awoken, tends to fall back asleep after being aroused) *Obtundation* (impaired consciousness characterised by ↑ sleepiness) *Stupor* (insensitivity bordering on unconsciousness from which patient is not easily awoken – normally only a painful stimulus provokes a response) *Coma* (unrousable unresponsiveness characterised by closed eyes, absent reflex responses and motor activity but preserved circulatory function and breathing drive) • Quantify with GCS
Mood and affect	• Remember that mood is the patient's subjective assessment of their emotions, while affect refers to the clinician's objective assessment of the patient's emotions conveyed verbally and non-verbally • It is important to assess affect during the MSE because changes are characteristic of many conditions: • Schizophrenia = blunted, inappropriate affect • Mania = exaggerated, blunted affect • Severe depression = fixed and/or constricted affect	• Mood should be described using the patient's own words • Most psychiatric considerations are associated with some degree of mood alteration • Depression commonly involves feelings of sadness, or nothing at all • Mania commonly involves feelings of ecstasy • Patients with social anxiety disorder may describe feeling frightened or embarrassed when exposed to a large group of people • Describe affect covering the following: • Quality • Congruency • Range • Mobility • Appropriateness to situation
Speech	• *Mutism*: either structural or motor dysfunction or result of a patient's unwillingness to speak (e.g. akinetic mutism in which the patient is in a wakeful state of apathy, indifferent to pain, thirst or hunger) • *Dysarthria*: impaired articulation of words due to motor dysfunction • *Echolalia*: involuntary repetition of another's speech • *Palilia*: involuntary repetition of words/phrases with increasing rapidity • *Alogia/poverty of speech*: impaired thinking that manifests with reduced speech output • *Pressured speech*: accelerated thoughts that are expressed as rapid, loud and voluminous speech • *Neologisms*: new words created and understood by the speaker • *Word salad*: incoherent thinking expressed as a sequence of words with no logical connection	• Speech is characterised by: • Rate (rapid, normal, slow, pressured) • Volume (loud, normal, soft, whispered) • Quantity (logorrhoeic, talkative, responsive, reserved) • Articulation/fluency (incomprehensible, stuttered, slurred, mumbled, clear, articulated) • Speech latency (increased, decreased, no latency) • Speech is very important and characteristic of many psychiatric conditions: • Patients with depression may have soft speech with increased latency • Those in a manic state are often logorrhoeic and speak loudly and extremely fast • Schizophrenic patients may have disorganised, incomprehensible speech

Advanced Clinical Practice at a Glance, First Edition. Edited by Barry Hill and Sadie Diamond Fox.
© 2023 John Wiley & Sons Ltd. Published 2023 by John Wiley & Sons Ltd.

Table 10.1 (Continued)

Component	Clinical significance/important clues	Specific considerations
Thought process	• *Circumstantial*: long-winded and multiple deviations from central topic. • *Tangential*: non-linear thought with gradual deviation from central topic • *Derailment*: incoherent, illogical with sudden and frequent changes of topic • *Flight of ideas*: quick succession of thoughts normally expressed as continuous rapid speech and abrupt changes in topic • *Clang associations*: the use of words based on rhyme patterns rather than meaning • *Preservation*: inappropriate repetition/persistence of behaviour, speech or sounds • *Thought blocking*: abrupt ending of thought process expressed as sudden interruption in speech	• Schizophrenia, bipolar disorder, epilepsy, intellectual disability, developmental delay • Schizophrenia, anxiety, delirium • Schizophrenia • Manic phase of bipolar disorder • Schizophrenia, manic states • Psychoses, epilepsy, dementia, Parkinson disease, traumatic brain injury, stroke • Schizophrenia
Thought content	• Normally evaluated based on presence of delusions, obsessions, compulsions, phobias and homicidal/suicidal ideation • *Delusions* are fixed, false beliefs (unrelated to religious beliefs of culture) that are maintained, despite being contradicted by reality or rational arguments • *Suicidal ideation* is any type of thought that an individual has regarding their own life. Can range from brief consideration of the act to concrete planning of time, place and/or method. Risk can be assessed with the help of Joiner's Triad (Figure 10.1) • *Homicidal ideation* are thoughts regarding ending someone else's life • *Obsessions* are persistent, intrusive and unpleasant thoughts/urges that cause severe distress	• Important because lots of psychiatric conditions are associated with various disturbances of thought content, some of which are pathognomic • Make sure to consider the patient's individual cultural, social, religious and educational background in the context of thought content • See Table 10.2 for common delusions and how to assess for them • Compulsions can be assessed by asking the patient if there is something they constantly think about and whether they engage in any specific behaviour to get rid of the persistent thoughts
Perceptual disturbances	• Some physical or mental disorders can cause disruptions to a patient's perception causing hallucinations, illusions, dissociation and agnosia • *Dissociation* is a psychological defence mechanism that is a natural protective response to a traumatic or stressful experience • *Agnosia* is characterised by impaired recognition of sensory stimuli	• See Table 10.3 for common hallucinations and how to assess for them – *remember that hallucinations are not always pathological and must be taken in context of the clinical assessment* (auditory verbal hallucinations, for example occur in around 13% of adults in the United States general population) • Dissociation can be assessed by asking the patient if they feel detached from themselves or others • See Table 10.4 for the different types of agnosia and their causes
Insight and judgement	• *Insight* refers to the patient's awareness and understanding of their current medical condition • *Judgement* refers to the patient's ability to make considered decisions	• Can the patient recognise that they have a medical condition, be compliant with treatment, and relabel unusual mental events as pathological? • Judgement can be assessed by asking the patient to elaborate on a hypothetical situation or interpret a well-known idiom

ACP, advanced clinical practitioner; AEIOU-TIPS, Alcohol, Epilepsy, Insulin, Uremia, Trauma, Infection, Psychiatric, Stroke/Shock; GCS, Glasgow Coma Scale.

Figure 10.1 Joiner's interpersonal theory of suicide. Source: Adapted from Romero AJ, Edwards LM, Bauman S, Ritter MK (2014) What drove her to do it? Theories of depression and suicide. In: *Preventing Adolescent Depression and Suicide Among Latinas: Resilience Research and Theory*. Springer International Publishing, New York, pp.11–20.

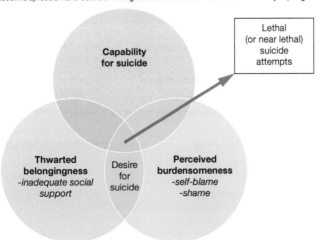

Table 10.2 Common delusions and example questions

Type of delusion	Description	How to assess
Persecutory	The patient thinks they're being persecuted – cheated on, harassed	Does the patient feel wronged or threatened by anyone?
Paranoia	An exaggerated distrust of people and is highly suspicious of motives	Does the patient think an individual or group of people is 'out to get them'?
Erotomania	The patient believes people are in love with them (e.g. having relationship with a famous person)	Does the patient have a special relationship with someone, sending them secret messages?
Grandiosity	The patient believes they are special or have special powers	Does the patient believe they have special abilities?
Somatic	The patient may believe that there is something wrong with their body's function or appearance	Does the patient think there is something wrong with their body?
Delusion of reference	The patient believes that a wide variety of natural events refer to them personally	Does the patient believe that the TV or radio is talking about them or trying to send them messages?
Religious delusions	The patient believes they are God, or have divine powers	Does the patient believe they are in contact with a religious figure?
Jealousy	The patient believes their partner is unfaithful with no evidence or justification	N/A
Delusion of guilt	The patient feels they and their families may be punished due to a perceived sin	Does the patient think they are being punished for something?

Table 10.3 Common hallucinations

Type of hallucination	Description	Aetiology/epidemiology
Auditory	Perceptions of hearing in the absence of external stimuli	• Most common
Visual	Visual perceptions in the absence of external stimuli	• The most common hallucination in those with dementia or delirium
Olfactory	Perception of an odour (normally unpleasant) when there is no odorant in the environment	• The most common hallucination in those with focal-onset temporal lobe seizures
Gustatory	Spontaneous perceptions of taste sensations (sweet, sour, bitter, umami, salty) in the absence of any food or drink	• Rare
Somatic	A perception of being touched in the absence of any sensory stimuli	• Common in alcohol withdrawal and intoxication • A symptom of delusional parasitosis
Synaesthesia	A perception of being able to hear colours, feel sounds and/or taste shapes	• There is no clear aetiology, however recent discussions posit a theoretical link between neurodivergence pathologies such as autism and synaesthesia

Table 10.4 Types of agnosia and their causes

Type of agnosia	Description	Aetiology/epidemiology
Visual	Unable to recognise visually presented objects despite normal vision	• Lesion in the visual association cortex (occipital lobe) • Lesion in the ventral visual stream (temporal lobe)
Auditory	Unable to recognise sounds despite normal and intact hearing	• Lesion in the auditory ventral stream (anterior superior temporal gyrus)
Tactile (astereognosis)	Unable to recognise objects by touch without visual input	• Lesion in the contralateral parietal lobe
Visuospatial dysgnosia	Unable to localise and orient oneself	• Damage to right posterior parietal lobe
Prosopagnosia	Unable to recognise familiar faces but can still name individual parts (e.g. nose, ears)	• Bilateral lesions or large unilateral lesions of the ventral occipitotemporal cortex (fusiform gyrus)
Autotopagnosia	Unable to localise parts of the body	• Damage to left posterior parietal area of the cortex

Mental health and well-being present a unique challenge to clinicians, with increasingly alarming year-on-year increases in demand for services, admissions for self-harm and referrals to specialist mental health services. Indeed, some commentators estimate that approximately 14% of the global disease burden can be attributed to neuropsychiatric disorders. Thus, taking an effective and cogent history together with an appropriate examination is a critical skill for advanced clinical practitioners (ACPs) across both primary and secondary care.

The psychiatric interview

An effective history, as for most specialties, is integral to determining a possible aetiology, choosing appropriate investigations and forming a clinical impression/diagnosis. However, the psychiatric history differs from a standard medical assessment slightly due to having a greater emphasis on the history component. Furthermore, a large element of the examination is undertaken during the history component rather than as a discrete set of procedures afterwards. As such, obtaining a collateral history may be necessary and while a history may be taken from the patient alone, information from their friends, family or other healthcare professionals may offer additional important keys in establishing a clinical impression.

It is essential to establish a therapeutic alliance as this forms the groundwork of history taking because initially the patient will be making a decision as to your trustworthiness and as a corollary, instituting a therapeutic relationship is one of the key aims of the psychiatric interview. This is followed by eliciting the symptoms, history and background information at the same time as examining the patient's mental state by means of the Mental State Examination (MSE), and concluding by providing information, reassurance and advice to them.

Ensure that due attention is paid to potential risks. While violence against medical professionals is still relatively uncommon, it is recognised that violence against healthcare staff in emergency departments is happening. Therefore, before the interview (if possible) speak to someone who knows the patient and establish whether it is safe to interview them alone. If there is any doubt, do not interview by yourself or out of the sight/hearing of another staff member. Conduct the interview in a quiet room alone and ensure you are sitting between the patient and the door in case you need to exit quickly.

Components of the psychiatric history

While most ACPs will not be expected to diagnose psychopathologies, obtaining salient points during the history allows senior clinical staff or psychiatric specialists during feedback/referral to form suitable differentials and help formulate ongoing plans and review. Key components of the psychiatric history include the following.

- *Presenting complaint*: why the patient is here, and have they been referred? If so, by whom?
- *History of presenting complaint*: include the course of the illness, from the earliest time the patient noticed it up to their current presentation. Remember to establish the severity of the illness, any periodicity, patterns and associated symptoms/factors together with a review of systems.

- *Past medical history*: include accidents, operations and any emotional responses to previous illnesses. With patients who are/were able to bear children, include information relating to menstrual problems, pregnancies, miscarriages, terminations and menopause.
- *Past psychiatric history*: direct questions may be required as the patient may not volunteer information. Remember to include any previous self-harm or suicide attempts. Include any previous formal assessments and/or treatments under the Mental Health Act 1983.
- *Past drug history*: remember to ask about herbal medications, illicit drugs, alcohol, tobacco, caffeine and prescribed medications.
- *Personal history*: birth and early developmental history, any major childhood events, education, occupational history, relationship(s), marriage, children, major adulthood events.
- *Social history*: current employment, financial status, housing, benefits, stressors.
- *Personality*: includes how the patient may normally deal with stress. How do they define their personality? Do they like being in the company of people or do they like being alone? Do they trust others? This may be elicited when obtaining collateral information from someone who knows the patient well.
- *Forensic history*: does the patient have any violent or sexual offences? This helps form part of a risk assessment. Do they ever suffer with homicidal ideation? This element of the history can be inflammatory and so it may be useful to explain that ill health can occasionally result in problems with law enforcement.

Mental State Examination

Examination of the psychiatric patient largely takes place during the history-taking phase through the MSE, which is a framework derived from a 1912 conceptual framework by German philosopher and psychiatrist Karl Jaspers that outlines a systematic objective examination of the patient's thinking, emotion and behaviour by eliciting objective clinical signs and is therefore a core fundamental skill for the ACP. It is used to aid assessment for mental health presentations, and is useful due to both its systematic nature and its objective evaluation of the *current* state of the patient. This is important because it also provides a documented baseline which allows mental health professionals to conduct serial MSE reassessments of the patient and therefore response to treatment. It should be remembered that just as a patient presenting with an orthopaedic pathology may require specialist review, so too should the patient presenting with a psychopathology (if appropriate) and the use of the MSE alone should *not* replace specialist review as inaccurate assessment could affect care and the patient's journey.

The MSE comprises nine key components: appearance, behaviour, sensorium and cognition, mood and affect, speech, thought process, thought content, perceptual disturbances, and insight and judgement. Remember that some patients have social or cultural practices or beliefs that may run counter to yours and so evaluating any pathology should be done with metacognition of your own cognitive biases. Table 10.1 outlines the key components of the MSE with any associated clinical significance and specific considerations.

History taking for patients who lack mental capacity

Table 11.1 Core principles of the MCA 2005

Principles	Application to clinical practice
1. A person must be assumed to have capacity unless it is established that they lack capacity	Every person from the age of 16 has a right to make their own decisions if they have the capacity to do so. Practitioners and carers must assume that a person has capacity to make a particular decision at a point in time unless it can be established that they do not
2. A person is not to be treated as unable to make a decision unless all practicable steps to help him to do so have been taken without success	People should be supported to help them make their own decisions. No conclusion should be made that a person lacks capacity to make a decision unless all practicable steps have been taken to try and help them make a decision for themselves
3. A person is not to be treated as unable to make a decision merely because he makes an unwise decision	People have the right to make a decision that others would see as 'unwise'. This does not automatically mean they lack capacity and they should not be treated as such
4. An act done or decision made, under this Act for or on behalf of a person who lacks capacity must be done, or made, in his best interests	If the person lacks capacity any decision that is made on their behalf or subsequent action taken must be done using best interests, as set out in the Act
5. Before the act is done, or the decision is made, regard must be had to whether the purpose for which it is needed can be as effectively achieved in a way that is less restrictive of the person's rights and freedom of action	As long as the decision or action remains in the person's best interests, it should be the decision or action that places the least restriction on their basic rights and freedoms

Figure 11.1 Interviewing the person without capacity

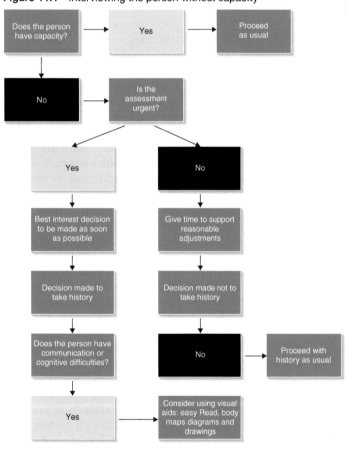

Figure 11.2 Advanced communication skills used whilst interviewing people who may lack capacity

Verbal Communication: Be respectful, use direct questions, use short clear sentences, use simple words with no jargon, let people know what you are about to do

Non-verbal Communication: adopt an open expression, smile, do nothing sudden or unexpected to help people anticipate what you are about to do

Other sources of information and collaborators in the interview process: carers, family, medical notes, hospital passports

Active listening: Listen carefully and ask the person to repeat if unclear, Look for non-verbal expression of pain or discomfort

Environment: Make sure the person is physically and mentally comfortable; think about noise, bright lights and distractions, consider giving extra time, e.g. double appointments

Advanced Clinical Practice at a Glance, First Edition. Edited by Barry Hill and Sadie Diamond Fox.
© 2023 John Wiley & Sons Ltd. Published 2023 by John Wiley & Sons Ltd.

The Mental Capacity Act (MCA) 2005 has been in force since 2007 and applies to England and Wales. It applies to young people over the age of 16 and adults. The primary purpose of the MCA 2005 is to promote and safeguard decision making within a legal framework and utilizes five key principles (Table 11.1). Everyone working with (or caring for) any person from the age of 16 who may lack capacity must comply with the Act.

A person is said to have mental capacity when they can make and communicate their own decisions. People may lack capacity for many reasons including dementia; severe learning or neurodevelopmental disability; brain injury; mental illness; stroke; or intoxication (Figure 11.1).[1] Nevertheless, a person should not be assumed to lack capacity to make a specific decision just because they have one of these conditions. Healthcare professionals must assume a person has the capacity to decide themselves unless it is proved otherwise. If healthcare professionals are going to decide for someone who does not have capacity, it must be in their best interests and any treatment or care provided must be the least restrictive course of action in terms of their basic rights and freedoms.

Capacity is time and decision specific. Healthcare professionals can only decide that a person lacks capacity at that time and for that decision. Therefore, it must be clear what specific decisions are needed from the history that is being taking. A person cannot be said to lack capacity generally; they may only be said to lack capacity to make that decision at the specific time they are assessed.

The MCA sets out a two-stage test of capacity.

1 Does the person have an impairment of their mind or brain?
2 Does the impairment mean the person is unable to make a specific decision when needed?

A person is unable to make a decision if they cannot:
- understand the information relevant to the decision
- retain that information
- use or weigh up that information as part of the decision-making process
- communicate their decision.

Before it is decided if a person lacks capacity, the health professional must have taken steps to enable them to try to make the decision themselves.

If the healthcare professional moves to a capacity assessment and a patient is found to lack capacity to consent for history taking and the situation is not urgent, then delaying the decision until such a time as the person could make the decision for themselves should be considered.

It may be that the person's incapacity is temporary, or that with the right support and information presented to them in a way that they can understand, they could make the decision if they are given more time. For example, if a person with dementia has a 'good' time of day when they are more cognitively able, then asking for consent could wait until that time.

Taking steps to enable them to make a decision themselves might also mean presenting information to the person in more accessible ways. This could include using an easy-read or pictorial format, recording conversations, using videos or taking more time to explain what the history taking will look like.

If the decision is more urgent, or the person is still not going to be able to make that decision for themselves in the future even with additional support and information, then a best interest decision-making process needs to be followed, under Section 4 of the Mental Capacity Act.[1] A decision maker must be identified – this is normally the same person who assessed capacity, unless there is a court-appointed deputy, or they are not best placed to make the decision. A practitioner or team that is responsible for providing health or social care to the individual could act as the decision maker in this instance.

The best interest decision MUST:
- encourage participation of the person
- identify all relevant circumstances
- find out the person's views
- avoid discrimination
- assess whether the person might regain capacity
- consult others
- avoid restricting the person's rights
- in the case of life-sustaining medical treatment, make no assumptions about the quality of the person's life and ensure that decisions are in no way motivated by a desire to bring about the person's death.

Unless there is a clear reason why this should not be the case (e.g. safeguarding concerns or clearly expressed preferences by the individual), it is important to involve family and paid carers in the process. These are the people who often know the person best, holding information about the individual and their needs and wishes.

It should be borne in mind that making a best interest decision for an individual does not mean they should be excluded from the process. They should very much remain at the heart of it and be included as much as is possible or desirable. In fact, the decision should be what the person would have chosen for themselves if they had capacity.

As such, it is important to gather as much information about the individual as possible, as well as from friends, family and carers; the person may have an advocate who should be included or may require an independent mental capacity advocate (IMCA).

More formal documentation such as care notes, etc. should also be considered as a source of information. Adults with a learning disability may have a hospital passport, which contains detailed information about their health needs and their communication needs.

Taking a history from a person who lacks capacity requires excellent communication skills and clinical observations skills, as the individual's ability to self-report may be compromised (Figure 11.2). Consider allowing more time for the assessment, or perhaps breaking it down into smaller stages and splitting these over a few days. The healthcare professional may also wish to consider where the history taking takes place, choosing somewhere where the person is comfortable and relaxed, and allowing supporters or family members to be with the person during the assessment.

Although taking a history from a person who lacks the capacity to consent to it may be more complicated, it is crucial that they receive a full assessment, to begin to address the health inequalities experienced by many who are more likely to lack capacity to make certain decisions, such as those who are mentally unwell or have a learning disability.

12 Dermatology history taking and physical examination

Table 12.1 Common skin, hair and nail presentations. Source: Based on British Society of Dermatologists.[1]

Skin	Nails	Hair
Rash	Clubbing	Alopecia
Pruritus	Koilonychia	Hirsutism
Lesions – an area of altered skin which may be discrete, confluent, linear, target-like, annular or discoid	Onycholysis	Hypertrichosis
Erythema	Pitting	
Purpura		
Hypo/hyperpigmentation		
Lumps		
Ulcers		
Comedones (blackheads or whiteheads)		
Papules		
Nodules		
Vesicles		
Bullae		
Pustules		
Wheals		
Furuncles/boils		
Carbuncles		
Excoriation		
Lichenification		
Scales		
Crust		
Scars		
Fissures		
Striae		
Naevus/mole – a localised malformation of tissue structures		
Skin colouration changes		

Incidental observations may occur during clinical presentations with other primary conditions across all categories.

Figure 12.1 Common skin eruptions. Source: Davey P (2014) *Medicine at a Glance*, with permission of John Wiley & Sons

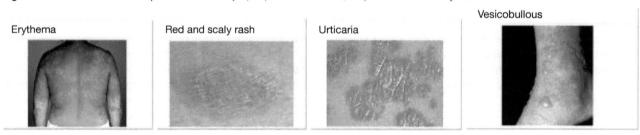

Erythema   Red and scaly rash   Urticaria   Vesicobullous

Table 12.2 Essential elements of a dermatological history

Onset of symptoms
Rate of progression
Associated symptoms, i.e. itchiness, discharge, pain
Systemic upset – fever, rigors
Immune status – diabetes, HIV, steroids
Recent trauma/surgery
Recent antibiotic therapy
Foreign travel
Animal exposure

Advanced Clinical Practice at a Glance, First Edition. Edited by Barry Hill and Sadie Diamond Fox.
© 2023 John Wiley & Sons Ltd. Published 2023 by John Wiley & Sons Ltd.

Figure 12.2 Clinical presentations of cutaneous adverse drug reactions. DRESS, drug rash with eosinophilia and systemic symptoms; MPE, maculopapular exanthema; SJS, Stevens–Johnson syndrome; TEN, toxic epidermal necrolysis. Source: Chung WH *et al.* (2016) Severe cutaneous adverse drug reactions. *Journal of Dermatology*, **43**, 758–766, with permission of John Wiley & Sons

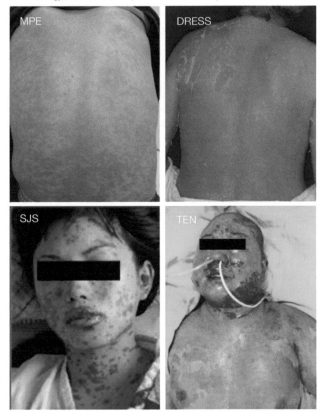

Table 12.3 Essential elements of a dermatological examination

Vital signs
Anatomical site and distribution – mark the side to assess for spread of erythema
Type of rash, e.g. raised, erythema, exudative, crusting, vesicular/bullous
Skin colour
Local lymphadenopathy
Lymphangitis – erythema travelling up the lymphatic system
Presence of gas under tissues
Evidence of precipitating breakdown of normal skin barriers, e.g. trauma or fungal infection

Figure 12.3 Acute phase fulminant meningococcemia and purpura fulminans. Source: Wick JM *et al.* (2013) Meningococcemia: the pediatric orthopedic sequelae. *AORN Journal*, **97**, 559–578, with permission from Elsevier

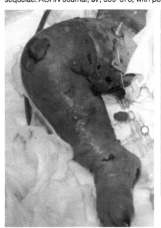 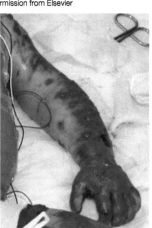

Prevalence of dermatological conditions

Dermatological conditions are common (10–15% of general practice consultation) and present to clinicians in all specialties. Affecting up to one-third of the population at any one time, they can have a serious impact on quality of life and contribute to approximately 2% of the total NHS health expenditure. Skin disorders can be due to many factors such as allergy, trauma, infection, tumour or environmental stresses. They may also be degenerative, congenital or secondary to another illness or disease within another organ system (e.g. acne can be attributed to hormonal imbalance in the endocrine system but appears as lesions on the skin).

Presentation of dermatological conditions

Due to the large number of dermatological conditions that can present with an array of skin, hair and nail changes, it is difficult to be prescriptive when describing how to take a good dermatological history. To ensure the history is focused and relevant, it may be appropriate to examine the area of concern prior to undertaking a detailed enquiry. Common presentations are summarised in Table 12.1[1] and can be viewed in Figure 12.1.

History of presenting complaint and past medical history

An accurate history is vital in establishing the correct diagnosis in conditions affecting the skin. Use a standard structure to your history taking (Table 12.2) for essential points. The following questions should also be considered during the consultation.

- Previous skin diseases/problems?
- Atopic symptoms (eczema, asthma, hay fever suggest atopy).
- Medical disorders which may involve the skin include diabetes, connective tissue disease, inflammatory bowel disease, SLE (any medical condition which may have skin manifestations).
- Recent trauma/surgery.
- Where is it? When was it first noticed? Were there any precipitants (e.g. medication, sunlight, allergen potential, diet)?
- Common presenting symptoms include rash (scaly, blistering, itchy), a lump or lesion, pruritus (itch).
- Has it spread or changed since onset?
- Do the symptoms vary with time?
- Any preceding symptoms (e.g. illness, new medication)?
- Any aggravating or relieving factors (e.g. exercise or heat precipitation)?
- Any treatments tried (e.g. topical, or oral medications)?
- Any associated symptoms (e.g. joint or muscle pain, fever, weight loss, fatigue)?
- What is the impact of the presentation on quality of life?

Drugs

A detailed and accurate drug history is paramount. If a dermatological condition is suspected, there are several drugs that may affect precipitation of disease onset, contribute to subsequent recognised complications or aid in differential diagnosis,

- Antibiotics
- Immunosuppression and steroids can increase the risk of skin cancer
- Common drug eruption culprits: anticonvulsants, sulphonamides, penicillins, allopurinol, non-steroidal analgesics (NSAIDs)

Allergies

- Cutaneous (Figure 12.2) and non-cutaneous drug reactions: *always* ascertain the extent/effect of an allergy (i.e. mild/localised, severe/systemic, life-threatening). Simply writing 'rash' is *not* sufficient and potentially negligent! Be specific as to the extent and nature of the reaction and document this clearly.
- Prescribed or self-medicated drugs including creams.
- Foods or substances such as latex/metals/hygiene products.
- Remember to ask about the nature of any allergic reaction claimed.
- Has the patient undergone any patch testing or IgE responses?

Family and social history

Pertinent dermatology-related familial history includes:

- psoriasis
- skin cancer
- atopic disease.

Social history

Pertinent dermatology-related familial history includes:

- occupation (consider sun exposure, wet work, chemical and plant exposure)
- hobbies
- pets (including pets of close family or friends that the person may be in contact with)
- living conditions: shared living space, damp
- recent travel: vaccines taken before travel, sun exposure
- insect bites
- risk factors for STDs
- recent exposure to infectious conditions (e.g. chickenpox).

Psychosocial impact

Skin conditions can influence psychosocial functioning and reduce a person's quality of life, resulting in depression. Early interventions such as coping strategies, self-help and cognitive behavioural therapy (CBT) can reduce this risk.

Review of systems

A functional enquiry into the possibility of any associated systemic disease should be undertaken, such as coeliac disease, parasitic infection, systemic lupus erythematosus (SLE) or psoriatic arthropathy. This line of enquiry may prompt you to perform a general examination of all or some other body systems.

Ensure that you enquire about the patient's immune status (diabetes, HIV, steroids) and if they have any features of systemic upset (fever, rigors).

Examination

A systematic check of the nails, scalp, hair and mucous membranes should also be included as part of your dermatology assessment (Table 12.3). Accurate diagnosis of skin disease is usually based on visual pattern recognition developed through experience rather than analytical rule-based approaches. You need to familiarise yourself with the patterns of skin conditions and then test the hypotheses for best fit with history and examination.

Examination key points

- Is the patient well or unwell? Serious skin conditions affecting larger areas of skin can lead to life-threatening fluid loss and secondary infections so obtain vital signs and consider sepsis.
- Ensure that you examine the whole organ; this means ensuring the patient is adequately exposed after gaining consent (consider chaperone requirement).
- Review the skin condition in the context of the whole patient and examine other systems as indicated if you are considering systemic disease manifestation (e.g. SLE, malignancy).
- What is the skin abnormality – rash, ulcer, lump, discolouration?
- Where is the skin abnormality?
- Are there any secondary skin changes – scale, crust, erosion, atrophy, scar, excoriation, fissure, lichenification?
- What is the extent, shape and pattern of the distribution – localised, generalised, symmetrical/asymmetrical, areas of exposure, skin creases, follicular?
- Palpate for temperature, mobility, tenderness and depth and regional lymph nodes if appropriate.

Investigations

Following examination, specific investigations may be required to enable an accurate diagnosis.

- Skin biopsy for histology examination in the laboratory.
- Mycology to confirm fungal infection (skin scraping, nail clippings, hair plucking).
- Patch testing if suspecting contact allergy.

Documentation

A picture (or diagram) can aid your documentation. Ensure that you note size/shape/surrounding features. Documentation should include relevant history, PMH, drug history and allergies.

Dermatological emergencies

Identification of these life-threatening situations and prompt management are vital, particularly if this is the first presentation.[1]

- Anaphylaxis and angio-oedema
- Toxic epidermal necrolysis (see Figure 12.2)
- Stevens–Johnson syndrome (see Figure 12.2)
- Acute meningococcaemia (Figure 12.3)
- Erythroderma
- Eczema herpeticum
- Necrotising fasciitis

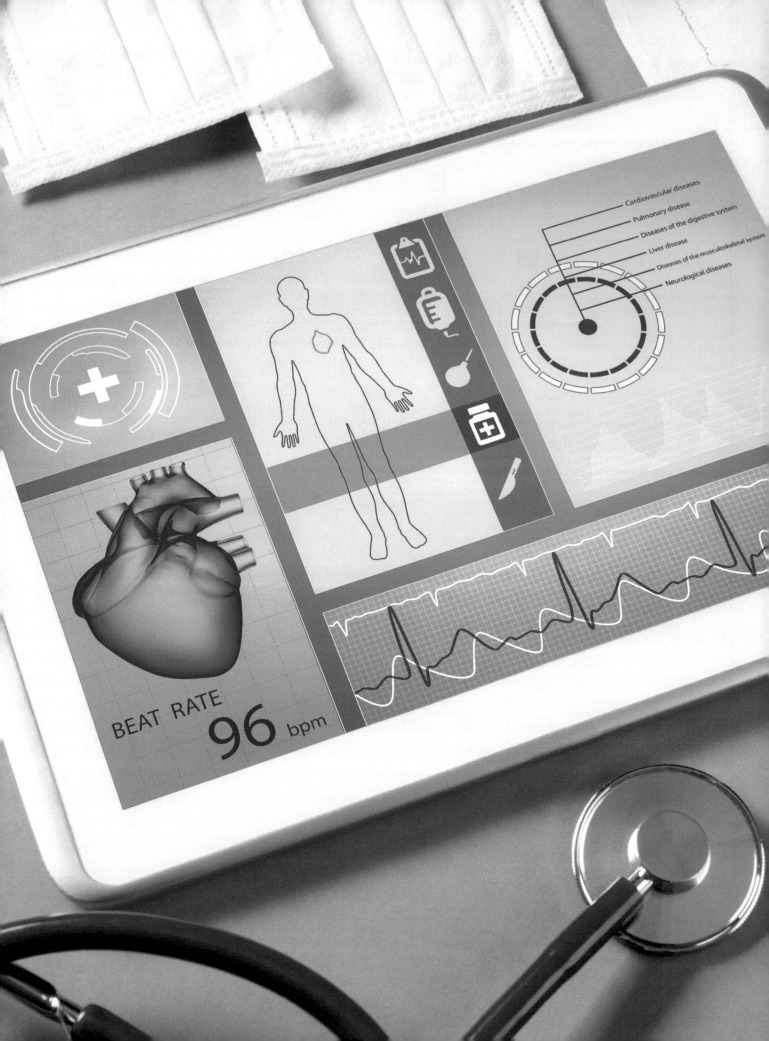

Cardiovascular diseases
Pulmonary disease
Diseases of the digestive system
Liver disease
Diseases of the musculoskeletal system
Neurological diseases

BEAT RATE
96 bpm

13 Neurological history taking and physical examination

Figure 13.1 Cranial nerve examination. Source: Gleadle J (2012) *History Taking and Clinical Examination at a Glance*, 3rd edn. Wiley-Blackwell, Chichester

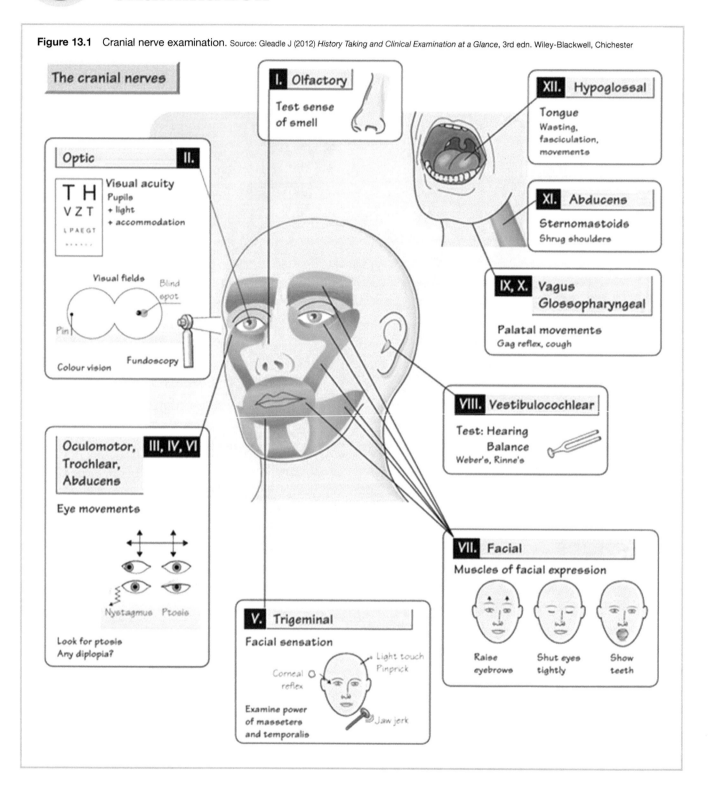

Prevalence of neurological disorders

A recent study by the Global Burden of Disease and Injuries Collaborators, one of the largest epidemiological studies to date, has demonstrated multiple risks associated with the development of neurological disorders worldwide.[1] Stroke is the third leading cause of disability-adjusted life-years (DALYs), a measure which combines the years lost due to disability, illness and early death.

Vascular, neoplastic, inflammatory, degenerative, demyelination and infective are the most common aetiologies of neurological compromise, all of which provide potential targets of manipulation with pharmacological and non-pharmacological therapies if diagnosed in a timely manner.

Presentation of neurological disorders

Neurological compromise may manifest as:
- altered mental state such as confusion, personality changes, changes in memory
- psychological changes such as agitation, tearfulness, depression or elation
- sleep disturbance
- headache, migraine, vertigo or dizziness
- head trauma
- olfactory changes such as loss of olfactory sensation, altered olfaction (smell)
- altered vision such as blurring or diplopia
- hearing changes such as loss or tinnitus
- changes in ability to speak or tone of voice
- problems with swallowing, nausea or vomiting, altered taste and smell
- peripheral sensory symptoms such as numbness and paraesthesia
- shaking and tremors, fits or seizure activity
- changes in urination and bowel habits, and pain.

Ask the patient further questions about the presenting complaint. Mnemonics can be used to elicit further detail using a systematic assessment approach.

Past medical history (PMH)

Specific questions should be asked about relevant past medical history that may indicate relevant and significant neurological conditions. These include:
- ischaemic stroke
- haemorrhagic stroke
- epilepsy
- migraines
- multiple sclerosis
- chronic inflammatory demyelinating polyneuropathy
- Alzheimer disease
- Parkinson disease
- motor neuron disease
- myaesthenia gravis
- myotonic dystrophy.

Drug history (DH)

A full drug history should be taken, including over-the-counter, recreational and herbal drugs. Allergies and adverse drug reactions (ADRs) should include type of agent and reaction, severity and whether dose dependent.

Family history (FH)

Ask whether anyone in the family has had any neurological conditions in the past. Attempt to determine whether any conditions have a clear pattern of transmission – autosomal dominant, autosomal recessive or X-linked.

Inherited neurological disorders include dementias such as:
- familial Alzheimer disease
- ataxia such as Friedreich ataxia, ataxia-telangiectasia, spinocerebellar ataxia
- hereditary neuropathies such as Charcot–Marie–Tooth
- hereditary neuropathy with liability of pressure palsies
- muscular dystrophies, such as Duchenne, Becker, facioscapulohumeral, myotonic dystrophy, spinal muscular atrophy
- inherited forms of epilepsy
- hereditary spastic paraplegia
- Huntington disease
- neurofibromatosis
- tuberous sclerosis
- mitochondrial disorders.

Social history (SH)

Practitioners should explore the patient's birthplace, education, occupation, functional status, diet, sleep, tobacco, alcohol and/or illicit drug use, sexual history and religion, which may be important factors related to the current illness. This information may be key to developing an appropriate differential diagnosis.

Review of systems (ROS)

The ROS may detect health problems of which the patient may not complain, but which require attention in relation to the history of presenting illness (HPI). Pertinent positives and negatives should go in the HPI. List systems reviewed. For a complete work-up, the requirement is to review systems from the following categories: head, ears, eyes, nose, throat (HEENT), respiratory, cardiovascular, gastrointestinal, genitourinary, integument/breast, hematological/lymphatic, musculoskeletal, behavioural/psychological, endocrine, allergic/immunological. The neurological review of systems should include seizures or unexplained loss of consciousness, headache, vertigo or dizziness, loss of vision, diplopia, difficulty hearing, tinnitus, difficulty with speech or swallowing, weakness, difficulty moving, abnormal movements, numbness, tingling, tremor, problems with gait, balance or co-ordination, difficulty with thinking or memory, problems sleeping or excessive sleepiness, depressive symptoms.

Physical examination

Examination of the cranial nerves includes testing of the olfactory, optic, oculomotor, trochlear, abducent, trigeminal, facial, vestibulocochlear, glossopharyngeal, vagus, accessory and hypoglossal nerves. See Figure 13.1.

Examination of the sensory system includes light touch and pinprick (sharp touch), temperature, proprioception (joint position sense), vibration sense and two-point discrimination. The sensory exam should be limited, focused and guided by the localisation hypothesis the practitioner developed prior to physical examination.

Examination of the motor system includes inspection of tone, power, deep tendon reflexes (DTRs), superficial tendon reflexes and co-ordination. Co-ordination should include fine finger movements, finger-to-nose manoeuvre, rapid alternating movements and heel-to-shin testing. It may also be useful to assess for Romberg sign. Gait & Station should be performed if the level of consciousness, strength and co-ordination allows the patient to stand safely with assistance. The minimum expected is natural gait, noting posture, stance, speed, stride length, arm swing and turns. In younger patients in whom subtle abnormalities are expected, the clinician may consider assessing tandem gait, heel walking and toe walking.

Concept mapping in neurological disorders

Findings from the HTPE exercise of those presenting with neurological complaints may be explored utilising a concept map (see Chapter 8).

Summary

The practitioner should provide a short summary of the history, including name and age of the patient, presenting complaint and relevant medical history, give a differential diagnosis and a brief investigation and management plan. Disclosure by patients of their ideas, concerns and expectations about diagnosis and/or treatment, brought together in the ICE acronym, is a part of 'gathering information' within the communication framework and exemplifies a patient-centred approach. Not only may this disclosure provide more insight into the reasons for an encounter (consultation or home visit), but it may also be a clue to establishing the right diagnosis. Additionally, it influences the process of shared decision making and will hopefully enhance patient compliance. The disclosure of the patients' ideas, concerns and expectations is paramount in a patient-centred consultation.

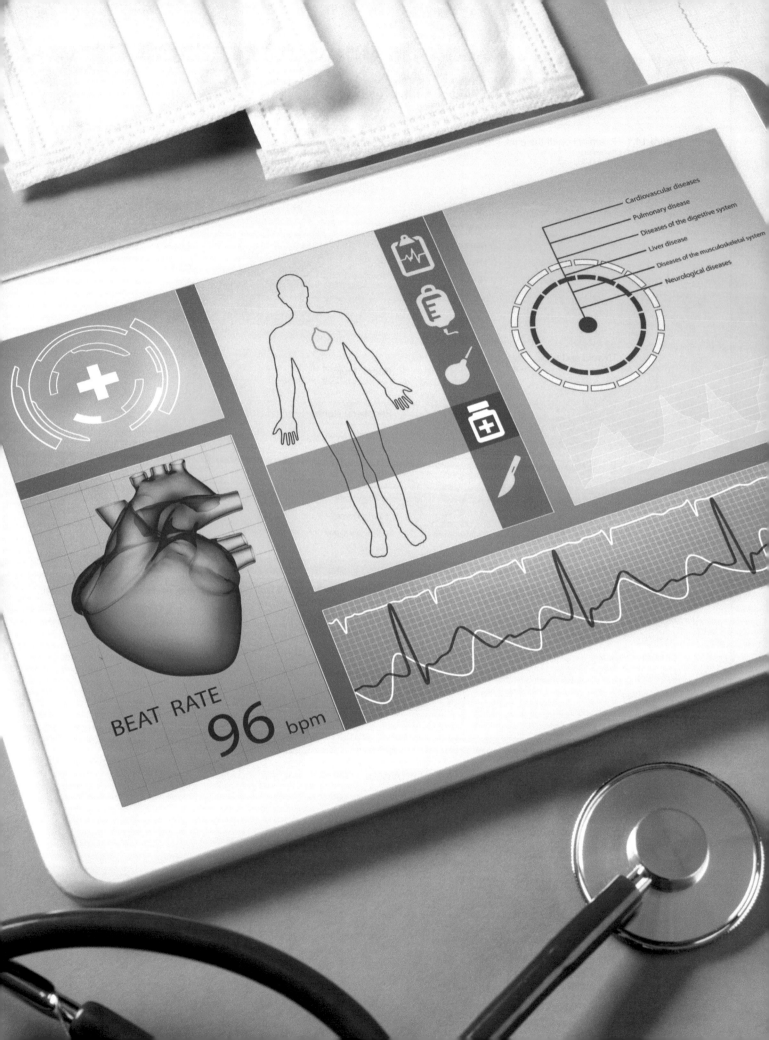

14 Ear, nose and throat history taking and physical examination

Figure 14.1   Examination of the ears, nose, throat and neck. Source: Gleadle J (2012) *History and Clinical Examination at a Glance*, p.60. Wiley-Blackwell, Chichester

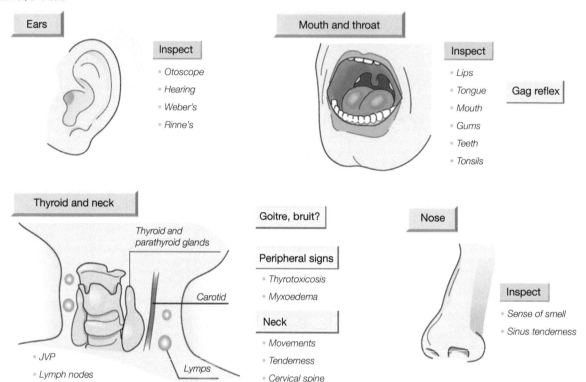

Ears

Inspect
- Otoscope
- Hearing
- Weber's
- Rinne's

Mouth and throat

Inspect
- Lips
- Tongue
- Mouth
- Gums
- Teeth
- Tonsils

Gag reflex

Thyroid and neck

Thyroid and parathyroid glands

Carotid

Lymps

- JVP
- Lymph nodes

Goitre, bruit?

Peripheral signs
- Thyrotoxicosis
- Myxoedema

Neck
- Movements
- Tenderness
- Cervical spine

Nose

Inspect
- Sense of smell
- Sinus tenderness

Table 14.1   ENT assessment checklist

	Ear	Nose	Throat
External			
Swelling	/	/	/
Bruising	/	/	
Deformity	/	/	
Inflammation	/	/	/
Discharge	/	/	/
Wounds	/	/	/
Scarring	/	/	
Symmetry	/		
Shape	/	/	
Foreign body	/		
Internal			
Swelling	/	/	/
Inflammation	/	/	/
Discharge	/	/	/
Foreign body	/	/	/
Lesions	/	/	/

Figure 14.2   Labelled diagram of the tympanic membrane. Source: Ludman HS, Bradley J (eds) (2007) *ABC of Ear, Nose and Throat*, p2. Blackwell, Oxford

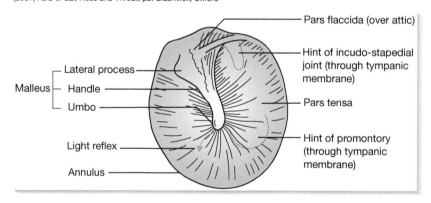

Pars flaccida (over attic)

Hint of incudo-stapedial joint (through tympanic membrane)

Lateral process

Malleus
- Handle
- Umbo

Pars tensa

Hint of promontory (through tympanic membrane)

Light reflex

Annulus

Ear, nose and throat (ENT) complaints are a common occurrence seen by advanced practitioners in both primary and secondary care. Being able to ascertain what conditions are life-threatening, urgent or minor can be accomplished by careful history taking and assessment. History taking should include when it started, any direct trauma, unilateral or bilateral problem, severity and radiation of pain. Each area has a similar 'look and feel' approach which helps to give a strong indicator to the problem (Figure 14.1, Table 14.1).

Due to the vast number of diagnoses that can be made, a few significant differentials for each area are discussed, highlighting red flags for each area.

Ear

Assessment of the ear will always begin with what you can visualise. Don't forget that ear pain can be referred from dental pathology or the temporomandibular joint (TMJ).

An otoscope should be used to examine the tympanic membrane to ensure it is intact (Figure 14.2). This can be assumed if a cone of light and handle of malleolus are seen. The canal can sometimes be impacted with cerumen (wax) which can obscure the ear drum.

Otitis media can be both acute and chronic and is common in children following a URTI. Symptoms include fever, earache, irritability, lethargy and reduced hearing. On examination with an otoscope, the tympanic membrane will show inflammation and loss of light reflex and a bulging drum.

Perforated tympanic membrane often occurs after direct penetrating injury but can occur after an ear infection. There will be discharge of fluid from the ear. This condition heals spontaneously and does not need antibiotics but should be re-examined in 6 weeks by the GP to ensure it has healed.

Mastoiditis is an uncommon presentation but can follow an episode of acute otitis media. It is a bacterial infection of the mastoid air cells that surround the inner and middle ear. It should be suspected if there is pain, redness and swelling over the mastoid process and often the pinna is pushed downwards. This is an ENT emergency and needs to be treated with intravenous antibiotics. It will require a CT scan of the mastoid area to determine the extent of infection.

Ramsay Hunt syndrome (herpes zoster oticus) occurs when the facial nerve is affected by shingles. Patients will present with severe pain, vesicles in the ear canal and/or on the face, often accompanied by facial palsy. The early prescribing of antivirals can help prevent permanent damage to the facial nerve.

Laceration to the pinna, should be sutured with fine sutures. Laceration to the cartilage requires suturing with fine absorbable sutures prevent necrosis.

Auricular haematoma, 'cauliflower ear', occurs after direct trauma to the ear and produces swelling in the cartilage. It should be aspirated with a large-bore needle. A firm pressure dressing is then applied for 24 hours. These haematomas tend to refill and may need further aspiration to help prevent deformity.

Foreign body in the ear can either be internal or external and can cause infection. An internal foreign body can be removed with a hook under direct vision but requires a compliant patient. Live insects should be drowned with olive oil, which helps bring the insect to the surface. After removal of the foreign body, the ear should be re-examined to ensure there is no further damage. External foreign body can be removed after local anaesthesia infiltrated either locally or as a greater auricular nerve block. Antibiotics may be required for infected wounds.

It is important to note that medications such as aminoglycosides, NSAIDs, furosemide and quinine, to name a few, can affect hearing, so always complete a full drug history.

Red flags include dizziness, profuse bleeding from the ear, mastoid tenderness, sudden onset of deafness and discharge from the ear accompanied by confusion.

Nose

Patients may present with a problem to their nose either caused by trauma or illness. The equipment used to look up the nose is an otoscope and thudicum nasal speculum. Utilising these pieces of equipment will provide clear vision inside the nose and assist in diagnosing the presenting complaint.

Foreign body in the nose may cause an offensive, unilateral discharge. To remove, try to get the patient to blow their nose whilst occluding the unaffected nostril. A fine-bore suction catheter attached to wall suction can also work. Objects that cause concern include button batteries and magnets as they can cause necrosis, so should be promptly removed by specialists.

Most epistaxis stops spontaneously but if persistent, an assessment of haemodynamic status should be carried out. Direct visualisation can establish the area of bleed, normally Little's area. The area should be cautiously cauterised with a silver nitrate stick for 10–15 seconds. Excessive cautery should be avoided and never cauterise both sides of the septum as this can cause septal necrosis. If bleeding persists, nasal tampons can be inserted to stall the bleed and the patient should be referred to ENT.

Nasal fractures are commonly caused by a blow to the face or a direct fall, and are rarely an emergency. There is likely to be swelling and tenderness, +/- deformity. Patency of both nostrils should be established. Observation of septal haematoma should be undertaken as this can cause necrosis and obstruction. Follow up as per local policy.

Red flags include haemorrhagic shock, recurrent unilateral epistaxis, nasal obstruction, facial numbness, diplopia, and if the patient is on anticoagulant therapy.

Throat

Tonsilitis is an infection of the tonsils classified as acute, recurrent or chronic and can be caused by virus or bacteria. On inspection, tonsils will be inflamed, with a white or yellow coating, ulcers in the throat, fever, headache, and swollen glands in the neck. The most common bacterium causing tonsilitis is *Streptococcus*. Antibiotics may be required for a 10-day course. If no pus is evident, just inflammation, the cause is probably viral.

Peritonsillar abscess ('quinsy') is a condition in which pus forms between the tonsil capsule and superior constrictor muscle. There is severe, unilateral sore throat, with dysphagia, drooling and severe pain. Treatment is with intravenous antibiotics and incision and drainage of abscess, by ENT specialist

Epiglottis can be caused by bacterial, fungal or viral infection, most often by *Streptococcus* or *Haemophilus influenzae*. It is treated as an emergency as the epiglottis can become swollen and block the airway. Key features to look for include dysphagia, dysphonia, drooling and distress. Treatment includes sitting the patient up, administration of antibiotics, steroids and fluids.

Red flags in throat examination include a patient who is severely short of breath, is unable to talk in full sentences, drooling, hoarse voice and stridor.

15 Lymph node assessment

Figure 15.1 Structure of the lymph node.

Source: Peckham M (2011) *Histology at a Glance*. Wiley-Blackwell, Chichester

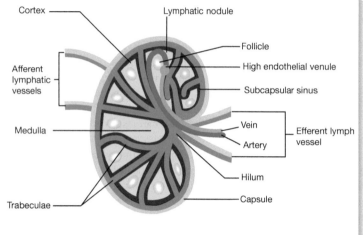

The medulla contains medullary cords and sinuses (not shown in diagram). Afferent lymph drains into cortical sinuses, through into medullary sinuses before leaving via efferent lymph vessels

Table 15.2 MIAMI for differential diagnosis of lymphadenopathy

Malignancies	Kaposi sarcoma, leukaemias, lymphomas, metastases, skin neoplasms
Infections	*Bacterial*: brucellosis, chancroid, cutaneous infections (staphylococcal or streptococcal) syphilis, tuberculosis, typhoid fever *Viral*: adenovirus, hepatitis, herpes zoster, HIV, rubella, infectious mononucleosis *Granulomatous*: cryptococcosis, histoplasmosis, silicosis *Other*: fungal, helminthic, Lyme disease, toxoplasmosis
Autoimmune disorders	Dermatomycosis, rheumatoid arthritis, Still disease, systemic lupus erythematosus
Miscellaneous/ unusual conditions	Sarcoidosis, Kawasaki disease, angiofollicular lymph node hyperplasia
Iatrogenic causes	Medications, serum sickness

Table 15.1 Medications that can cause lymphadenopathy

Allopurinol	Phenytoin
Atenolol	Primidone
Captopril	Pyrimethamine
Carbamazepine	Quinidine
Gold	Trimethoprim/sulfamethoxazole
Hydralazine	Sulindac
Penicillins	

Lymph nodes are present throughout the body and may be superficial or deep. Specific collections of lymph nodes are present in the neck, axillae and inguinal regions and form part of the lymphatic system.

The lymphatic system is a unidirectional circulatory system, with capillaries closely interlinked with the blood vessels. Fluids composed of fatty acids and waste products leak out of the capillaries into the interstitial spaces. They are absorbed by the lymphatic vessels and transported towards the two main lymph ducts in the body. Lymph fluid is filtered through lymph nodes interpolated along these thin vascular channels.

Lymph nodes are small oval-shaped balls of lymphatic tissue typically 1–2 cm long (Figure 15.1) and are surrounded by a fibrous capsule that encircles the internal cortex and medulla. The cortex is predominantly composed of collections of B and T lymphocyte cells. The medulla contains plasma cells, macrophages and B cells, as well as sinuses (vessel-like spaces that the lymph flows into). Inside each sinus cavity is a nodule which is the site of B cell proliferation when antigens to the lymphocytes are presented. This activates the adaptive immune response, causing the nodes to enlarge (reactive lymphadenopathy).

Lymphadenopathy

Lymphadenopathy describes the clinical condition of lymph nodes that are abnormal in size (greater than 1 cm) or consistency. This occurs when there is increased lymph flow into the nodes with fluid containing a greater amount of debris, causing inflammation to occur as more neutrophils and macrophages enter the node to remove this debris (lymphadenitis). However, cancer cells can also enter and proliferate in these cells abd in doing so, gain access to the rest of the circulatory system, thus spreading cancer or bacterial infection. However, lymphadenopathy is generally benign and self-limiting in most patients.

Assessing lymphadenopathy

History
A thorough history should be taken to explore potential aetiology, including the patient's age, duration, exposure, associated symptoms and location (generalised or localised). Also include environmental, sexual, occupational, travel-related and insect exposure. Chronic use of medications (Table 15.1), immunisation status, infectious contacts and a history of recurrent infections are commonly associated with persistent lymphadenopathy.

Examination sequence
A complete lymphatic examination should be performed to rule out generalised lymphadenopathy, followed by a focused lymphatic examination, differentiating between normal and pathological nodes with consideration of lymphatic drainage patterns.

Pathological lymphadenopathy is of importance for diagnosis and prognostication in the staging of lymphoproliferative and other malignancies.

For palpable nodes, consider the following characteristics.
- *Site*: location in relation to other anatomical structures.
- *Size*: nodes are considered normal if they are <1 cm in diameter.
- *Shape*: regular or irregular.
- *Consistency*: palpate enlarged lymph nodes and apply slight pressure to assess consistency. Normal nodes feel soft. Enlarged lymph nodes can be soft (fluctuant), rubbery (Hodgkin disease), matted (tuberculosis), hard (as in metastatic cancer) or variable.
- *Tenderness*: this occurs when a node increases in size, causing the capsule to stretch and causing pain due to acute viral or bacterial infection.
- *Attachment*: palpate nodes to ascertain if they are fixed to the skin, deep fascia or muscles. Primary malignant growth or secondary carcinoma is often fixed to the surrounding areas.
- *Overlying skin changes*: such as scars, swellings or skin changes.

General principles
- Inspect for visible lymphadenopathy or irregularities.
- Palpate one side at a time using the palmar aspect of 2–3 fingertips and compare with nodes on the contralateral side.

Cervical nodes
The deep cervical chain is mainly obscured by the overlying sternomastoid muscle, but the tonsillar and supraclavicular nodes may be palpable. Differentiation should be made from the submandibular gland, which is larger and has a lobulated, irregular exterior whereas nodes are normally round or ovoid, and smooth. The tonsillar, submandibular and submental nodes drain aspects of the mouth, throat and face.

- Ensure the patient is sitting and examine from behind. Ask the patient to tilt their chin slightly downwards and to relax their hands on their lap.
- Using a systematic approach, palpate for the submental, submandibular, tonsillar, parotid, pre- and postauricular, superficial cervical, deep cervical, posterior cervical, occipital and supraclavicular nodes.

One side at a time should be examined when palpating the anterior cervical chain to ensure that cerebral blood flow (due to carotid artery compression) is not compromised.

Axillary nodes
Lymphatics drain towards the axilla from most of the breast. The most palpable are the central nodes which lie along the chest wall, between the anterior and posterior axillary folds. Three other groups of lymph nodes drain into the central nodes; however, these are only occasionally palpable.
- Pectoral nodes
- Subscapular nodes
- Lateral nodes

Lymph drains from the central axillary nodes to the infraclavicular and supraclavicular nodes. However, malignant cells from a breast cancer may not follow the traditional direction of draining from the breast into the axilla and may instead spread directly to the infraclavicular nodes or deep into the channels within the chest.
- Ensure the patient is lying down at a 45° angle.
- Check to see if the patient has any shoulder pain before moving the arm.
- When examining the right axilla, use the left hand and vice versa for the left axilla.
- Examination should cover the pectoral (anterior), central (medial), subscapular (posterior), humoral (lateral) and apical groups of lymph nodes.

Epitrochlear nodes
Epitrochlear lymphadenopathy is rare and is usually obvious when present. This can be associated with metastatic melanoma.

Support the patient's left wrist with your right hand, hold their partially flexed elbow with your left hand and use your thumb to feel for the epitrochlear node. Do the same on the other side.

Inguinal nodes
- Ensure the patient is lying down.
- Palpate over the horizontal chain (lies just below the inguinal ligament) and then over the vertical chain along the line of the saphenous vein.

Causes of lymphadenopathy
The mnemonic MIAMI provides a comprehensive format for considering differential diagnoses (Table 15.2). Generalised lymphadenopathy occurs in a number of conditions and therefore lymph node assessment should form part of a wider general physical assessment.

16 Endocrine history taking and physical examination

Table 16.1 Common clinical symptoms and features of endocrine conditions and their differential diagnosis

Clinical symptom or feature	Differential diagnosis
Weight or appetite changes	*Weight loss* – Diabetes, hyperthyroidism, Addison's *Weight gain* – Diabetes, hypothyroidism, Cushings's, hyperparathyroidism
Sweating, flushing	Hyperthyroidism, phaeochromocytoma, acromegaly
Lethargy	Hypothyroidism, Addison's, diabetes
Altered bowel habit	Hyperthyroidism, Addison's, hypothyroidism
Polyuria, polydipsia	Diabetes, hyperparathyroidism, Cushings's, acromegaly, phaeochromocytoma, hyperthyroidism
Hypertension	Hyperparathyroidism, Cushings's, phaeochromocytoma, hypothyroidism
Skin, hair and nail changes	Polycystic ovary syndrome (PCOS), Cushing's, Addison's, acromegaly, hypopituitarism, hypothyroidism, hypoparathyroidism
Neck swelling	Graves' disease, thyroiditis
Erectile dysfunction, loss of libido	Hypogonadism, diabetes, hypopituitarism
Gynaecomastia, galactorrhoea	Hyperthyroidism, hyperprolactinaemia
Amenorrhoea	Hyperprolactinaemia, thyroid dysfunction, PCOS
Altered facial appearance	Acromegaly, Cushing's, hypothyroidism

Figure 16.1 Clinical examination findings and features of common endocrine conditions. Source: Alexandra Gatehouse

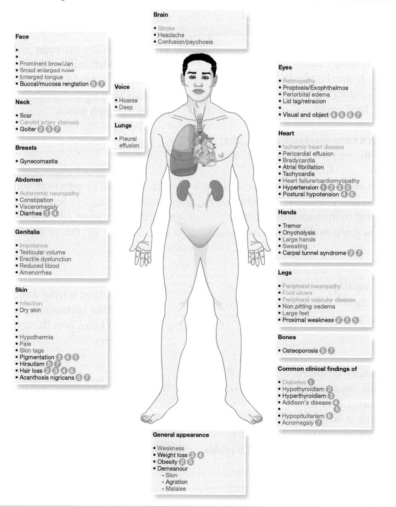

Advanced Clinical Practice at a Glance, First Edition. Edited by Barry Hill and Sadie Diamond Fox.
© 2023 John Wiley & Sons Ltd. Published 2023 by John Wiley & Sons Ltd.

Chapter 16 Endocrine history taking and physical examination

Prevalence of endocrine conditions

Diabetes mellitus and thyroid disease are the most common endocrine conditions. There are 4.9 million adults in the UK diagnosed with diabetes, with ongoing evidence that this will continue to rise due to genetic, lifestyle and environmental risk factors. Approximately 2% of the UK population have been diagnosed with hypothyroidism or hyperthyroidism. Other less common conditions include Addison disease, Cushing syndrome, hypopituitarism and acromegaly.

Presentation of endocrine disorders

Clinical features of endocrine pathology may be varied and nonspecific, in addition to affecting multiple anatomical sites and organ systems. Diagnosis of endocrine conditions may be incidental or secondary to investigations of other disease processes, and challenging due to potential coexistence with other endocrine pathology. Several conditions share common clinical symptoms and may go unrecognised because of focused management of single-organ dysfunction. The nature of the presenting symptoms requires careful questioning, exploration and consideration to rule out alternative diagnoses.

An appreciation of the common symptoms associated with endocrine conditions is essential.

These symptoms and clinical features may assist in the differential diagnosis of an endocrine condition (Table 16.1).

Past medical history

Specific questions should be asked relating to relevant past medical history that may indicate relevant and significant endocrine conditions. This includes previous surgery, radiotherapy, vascular disease, neuropathy, nephropathy, retinopathy, diabetes and thyroid treatment.

Drugs

A detailed and accurate drug history is vital. If an endocrine condition is suspected, there are several drugs that may be significant in terms of precipitation of disease onset, contribution to subsequent recognised complications or aiding in differential diagnosis.

- Diabetic or diabetogenic medications (cyclosporine, steroids)
- Hormone replacement therapy – thyroxine, oestrogren, testosterone, growth hormone
- Steroid replacement – Cushing syndrome, Addison disease
- Amiodarone – hypothyroidism, hyperthyroidism
- Lithium – hypothyroidism
- Chronic opioid dependence – hypogonadism
- Alcohol – pancreatitis, hypogonadism
- Benzodiazepines – pituitary gland damage leading to disruption of metabolism, growth and stress adaptation

Family history

Pertinent endocrine-related familial history includes the following.
- Diabetes – type 1 and type 2
- Congenital adrenal hyperplasia
- Autoimmune conditions such as thyroid disease or Addison disease (primary adrenocortical insufficiency)
- Phaeochromocytoma
- Multiple endocrine neoplasia (MEN) syndrome tumours
- Malignancy

Clinical examination

An overarching critical review of the patient's history and clinical examination is crucial in identifying the underlying endocrine pathology. The clinical manifestations of common endocrine conditions, as previously stated, are widely varied across numerous anatomical sites and organ systems. Specific clinical examination findings associated with these disease processes are depicted in Figure 16.1.

Clinical investigations

Clinical investigations aim to measure serum hormone levels, assessing undersecretion or oversecretion depending upon the clinical syndrome. Stimulation tests may confirm suspected hormone deficiencies, whilst suppression tests may determine if hormone excess is intrinsic. They can be summarised as follows.
- Urinalysis
  - Glucosuria present : diabetes mellitus
  - Ketones present: diabetic ketoacidosis
- Capillary blood glucose: high in diabetes
- Serum HbA1c – an average of serum blood glucose levels over 2–3 months, ideally 48 mmol/mol or less. If raised, increased risk of developing type 2 diabetes
- Serum thyroid function tests – including TSH, T_3 and T_4
  - High TSH with low T_4 in hypothyroidism
  - High TSH with normal T_4 in treated hypothyroidism or subclinical hypothyroidism
  - Low or undetectable TSH in hyperthyroidism, high T_3 or T_4
  - Low TSH with normal T_3 and T_4 in subclinical hyperthyroidism
- Serum calcium
  - High in hyperparathyroidism
  - Low in hypoparathyroidism
- Serum PTH
  - High in hyperparathyroidism
  - Low in hypoparathyroidism
- Serum cortisol
  - High in Cushing syndrome with no diurnal rhythm, no cortisol suppression with dexamethasone suppression test
  - Low in Addison syndrome, reduced response on short synacthen test
- Plamsa and urine metenephrines: raised in the presence of phaeochromocytoma
- Serum gonadotrophins: high in hypogonadism

Radiological imaging, such as ultrasound, computed tomography (CT), radionuclide or positron emission tomography (PET), may be utilised in identification of endocrine tumours.

Endocrine 'red flags'

Throughout the patient consultation process, the practitioner may be alerted to what are termed 'red flags'. Some of these can be immediately life-threatening for the patient or a clinical indicator of a serious underlying pathology. Red flag symptoms/findings in those with a working diagnosis of an endocrine disorder may include, but are not limited to:
- severe electrolyte abnormalities
- congestive heart failure or major fluid overload
- bradycardia, tachycardia and/or arrhythmias
- altered conscious state
- hypothermia – temperature <35.5 °C
- tetany
- seizures
- rapid renal function deterioration
- pancreatitis

Endocrine emergencies

Identification of these life-threatening situations and prompt management are vital, particularly if this is the first presentation. Emergencies include diabetic ketoacidosis (DKA), hypoglycaemia and hyperosmolar hyperglycaemic syndrome (HHS). Other endocrine emergencies include Addisonian crisis, thyrotoxic crisis, phaeochromocytoma, myxoedema coma, hypopituitary coma, neuroleptic malignant syndrome, malignant hyperthermia and severe electrolyte disturbances.

Respiratory history taking and physical examination

Table 17.1 Common clinical symptoms and features of respiratory conditions and their differential diagnoses

Clinical symptom or feature	Differential diagnosis
Dyspnoea	Pneumonia Asthma Chronic obstructive pulmonary disease (COPD)
Wheeze	Asthma COPD Anaphylaxis
Haemoptysis	Lung cancer Pulmonary embolism Infection Connective tissue disease Arteriovenous malformation
Chest pain	Rib fracture Costochondritis Pleural disease – pneumothorax, serositis Secondary pleural disease – pulmonary embolism, pneumonia
Cough	Asthma COPD Bronchiectasis Infection

Figure 17.1 Process for performing a respiratory examination. Source: Gleadle J (2012) *History and Clinical Examination at a Glance.* John Wiley & Sons, Oxford

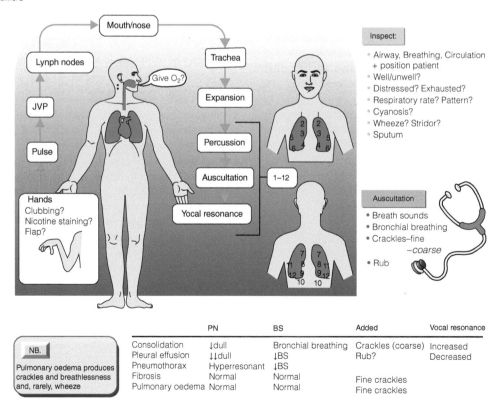

	PN	BS	Added	Vocal resonance
Consolidation	↓dull	Bronchial breathing	Crackles (coarse)	Increased
Pleural effusion	↓↓dull	↓BS	Rub?	Decreased
Pneumothorax	Hyperresonant	↓BS		
Fibrosis	Normal	Normal	Fine crackles	
Pulmonary oedema	Normal	Normal	Fine crackles	

NB.
Pulmonary oedema produces crackles and breathlessness and, rarely, wheeze

Prevalence of respiratory disorders

Respiratory disease is one of the biggest killers in the UK, encompassing diseases such as lung cancer and asthma. Approximately 1 in 5 of the UK population receive a lung disease diagnosis at some point in their lives. Respiratory disease accounts for a significant number of acute admissions to hospital year-on-year.

Bronchoconstriction, inflammation and loss of lung elasticity are some of the most common pathological processes that result in respiratory compromise, all of which provide potential targets for manipulation with pharmacological and non-pharmacological therapies if diagnosed in a timely manner.

Presentation of respiratory disorders

Clinical features of respiratory pathology may be varied and non-specific, in addition to affecting multiple anatomical sites and organ systems. Diagnosis of respiratory conditions may be incidental or secondary to investigation of other disease processes, and can be challenging due to the potential coexistence of other pathologies, particularly those of the cardiovascular system. Several conditions share common clinical symptoms and may go unrecognised as a result of focused management of single-organ dysfunction. The nature of the presenting symptoms requires careful questioning, exploration and consideration to rule out alternative diagnoses.

An appreciation of the common symptoms associated with respiratory conditions is essential and these include:
- weight or appetite changes
- shortness of breath
- wheeze
- cough with or without expectorant
- haemoptysis
- pain – tracheal, mediastinal, chest wall, pleuritic
- daytime somnolence
- tremor.

These symptoms and clinical features may assist in the differential diagnosis of a respiratory condition (Table 17.1).

Past medical history

Specific questions should be asked relating to past medical history that may indicate relevant and significant respiratory conditions.
- Eczema, hay fever, childhood asthma/recurrent childhood wheeze – all recognised links to asthma (the 'atopic triad').
- *Airway diseases*: asthma, chronic obstructive pulmonary disease (COPD), bronchiectasis.
- *Lung tissue diseases*: pulmonary fibrosis, sarcoidosis, cystic fibrosis.
- *Infectious diseases*: whooping cough, measles, pneumonia, pleurisy – all recognised links to connective tissue disorders (i.e. rheumatoid arthritis). Tuberculosis (TB) – recognised link to reactive disease or result in lung abscess/cavity.
- *Lung circulation/systemic diseases*: cor pulmonale, pulmonary hypertension, congestive heart failure, pulmonary embolism, alpha-1 antitrypsin deficiency.
- *Neuromuscular disorders*: motor neuron disease.
- Recent travel, immobility, surgery, cancer, pregnancy – recognised links to pulmonary embolism (PE).
- Loss of consciousness, neuromuscular disorders, spinal injury – recognised links to aspiration, pneumonia.

Drug history

A detailed and accurate drug history is essential. If a respiratory condition is suspected, there are several drugs that may precipitate disease onset, contribute to subsequent recognised complications or aid in differential diagnosis.
- Inhalers
- Steroids – long-term use can result in bone loss and osteoporosis
- Xanthines – therapeutic monitoring required due to risk of arrhythmias
- Antibiotics – recent use, duration, whether they are included in a 'rescue pack' and how many courses have been taken in a 1-year period (this can indicate the stability of disease)
- Beta-blockers and NSAIDs – can cause bronchoconstriction
- ACE inhibitors – can cause dry cough
- Oestrogen-containing drugs – increased risk of PE
- Amiodarone and methotrexate – can cause pleural effusion and interstitial lung disease (ILD)

Family history and social history

Pertinent respiratory-related familial and social history includes the following.
- Predisposition is higher in asthma, hay fever, cystic fibrosis and lung cancer in first-degree relatives.
- Recessive inheritance is found in alpha-1 antitrypsin deficiency.
- Current housing conditions.
- Ability to carry out activities of daily living and to what extent.
- Smoking – pack-year history.
- Occupation – coal mining, farming and those who work in shipyards, construction and plumbing may have been exposed to asbestos and therefore have an increased risk of developing mesothelioma.
- Exercise tolerance – an indirect way of assessing someone's cardiopulmonary reserve. It is essential to ascertain this when taking a history as premorbid physiological reserve is a good prognostic marker of recovery from acute illness.

Clinical examination

An overarching critical review of the patient's history and clinical examination is crucial in identifying the underlying respiratory pathology. The clinical manifestations of common respiratory conditions, as previously stated, are widely varied across numerous anatomical sites and organ systems. Figure 17.1 details the process for performing a respiratory examination. The significance of clinical features with regard to sensitivity, specificity and the likelihood ratio that the finding is present in each respiratory condition is represented in.[1,2]

Concept mapping in respiratory disorders

Findings from the HTPE exercise of those presenting with respiratory complaints may be explored utilising a concept map (see Chapter 8).

Respiratory red flags

Throughout the patient consultation process, the practitioner may be alerted to what are termed 'red flags'. Some of these can be immediately life-threatening for the patient or may be a clinical indicator of a serious underlying pathology. Red flags warn the practitioner of a symptom associated with a potentially life-threatening condition and must be acted upon accordingly. Red flag symptoms/findings in those with a working diagnosis of a respiratory disorder may include, but are not limited to:

- fever
- cough >3 weeks, particularly in smokers
- nasal flaring/grunting in babies
- recession of intercostal muscles in young children
- haemoptysis
- persistent hoarseness >3 weeks
- persistent sore throat
- persistent palpable neck lumps
- persistent unilateral enlarged tonsil
- difficulty completing sentences.

Respiratory emergencies

Identification of these life-threatening situations and prompt management are vital, particularly if this is the first presentation. Such emergencies include, but are not limited to:

- respiratory arrest
- severe hypoxia or hypercapnia resulting in secondary organ dysfunction
- upper airway obstruction – stridor, anaphylaxis, croup, Ludwig angina, foreign body obstruction
- lower airway obstruction – status asthmaticus, bronchiolitis
- disordered work of breathing – raised intracranial pressure, acute neuromuscular disorders, bradypnoea secondary to drug overdose or spinal injury
- lung tissue and vascular disease – pulmonary oedema, massive haemoptysis
- pleural disease – tension pneumothorax.

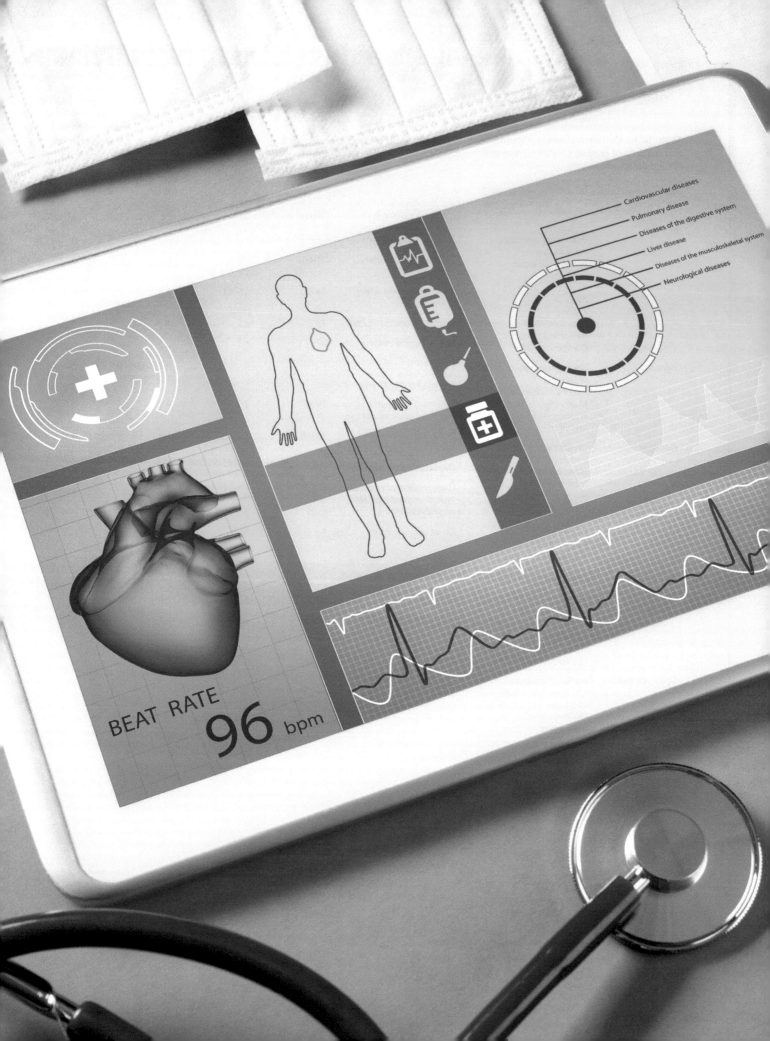

18 Cardiovascular history taking and physical examination

Table 18.1 Common clinical symptoms and features of cardiac conditions and their differential diagnoses

Clinical symptom or feature	Differential diagnosis
Chest pain	Pneumonia Pulmonary embolism Atrial fibrillation Acute myocardial infarction Angina/coronary artery disease Anxiety Musculoskeletal causes Reflux oesophagitis Costochondritis
Syncope	Neurogenic: vasovagal situational Parkinson disease Multisystem atrophy Hypovolaemia Arrhythmia
Oedema	Chronic venous insufficiency Heart failure Liver failure Renal failure Diabetes Sepsis Burns Lymphoedema Ruptured Baker cyst
Palpitations	Arrhythmias Anxiety Pharmacological agents: cocaine, digitalis, theophylline, beta agonists Hyperthyroidism Hypoglycemia
Dysrhythmias	Cardiac ischaemia Structural heart disease Idiopathic fibrosis Prior ablations Pericarditis Thyrotoxicosis
Claudication	Aortic coarctation Arterial dissection Arterial embolism Thrombosis Vasospasm Trauma
Dyspnoea	Pulmonary disease (asthma, COPD, pneumonia) Respiratory muscle dysfunction Psychogenic dyspnoea Deconditioning/obesity

Table 18.2 Cardiac conditions and common clinical features featuring their diagnostic weightings[3]

Cardiac conditions and common clinical features	Sensitivity (%)	Specificity (%)	Likelihood ratio if the finding is	
			Present	Absent
Severe aortic stenosis				
Delayed carotid artery upstroke	31–91	68–93	3.5	0.4
Reduced carotid artery volume	44–80	65–81	2.3	0.4
Sustained apical impulse	78	81	4.1	0.3
Apical-carotid delay	97	63	2.6	0.05
S_4 gallop	29–50	57–63	Non-significant (NS)	NS
Aortic regurgitation				
Detecting mild aortic regurgitation or worse	54–87	75–98	9.9	0.3
Detecting moderate-to-severe aortic regurgitation	88–98	52–88	4.3	0.1
Coronary artery disease				
Classification of chest pain: Typical anginaAtypical anginaNon-anginal	50–91 8–44 4–22	78–94 — 14–50	5.8 1.2 0.1	— — —
Chest pain duration >30 min	1	86	0.1	NS
Age: <30 years30–49 years50–70 years>70 years	0–1 16–38 62–73 2–52	97–98 — — 67–99	NS 0.6 1.3 2.6	— — — —
Prior myocardial infarction	42–69	6699	3.8	0.6

Advanced Clinical Practice at a Glance, First Edition. Edited by Barry Hill and Sadie Diamond Fox.
© 2023 John Wiley & Sons Ltd. Published 2023 by John Wiley & Sons Ltd.

Figure 18.1 Cardiovascular examination. Source: Aaronson PI, Ward JPT, Connolly MJ (2013) *The Cardiovascular System at a Glance*, 4th edn. Wiley-Blackwell, Chichester

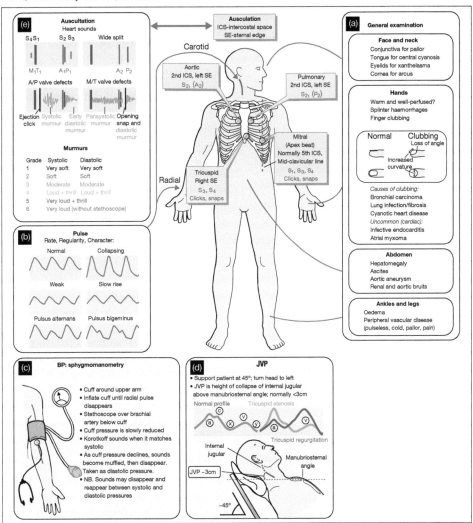

Figure 18.2 Concept map detailing the potential aetiology of oedema. Source: Irfan M (2019) *The Hands-on Guide to Clinical Reasoning in Medicine*. Wiley-Blackwell, Chichester

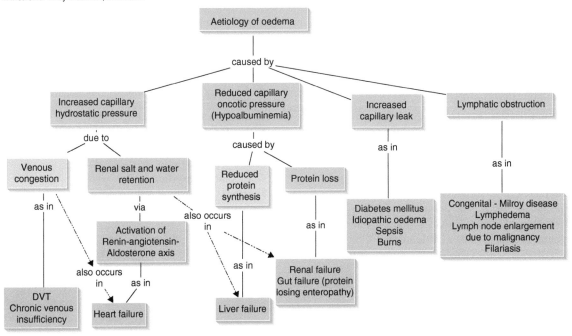

Presentation of cardiac disorders

The nature of the presenting symptoms requires careful questioning, exploration and consideration to rule out alternative diagnoses. An appreciation of the common symptoms associated with cardiac conditions is essential. Common clinical symptoms and features of cardiac conditions, their differential diagnoses and their diagnostic weightings are explored in Tables 18.1 and 18.2.

Drug history

A detailed and accurate drug history is essential. If a cardiac condition is suspected, there are several drugs that may precipitate disease onset, contribute to subsequent recognised complications or aid in differential diagnosis. The following major drug groups are known to have potentially cardiovascular toxic effects.

- Anthracyclines ('rubicins) – prolonged, high doses can cause cardiomyopathy
- Antipsychotics – increased risk of arrhythmias
- Non-selective beta agonists – cardiomyopathy, direct toxic effects upon cardiomyocytes, hypotension
- Non-steroidal anti-inflammatory drugs – hypertension, exacerbate heart failure, increase risk of MI in those already in 'at-risk' groups
- St John's wort – reduces effect of warfarin
- Androgens/anabolic steroids – cardiomyopathy, atheroscelorsis, hypertension and MI

Clinical examination

Cardiac assessment is a key part of the management of the acutely unwell patient. During the ABCDE approach, this would be more generalised, unless a specific cardiovascular abnormality was identified. A more detailed cardiovascular assessment needs to be carried out if any altered pathology was discovered, which could provide information to aid clinical management. Although technologies have advanced tremendously over the years, clinical examination remains a central tool within the assessment process. As with all other body systems, the main components of cardiovascular assessment are inspection, palpation, percussion and auscultation. There are specific features within the cardiac assessment that can help with differential diagnosis (Figure 18.1). In the acutely unwell patient, cyanosis, pallor and diaphoresis can all be indications of impending catastrophe.

Understanding the cardiac cycle can give you an indication of any abnormalities within the heart.

- *Atrial systole*: contributes to the last ~15–20% of the final ventricular volume. End-diastolic pressure (EDP) <10 mmHg, and is higher in the left ventricle than in the right due to the thicker and therefore stiffer left ventricular wall.
- *Ventricular systole*: ventricular pressure rises sharply during contraction. AV valves close as soon as this is greater than the atrial pressure. Results in first heart sound (S_1) (lub).

- *Ejection*: ventricular pressure exceeds that in the aorta or pulmonary artery. The outflow valves open and blood is ejected. Flow briefly reverses, causing closure of the outflow valve. There is a small increase in aortic pressure (dicrotic notch) resulting in the second heart sound (S_2) (dub).
- *Diastole*: immediately after closure of the outflow valves, the ventricles rapidly relax. This phase is twice the length of systole at rest, but decreases as the heart rate increases.

There are a number of clinical examination findings associated with CVD.

- *Cyanosis*: the colour of the skin depends on the colour of blood flowing through the dermal capillaries and subpapillary venous plexus, rather than the arteries and veins that lie too deep to cause colour alterations. Patients with central cyanosis typically present with discolouration/bluish tinge to their lips, tongue and sublingual tissues.
- *Diaphoresis*: excessive sweating which is abnormal in relation to the level of activity or environment. This can be caused by a variety of conditions, MI being one of them. If coupled with syncope, shortness of breath and chest pain, then cardiovascular causes must be ruled out.
- *Jugular venous pressure (JVP)*: normal range is 6–8 cmH₂O. A raised JVP can indicate impending cardiac failure (see Figure 18.1d).
- *Hepatojugular reflux/abdominojugular test*: hand pressed firmly over patient's midabdomen for 10 seconds, which increases venous return but displaces splanchnic venous blood towards the heart. In fit and healthy individuals, this should not change the central venous pressure (CVP). A positive abdominojugular test can indicate elevated left atrial pressures.
- *Additional or abnormal heart sounds*: caused by an obstruction to blood flow, the result is a turbulent sound that can be heard with a stethoscope. A valve that fails to close properly is known as incompetent and produces a swishing sound, resulting from blood regurgitating back through the partially close valve. A valve that fails to open as it should is known as stenotic and often produces a high-pitched sound or click.

Concept mapping in cardiac disorders

Findings from the HTPE exercise of those presenting with CVD may be explored utilising a concept map (see Chapter 8). Figure 18.2 shows a concept map for those presenting with oedema.

Cardiac red flags

- Central chest pain radiating to the neck, arms or shoulders, lasting for several minutes (usually >20 minutes)
- Chest pain associated with autonomic features like sweating, sickness, palpitations
- Chest pain on exertion
- Shortness of breath at rest
- Tachypnoea
- Orthopnoea
- Postural nocturnal dyspnoea

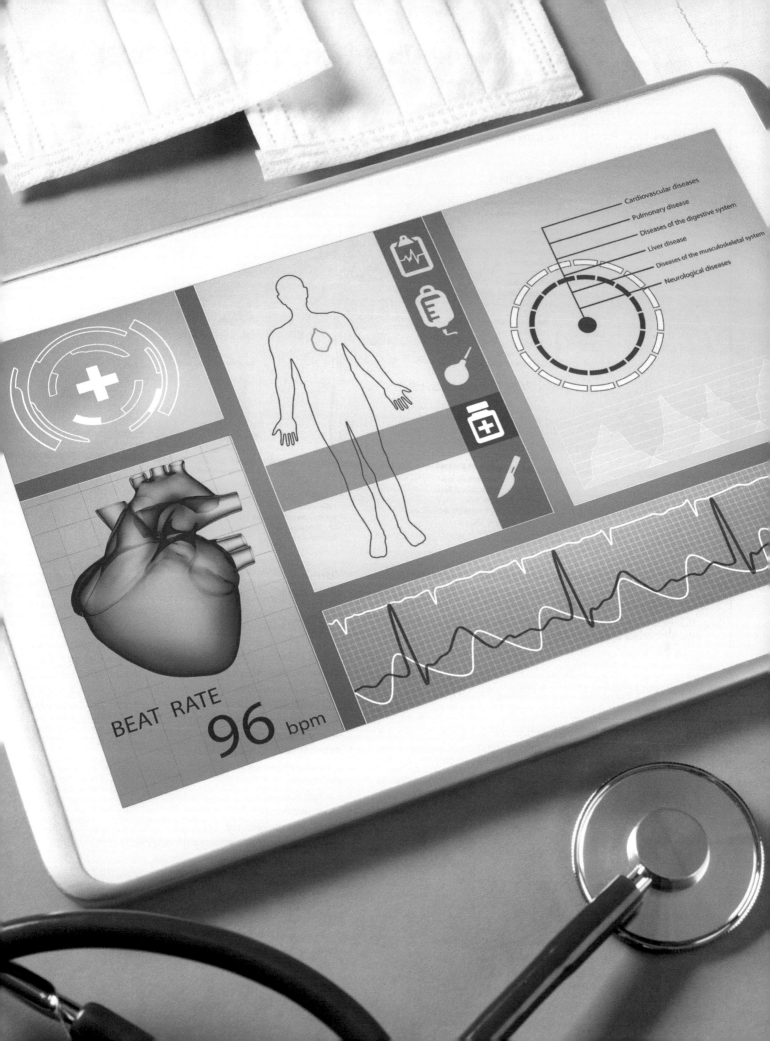

19 Abdominal history taking and physical examination

Figure 19.1 Process for performing an abdominal examination. Source: Gleadle J (2012) *History and Clinical Examination at a Glance*, p.42. Wiley-Blackwell, Chichester

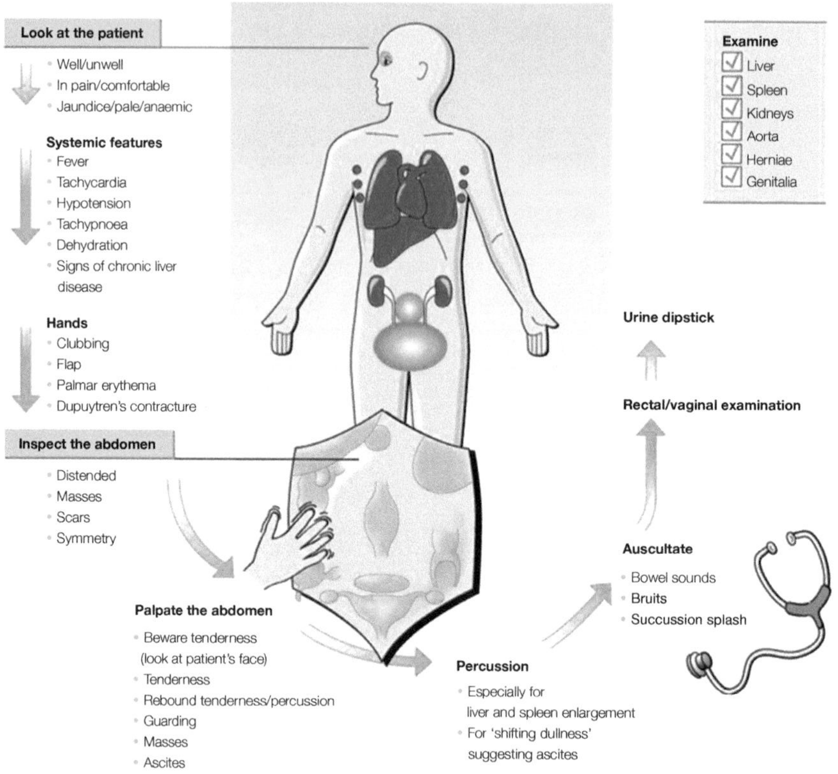

Look at the patient
- Well/unwell
- In pain/comfortable
- Jaundice/pale/anaemic

Systemic features
- Fever
- Tachycardia
- Hypotension
- Tachypnoea
- Dehydration
- Signs of chronic liver disease

Hands
- Clubbing
- Flap
- Palmar erythema
- Dupuytren's contracture

Inspect the abdomen
- Distended
- Masses
- Scars
- Symmetry

Palpate the abdomen
- Beware tenderness (look at patient's face)
- Tenderness
- Rebound tenderness/percussion
- Guarding
- Masses
- Ascites

Percussion
- Especially for liver and spleen enlargement
- For 'shifting dullness' suggesting ascites

Examine
- ☑ Liver
- ☑ Spleen
- ☑ Kidneys
- ☑ Aorta
- ☑ Herniae
- ☑ Genitalia

Urine dipstick

Rectal/vaginal examination

Auscultate
- Bowel sounds
- Bruits
- Succussion splash

The upper gastrointestinal tract lies above the ligament of Trietz, the lower gastrointestinal tract beneath. The abdomen is divided into nine regions and four quadrants. The abdominal organs receive their blood supply from the three major branches of the abdominal aorta: the coeliac trunk (foregut), superior mesenteric artery (midgut) and inferior mesenteric arteries (hindgut).

Presentation of gastrointestinal disorders

Abdominal history taking and physical examination can be complex owing to the multiple organs housed within the abdominal cavity. Therefore, clinical symptoms may go unrecognised as a result of focused management of single-organ dysfunction. An appreciation of the common symptoms associated with gastrointestinal disorders (GID) is essential. These include, but are not limited to:
- abdominal pain
- bloating
- vomiting
- jaundice
- aphthous ulceration
- gastro-oesophgeal reflux
- abdominal distension
- abdominal tenderness
- constipation
- diarrhoea
- steatorrhoea.

Past medical history

A comprehensive abdominal history should elicit the presence of any signs and symptoms of the gastrointestinal, renal or reproductive systems. A systematic clinical history should focus on local, systemic and other associated signs and symptoms which should be fully explored to stratify the risk of life-threatening illness. Past medical history relevant to gastrointestinal disease includes:
- diverticular disease
- non-alcoholic fatty liver disease
- liver cirrhosis
- gallstones
- Crohn's disease
- ulcerative colitis
- abdominal malignancy
- endoscopy and colonoscopy with dates and results
- iron deficiency anaemia
- B12 deficiency
- irritable bowel syndrome
- constipation
- abdominal surgery (e.g. cholecystectomy, bowel resection)
- previous bowel obstruction
- stoma formation.

Advanced Clinical Practice at a Glance, First Edition. Edited by Barry Hill and Sadie Diamond Fox.
© 2023 John Wiley & Sons Ltd. Published 2023 by John Wiley & Sons Ltd.

Drug history

A detailed and accurate drug history is essential. If a gastrointestinal condition is suspected, there are several drugs that may precipitate disease onset, contribute to subsequent recognised complications or aid in differential diagnosis.

- *Biphosphonates* – oesophagitis
- *Cardiac system agents* – gastro-oesophageal reflux disease due to inappropriate lower esophageal sphincter (LES) relaxation
- *Central nervous system agents* – xerostomia resulting in mucositis, inflammation, fissures, ulceration, burning sensation in the mouth, a sore tongue and gingivitis
- *Anti-infective medications* – erythematous or ulcerative reaction in the buccal mucosa, ageusia or dysgeusia, oesophageal ulcers
- *Antineoplastic agents* – gingival hyperplasia, mucositis, oesophageal ulcers
- *Sulfonamides* – Stevens–Johnson syndrome, a severe form of erythema multiforme

Family history and social history

Pertinent abdominal-related familial and social history includes:

- bowel cancer
- haemochromatosis
- inflammatory bowel disease
- hereditary non-polyposis colorectal cancer
- familial adenomatous polyposis
- smoking – increases risk of gastrointestinal malignancy and Crohn's disease
- recreational drug use – increases risk of hepatitis
- alcohol intake –increases risk of gastrointestinal malignancy and the development of alcoholic hepatitis/cirrhosis
- diet – biliary colic may be triggered by consumption of fatty foods. Consumption of gluten in coeliac disease may result in nausea, diarrhoea and abdominal pain.

Clinical examination

The clinical manifestations of gastrointestinal conditions are widely varied across numerous anatomical sites and organ systems. The process for performing an abdominal examination is detailed in Figure 19.1.

Differential diagnosis and concept mapping in gastrointestinal disorders

A commonly used aid is the VITAMIN C D E mnemonic to determine differential diagnoses.

- **V**ascular – oesophageal varix, abdominal aortic aneurysm, aortic dissection
- **I**nfective/Inflammatory – spontaneous bacterial peritonitis, Crohn's, colitis, inflammatory bowel disease (IBD), pancreatitis, intra-abdominal sepsis, pregnancy (complications of), biliary sepsis, cholecystitis
- **T**rauma – blunt force trauma – ruptured spleen, penetrating trauma
- **A**utoimmune – pancreatitis, IBD, Crohn's, pregnancy (complications of)
- **M**etabolic – diabetic ketoacidosis, hyperglycaemic hyperosmolar syndrome
- **I**diopathic/**I**atrogenic – bowel perforation, intra-abdominal collections, fistulae
- **N**eoplastic – adenocarcinoma, cholangiocarcinoma
- **C**ongenital – malformations, fistulae
- **D**egenerative
- **E**ndocrine – Addison disease, diabetic ketoacidosis, hyperglycaemic hyperosmolar syndrome

Findings from the HTPE exercise of those presenting with GID may be explored utilising a concept map (see Chapter 8).

Gastrointestinal red flags

- Absent bowel sounds
- Abdominal pain with associated fever
- Involuntary guarding
- Tenderness to percussion
- Haematemesis
- Haematochezia
- Melaena
- Unintentional weight loss
- Dysphagia/odynophagia
- Abdominal rigidity

Investigations

Laboratory tests

- *Serum samples* – full blood count, urea and aelectrolytes, clotting screen, C-reactive protein, amylase (or lipase) and group & save.
- *Septic screen* – if there are signs of infection, a full septic screen including blood cultures, urine culture, stool culture (if relevant) and ascitic tap if ascites is present.
- *Blood gas* – helpful to check serum lactate and assess metabolic state. In a woman of reproductive age, it is important to perform a beta-HCG test.
- *Tumour markers* – laboratory tests in patients presenting with more chronic symptoms can be tailored based on differential diagnosis to the presenting symptoms and signs. These may include tumour markers (CEA, CA19-9, CA125, AFP, PSA).
- *Disease-specific diagnostic tests* – coeliac serology, chronic liver disease screen, *H. pylori* serology, faecal calprotectin.

Radiology

- *X-ray* – an erect chest X-ray and an abdominal X-ray are often the first line of investigation in acute abdomen to look for evidence of pneumoperitoneum (Rigler sign) or bowel obstruction (e.g. dilated small bowel loop, toxic megacolon). Sometimes incidental normal variant may be confused with more serious pathology (e.g. Chilaiditi sign).
- *Ultrasound* – focused assessment with sonography in trauma (FAST) scan is a rapid screening bedside ultrasound scan performed in the emergency department to assess for blood in the four dependent areas (perihepatic, perisplenic, pelvis, pericardium) and can be useful in diagnosing a leaking aortic abdominal aneurysm (AAA). A formal transabdominal (transvaginal if indicated) ultrasound is requested in the acute abdomen setting commonly to investigate biliary causes (e.g. acute cholecystitis, acute cholangitis), gynaecological causes (ovarian torsion, ruptured ectopic pregnancy), testicular torsion and causes of abnormal liver biochemistry or renal function.
- *Computed tomography (CT)* – cross-sectional imaging remains the main diagnostic imaging test in many abdominal presentations. A CT abdomen and pelvis with contrast is the commonly performed scan, but discussion with radiologist is recommended where possible to ensure the correct choice of test is performed. A non-contrast CT of the kidneys, ureters and bladder (KUB) is preferred to detect ureteric calculi and a CT angiogram should be considered if vascular complication is suspected.

20 Genitourinary system history taking and physical examination

Table 20.1 GUS examination in males

- Inspection of anus and perineum
  Examination (with or without specimen collection for smears and cultures) of genitalia including:
- Scrotum (e.g. lesions, cysts, rashes)
- Epididymites (e.g. size, symmetry, masses)
- Testes (e.g. size, symmetry, masses)
- Urethral meatus (e.g. size, location, lesions, discharge)
- Penis (e.g. lesions, presence or absence of foreskin, foreskin retractability, plaque, masses, scarring, deformities)
  Digital rectal examination including:
- Prostate gland (e.g. size, symmetry, nodularity, tenderness)
- Seminal vesicles (e.g. symmetry, tenderness, masses, enlargement)
- Sphincter tone, presence of haemorrhoids, rectal masses

Table 20.2 GUS examination in females

- Inspection and palpation of breasts (e.g. masses or lumps, tenderness, symmetry, nipple discharge)
- Digital rectal examination including sphincter tone, presence of haemorrhoids, rectal masses
  Pelvic examination (with or without specimen collection for smears and cultures) including:
- External genitalia (e.g. general appearance, hair distribution, lesions)
- Urethral meatus (e.g. size, location, lesions, prolapse)
- Bladder (e.g. fullness, masses, tenderness)
- Vagina (e.g. general appearance, oestrogen effect, discharge, lesions, pelvic support, cystocoele, rectocoele)
- Cervix (e.g. general appearance, lesions, discharge)
- Uterus (e.g. contour, position, mobility, tenderness, consistency, descent or support)
- Adnexa/parametria (e.g. masses, tenderness, organomegaly, nodularity)
- Anus and perineum

Figure 20.1 History taking and physical examination of the GUS in male anatomy. Source: Gleadle J (2012) *History Taking and Clinical Examination at a Glance*, 3rd edn, p.56. Wiley-Blackwell, Chichester

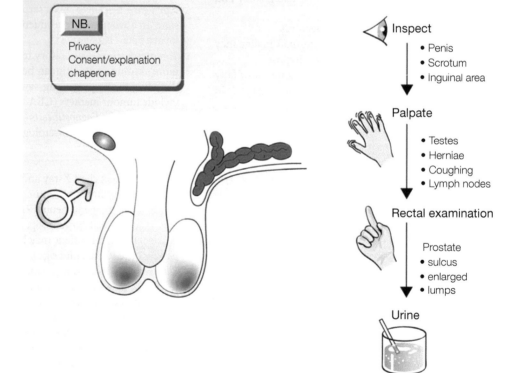

Advanced Clinical Practice at a Glance, First Edition. Edited by Barry Hill and Sadie Diamond Fox.
© 2023 John Wiley & Sons Ltd. Published 2023 by John Wiley & Sons Ltd.

Figure 20.2 History taking and physical examination of the GUS in female anatomy

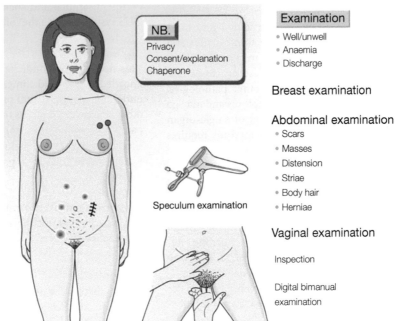

History
- Menstruation
- Bleeding
- Discharge

Sexual history
- Contraception
- Urinary symptoms
- Obstetric history

NB.
Privacy
Consent/explanation
Chaperone

Speculum examination

Examination
- Well/unwell
- Anaemia
- Discharge

Breast examination

Abdominal examination
- Scars
- Masses
- Distension
- Striae
- Body hair
- Herniae

Vaginal examination

Inspection

Digital bimanual
examination

Figure 20.3 History taking and physical examination of the pregnant patient

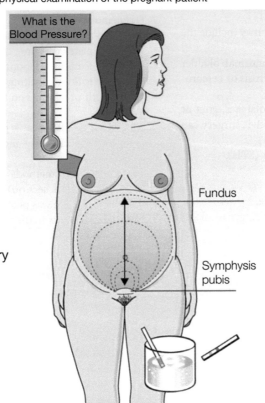

What is the
Blood Pressure?

History

Last menstrual period
Menstrual cycle

Any:
Bleeding
Anaemia
Hypertension
Diabetes
Infection
Vomiting
Thromboses

Past obstetric history
Gravidity
Parity
Mode of delivery
Complications

Past gynaecological
history

Fundus

Symphysis
pubis

Examination

Well/unwell
Anaemia
Fever
Blood pressure
Breast examination

Oedema
Cardiovascular examination
Respiratory examination
Urinalysis

Uterine swelling
Measure symphysis pubis–fundal
height
Tenderness
Fetal parts:
- Lie
- Liquor volume
- Presentation
- Engagement
- Fetal heart

Presentation of genitourinary system disorders

Clinical features of GUS pathology may be varied and non-specific, in addition to affecting multiple anatomical sites and organ systems. Diagnosis of GUS conditions may be incidental or secondary to investigations of other disease processes and challenging due to potential coexistence of other pathologies. Several conditions share common clinical symptoms and may go unrecognised because of focused management of single-organ dysfunction. The nature of the presenting symptoms requires careful questioning, exploration and consideration to rule out alternative diagnoses. An appreciation of the common symptoms associated with GUS disorders is essential and will inform the clinical practitioner in asking questions.

- Ask if the patient is experiencing any difficulty with voiding.
- Ask the patient about colour of their urine.
- Ask about history of urinary tract infections, burning, frequency, presence of blood in urine, sediment, odour with urine, and history of kidney, renal and genital health issues.
- Ask about nocturia and incomplete bladder emptying. In older males, alterations to urinary habits (frequency, urgency, nocturia) may suggest prostate disease.
- Ask the patient if they have any concerns about their sexual health.

Past medical history

Focused enquiry into GUS past medical history may include the following.
- *Neurological diseases* – these may cause abnormal bladder function, e.g. Parkinson disease, multiple sclerosis or cerebrovascular disease.
- Any previous kidney disease, hypertension, diabetes, gout or back injury may be relevant. Abdominal or pelvic surgery can cause denervation injury to the bladder.
- Any history of sexually transmitted infections (STIs).
- History of infertility.
- History of UTIs.
- Previous surgery, e.g. for urinary incontinence.
- Ureteric injury may occur following abdominal, gynaecological or spinal operations.

Drug history

A detailed and accurate drug history is essential. If a GUS condition is suspected, there are several drugs that may precipitate disease onset, contribute to subsequent recognised complications or aid in differential diagnosis. These include (but are not limited to):
- *diuretics (e.g. furosemide)* – a common cause of nocturia and can cause acute kidney injury
- *alpha-blockers* – commonly used to treat prostatic enlargement
- *nephrotoxic medications (e.g. ACE inhibitors, NSAIDs)* – may cause acute or chronic kidney injury
- *Antibiotics* – commonly required for recurrent UTIs and may be prescribed as prophylaxis
- *Antihypertensives* – these may affect erectile dysfunction in males.

Family history and social history

Pertinent familial and social history pointers that relate to the GUS system include the following.

Psychosexual history

This needs to be conducted sensitively. It requires experience, knowledge and good clinical judgement to recognise and define underlying psychosexual problems and differentiate them from other causes of symptoms (dyspareunia, low abdominal or pelvic pain, for example). A history should include enquiry about:
- relationship details, including issues of sexuality
- intercourse and sexual practices
- libido
- orgasm
- association of other symptoms
- if it seems relevant/there are cues, ask about previous negative sexual experiences.

Obstetric history in female patients
- Ask whether the patient has ever been pregnant.
- Record completed and unsuccessful pregnancies.
- Take details of gestation at time of any miscarriages or terminations.
- Note complications of pregnancy, particularly gestational diabetes, hypertension, HELLP syndrome, a condition related to pre-eclampsia and characterised by:
  - H aemolysis
  - EL (elevated liver) enzymes
  - LP (low platelet) count.
- Ask about features of labour which might encourage weakness of the pelvic floor, resulting in stress incontinence.
- Note length of labour and whether there was any prolonged pushing.
- Note size of babies – a larger baby, particularly if there was shoulder dystocia, may increase the chances of later stress incontinence.
- Ask whether any methods of assisted delivery were required (forceps, caesarean section).
- Ask whether there was postpartum haemorrhage.
- Note complications in the puerperium, e.g. depression.

Clinical Examination

An overarching critical review of the patient's history and clinical examination is crucial in identification of underlying GUS pathology. The clinical manifestations of common GUS conditions are widely varied across numerous anatomical sites and organ systems. A general clinical examination should detect conditions which may either present or complicate genitourinary disease. Examples include:
- hirsutism and/or acne, reflecting possible endocrine disorders
- anaemia, which commonly accompanies menstrual disorders
- conditions which are associated with menstrual symptoms
- thyroid disease
- Cushing's syndrome
- anorexia nervosa

- other chronic diseases
- breast examination
- lymphadenopathy, especially inguinal nodes
- assessment of secondary sexual characteristics.

Specific GUS examination in males and females is detailed in Tables 20.1 and 20.2. Figures 20.1 and 20.2 demonstrate GUS examination in those with male and female anatomy, respectively, and Figure 20.3 shows HTPE in the pregnant female.

Genitourinary system red flags

Throughout the patient consultation process, the practitioner may be alerted to 'red flags'. Some of these can be immediately life-threatening for the patient or may be a clinical indicator of serious underlying pathology. Red flags warn the practitioner of a symptom associated with a potentially life-threatening condition and must be acted upon accordingly. Red flag symptoms/findings in those with a working diagnosis of a GUS disorder may include, but are not limited to:

- pain (urination, testicular, menstrual, abdominal, lower back)
- genital ulcers
- dyspareunia
- urinary symptoms, i.e. pain, discharge, urgency, frequency, incontinence
- discharge
- abnormal bleeding or amenorrhoea (absence or cessation of menstruation)
- abnormal puberty.

21 Musculoskeletal system history taking and physical examination

Table 21.1 Types of musculoskeletal pain

Bone pain: injuries such as bone fractures or other musculoskeletal injuries cause bone pain. Less commonly, a tumour may cause bone pain

Joint pain: stiffness and inflammation often accompany joint pain. For many people, joint pain gets better with rest and worsens with activity

Muscle pain: muscle spasms, cramps and injuries can all cause muscle pain. Some infections or tumours may also lead to muscle pain

Tendon and ligament pain: ligaments and tendons are strong bands of tissue that connect joints and bones. Sprains, strains and overuse injuries can lead to tendon or ligament pain

Table 21.2 Referral, diagnosis and investigations of rheumatoid arthritis. Source: Modified from NICE (2020) NICE Guideline NG100. Rheumatoid arthritis in adults: management. www.nice.org.uk/guidance/ng100/chapter/Recommendations#investigations-following-diagnosis (accessed March 2022).

Referral from primary care

Refer for specialist opinion any adult with suspected persistent synovitis of undetermined cause. Refer urgently (even with a normal acute-phase response, negative anticyclic citrullinated peptide [CCP] antibodies or rheumatoid factor) if any of the following apply:
- the small joints of the hands or feet are affected
- more than one joint is affected
- there has been a delay of 3 months or longer between onset of symptoms and seeking medical advice

Investigations

If the following investigations are ordered in primary care, they should not delay referral for specialist opinion.

Investigations for diagnosis

Offer to carry out a blood test for rheumatoid factor in adults with suspected rheumatoid arthritis (RA) who are found to have synovitis on clinical examination

Consider measuring anti-CCP antibodies in adults with suspected RA if they are negative for rheumatoid factor

X-ray the hands and feet in adults with suspected RA and persistent synovitis

Investigations following diagnosis

As soon as possible after establishing a diagnosis of RA:
- measure anti-CCP antibodies, unless already measured to inform diagnosis
- X-ray the hands and feet to establish whether erosions are present, unless X-rays were performed to inform diagnosis
- measure functional ability using, for example, the Health Assessment Questionnaire (HAQ) to provide a baseline for assessing the functional response to treatment

If anti-CCP antibodies are present or there are erosions on X-ray:
- advise the person that they have an increased risk of radiological progression but not necessarily an increased risk of poor function, and
- emphasise the importance of monitoring their condition and seeking rapid access to specialist care if disease worsens or they have a flare

Figure 21.1 Physical examination of the MSK system. Source: Gleadle J (2012) *History Taking and Clinical Examination at a Glance*, 3rd edn, p.54. Wiley-Blackwell, Chichester

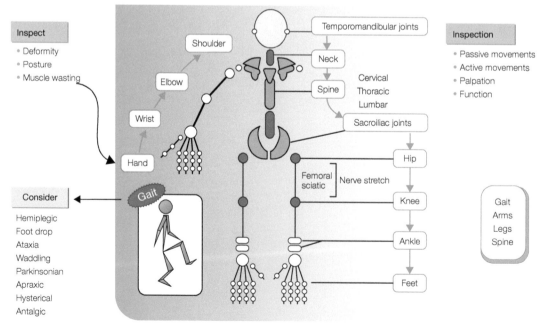

Table 21.3 MSK inspection

- Observe stance and note any abnormal curvature of the spine such as kyphosis, lordosis or scoliosis
- Ask the patient to walk away from you, turn and walk back toward you while you observe their gait and balance
- Ask the patient to sit
- Inspect the size and contour of the muscles and joints and if the corresponding parts are symmetrical. Notice the skin over the joints and muscles and observe if there is tenderness, swelling, erythema, deformity or asymmetry
- Observe how the patient moves their extremities and note if there is pain with movement or any limitations in active range of motion (ROM). Active range of motion is the degree of movement the patient can voluntarily achieve in a joint without assistance
- Inspect standing position (if appropriate) for postural abnormalities

Table 21.4 MSK palpation

- Palpation is typically done simultaneously during inspection
- As you observe, palpate each joint for warmth, swelling or tenderness
- If you observe decreased active range of motion, gently attempt passive range of motion by stabilising the joint with one hand while using the other hand to gently move the joint to its limit of movement
- Passive range of motion is the degree of range of motion demonstrated in a joint when the examiner is providing the movement
- Crepitus may be heard as joints move. Crepitus sounds like a crackling, popping noise that is considered normal if it is not associated with pain
- As the joint moves, there should not be any reported pain or tenderness
- Assess muscle strength
- Muscle strength should be equal bilaterally, and the patient should be able to fully resist an opposing force
- Muscle strength varies among people depending on their activity level, genetic predisposition, lifestyle and history

Prevalence of musculoskeletal system disorders

Musculoskeletal (MSK) conditions affect the joints, bones and muscles, and also include rarer autoimmune diseases and back pain. According to the World Health Organization,[1] MSK disorders comprise more than 150 conditions that affect the locomotor system of individuals (Table 21.1). They range from those that arise suddenly and are short-lived, such as fractures, sprains and strains, to lifelong conditions associated with ongoing functioning limitations and disability. Common MSK disorders include rheumatoid arthritis, osteoarthritis, gout, juvenile onset idiopathic arthritis, psoriatic arthritis and ankylosing spondylitis. Musculoskeletal conditions are typically characterised by pain (often persistent) and limitations in mobility, dexterity and overall level of functioning, reducing people's ability to work. The clinical management of painful musculoskeletal conditions uses a holistic approach incorporating education, psychological, physical and surgical interventions.

Presentation of musculoskeletal system disorders

Clinical features of MSK pathology may be varied and nonspecific, in addition to affecting multiple anatomical sites. Diagnosis of MSK conditions may be incidental or secondary to investigations of other disease processes, and challenging due to the potential coexistence of other pathologies, particularly those of the neurological system. Several conditions share common clinical symptoms and may go unrecognised because of focused management of single-organ dysfunction. The nature of the presenting symptoms requires careful questioning, exploration and consideration to rule out alternative diagnoses. Common symptoms associated with MSK conditions include weakness, stiffness, joint pain and swelling, and changes with mobility.

Musculoskeletal conditions include disorders that affect:

- joints, such as osteoarthritis, rheumatoid arthritis, psoriatic arthritis, gout and ankylosing spondylitis
- bones, such as osteoporosis, osteopenia and associated fragility fractures, traumatic fractures
- muscles, such as sarcopenia
- the spine, such as back and neck pain
- multiple body areas or systems, including regional and widespread pain disorders and inflammatory diseases such as connective tissue diseases and vasculitis that have musculoskeletal manifestations, for example systemic lupus erythematosus.

History of presenting complaint

Use the PRISMS acronym to explore key MSK symptoms.

- Pain
- Rashes, skin lesions and nail changes
- Immune system disorders
- Stiffness
- Malignancy
- Swelling and sweats

Past medical history

Specific questions should be asked relating to past medical history that may indicate relevant and significant MSK conditions as some conditions confer a higher risk of MSK pain, including the following.

- *Arthritis*: arthritis causes chronic joint inflammation. Many people who have arthritis experience joint pain and stiffness.
- *Fibromyalgia*: fibromyalgia is a chronic illness that causes all-over musculoskeletal pain and fatigue. Usually, people with fibromyalgia experience muscle, tendon or ligament pain.
- *Tunnel syndromes*: some conditions cause nerve compression or pinched nerves. Examples of these conditions include carpal tunnel syndrome, cubital tunnel syndrome and tarsal tunnel syndrome. Often, overuse injuries lead to these conditions.

Disease of the musculoskeletal system can manifest with muscular skeletal pain particularly of the joints (arthralgia), deformity, swelling, reduced mobility, reduced function and systemic features such as rash or fever.

Drug history

A detailed and accurate drug history is essential. If a MSK condition is suspected, there are several drugs that may precipitate disease onset, contribute to subsequent recognised complications or aid in differential diagnosis.

- Acetaminophens (e.g. paracetamol)
- Analgesics (e.g. NSAIDs, opiates)
- Corticosteroids (oral and injectables) (e.g. prednisolone) – long-term use can result in bone loss and osteoporosis
- Anti-TNF agents (e.g. infliximab)
- Biologics (e.g. rituximab)

Besides medications, there are several MSK treatments used to control pain, including:

- acupuncture
- chiropractic adjustment

- occupational therapy
- physical therapy
- splints
- therapeutic massage.

Family history and social history

Pertinent familial and social history pointers that relate to the MSK system should be discussed. A view of the general social context should be gained, enquiring about accommodation and any adaptations, support networks, abilities with the activities of daily living, and any carer involvement.

Clinical examination

An overarching critical review of the patient's history and clinical examination are crucial in identifying the underlying MSK pathology. The purpose of a routine physical exam of the musculoskeletal system is to assess function and screen for abnormalities (Figure 21.1). Most information about function and mobility is gathered during the patient interview, but the patient's posture, walking and movement of their extremities should be checked during the physical exam. An example of physical examination findings in the patient with rheumatoid arthritis can be seen in, and its referral, diagnosis and investigation guidance in Table 21.2. Typical MSK assessments include inspection and palpation (Tables 21.3 and 21.4).

Maintain a holistic assessment and be mindful of the patient's PMH. Some patients may have limited mobility and range of motion due to age-related degeneration of joints or previously diagnosed muscle weaknesses. Be considerate of these limitations and never examine any areas to the point of pain or discomfort. Support the joints and muscles as you assess them to avoid pain or muscle spasm. Compare bilateral sides simultaneously and expect symmetry of structure and function of the corresponding body area.[2]

Musculoskeletal system red flags

Serious pathology includes spinal infection, cauda equina, fracture and malignancy. Although they have a low incidence rate, these conditions should be considered as differential diagnoses when individuals present with back pain, particularly if the patient is not responding in an expected way or is starting to worsen. Identifying serious pathology early on is very important for several reasons.

- Prognosis improves with early diagnosis.
- Patients tolerate treatment better.
- Outcomes are better.
- Quality of life is better maintained.

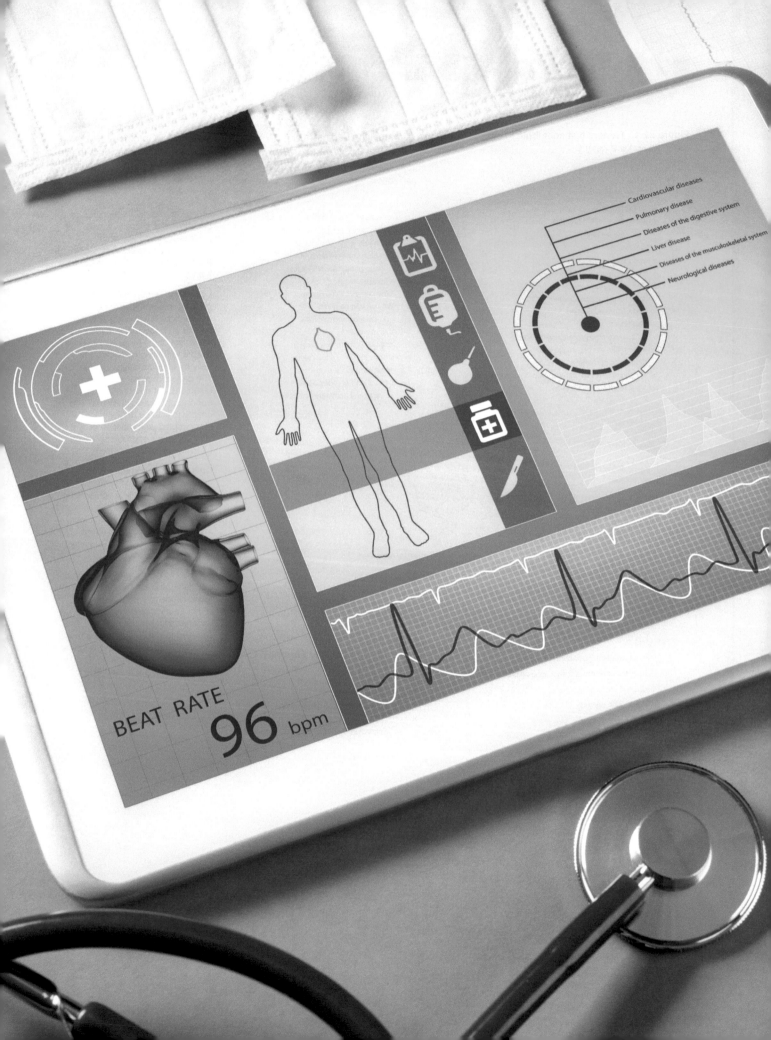

22 Dealing with difficult situations

Figure 22.1   Factors that contribute to difficult experiences in breaking bad news.
Source: Warnock *et al.* (2017).[3]

Situation

- Difficult subjects
  - Complex ethical situations
  - Transitions in care
  - Emotive events
- Unexpected news/events
  - Sudden death/deterioration
  - False early reassurance
  - Information not anticipated
- Context of communication
  - Not face to face
  - Unsuitable environment (event related)
- Tensions within the healthcare team
  - Situations mishandled by others
  - Disagreement over care/communication plan
  - Poor team communication

Organisation

- Time and staffing
  - Not enough time/competing demands
  - Staff not available e.g. inadequate staff levels, duty rotas, out of hours
- Relationships between departments
  - Poor communication transfer
- Information systems
  - Who can give information
  - When it can be given
  - Formal and informal "rules"
- Services available
  - Access to interpreter services
  - Delays in availability of tests, investigations and results
  - Lack of appropriate spaces e.g. private, free from interruptions

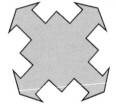

Individual

- Individual resources
  - Knowledge and skills
  - Confidence
  - Experience
- Balancing
  - Doing the right thing and paying a price
  - Taking responsibility and encountering challenges
  - Learning from reflection and doubting own practice
- Emotional consequences
  - Experiencing difficult emotions
  - Identification and personal engagement

Patients/relatives

- Reactions to news
  - Emotionally heightened
  - Non-acceptance, denial
- Family context
  - Issues around disclosure
  - Family dynamics
- Relationship breakdown with the healthcare team
  - Disagreement over the care plan
  - Challenging coping behaviours
- Communication barriers
  - Physical e.g. deafness, speech
  - Language
  - Comprehension: health related
  - Comprehension: emotional response, e.g. overwhelmed

Table 22.1   Common communication behaviours to avoid when responding to challenging behaviours. Source: Mesgarpour *et al.* (2021).[4]

Blocking – when a patient raises a concern but the healthcare professional fails to respond or changes the conversation, leading to the patient's most pressing concern not being addressed

Lecturing – when the healthcare professional provides large amounts of information without giving the patient an opportunity to respond or ask questions. The patient may be unable to follow the pace of the delivery of information and take it in. The patient may have specific questions but does not get an opportunity to ask. They may also be unable to listen if they are preoccupied with other emotions, such as worry, sadness or feeling overwhelmed

Collusion – when patients and healthcare professionals avoid discussing sensitive or contentious matters. This is also known as 'don't ask, don't tell'. In these situations, important conversations about prognosis, cure or end of life may not occur

Premature reassurance – when a clinician responds too quickly with reassurance to a patient concern, without sufficient exploration or understanding of the concern. This can lead to the patient feeling that they have not been 'heard' and that their concern has not been understood or addressed[2].

Healthcare professionals working in large healthcare organisations will experience difficult situations daily. These challenging interactions may arise due to discrepancies in staff or patient expectations, altered perceptions, stress, emotion and ineffective communication between the patient and healthcare practitioner.

Duty of care

The law imposes a duty of care on a healthcare practitioner in situations where it is foreseeable that the practitioner might cause harm to patients through their actions or omissions. This is the case regardless of the registered professional's role. It exists when the practitioner has assumed some sort of responsibility for the patient's care. This can be fundamental personal care or a complex procedure.

To discharge the legal duty of care, healthcare practitioners must act in accordance with the relevant standard of care. This is the standard expected of an ordinarily competent practitioner performing that task or role. Failure to discharge the duty to this standard may be regarded as negligence. When harm has come to a patient, the law determines who has a duty of care to that patient – and whether there was negligence – to attribute responsibility/liability for that harm.

Informed refusal

Informed consent is a familiar concept but it is potentially even more significant to recognise its opposite: informed refusal. A patient with capacity who has been fully informed of the risks has the right to refuse treatment. The difficulty for ACPs, particularly when a patient wishes to discharge against advice, is being sure the patient has been fully informed and understands the risks they take by refusing treatment. For informed consent or refusal to be valid, the patient needs to have all the material facts that may affect their decision. Clearly explain the condition, and what further tests or treatment need to be performed. Be sure to explain why these measures are necessary, and what might happen if the patient refuses.

Preventing a challenging interaction

To prevent and resolve challenging interactions, clinical practitioners must consider factors that might contribute to these situations. Two principal factors are the local healthcare setting in which the interactions take place, and the variation in clinical practices. Many healthcare settings are overworked and overstretched to meet demand, and this continuously affects meaningful interactions. Insufficient time for consultation or interaction with patients plays a key role, as healthcare system pressures are increasing along with patient numbers and expectations, against a background of economising. Primarily, it is important to consider that both patients and healthcare practitioners want a positive interaction to ensure the best possible health outcome, as time spent in consultations is valuable for both parties.

Handling a challenging interaction

The *British Medical Journal* states that a healthcare professional's reaction to a difficult interaction can make matters worse.[1] ACPs might find themselves making subconscious changes in behaviour, such as body language and degree of listening. Arguing, talking over the patient or interrupting the patient can lead to a decline in the interaction.

Recognising a difficult consultation is the first step towards dealing with the problem. Diagnosis and management of the interactional difficulty might be necessary before diagnosis and management of the patient's presenting complaint. To do this takes skill and being aware of the causes of difficult interactions, and using strategies to cope with them should assist both ACPs and patients in achieving a satisfactory outcome to a consultation.

Breaking bad news

It is proposed by Collini *et al.* that breaking negative news to patients and their families is a common occurrence for healthcare practitioners.[2] This challenging task requires patience and refined communication skills and must be approached with empathy for all parties involved.

Any news that provokes a negative reaction can be described as bad news, and this can differ depending on individual circumstances. Nevertheless, the news of death or dying is universally acknowledged as bad. Each patient, or their relative, will have preferences for how they want the news to be delivered, which depends on their individual circumstances, personality and culture. Despite this variation, there are some key areas where agreement occurs. These include ensuring privacy and adequate time without interruptions, clarity and honesty when delivering the information, and an empathetic and caring attitude. Empathetic communication is particularly important for patients' psychological reactions to bad news. In healthcare settings, death is often unexpected and sudden. This creates specific challenges for staff delivering bad news. It is often the first interaction between the healthcare professional and the patient or relatives, meaning there is sometimes very little time to build a relationship. Patients and their relatives may be unprepared for this bad news, which can provoke disbelief, shock, hostility and fear as well as grief.

Breaking bad news is challenging for clinicians (Figure 22.1), as it provokes negative emotions such as sadness, guilt and feelings of failure. It can be difficult to gauge a patient's preference for how much information they would like and how quickly, and clinicians may fear many aspects of the process – not doing it well enough, extinguishing hope, being wrong about the prognosis and the patient's emotional response. If in addition to these fears, a clinician does not feel confident in breaking bad news, they may avoid it or do it badly.

There are several common communication behaviours to avoid when responding to challenging behaviours (Table 22.1).

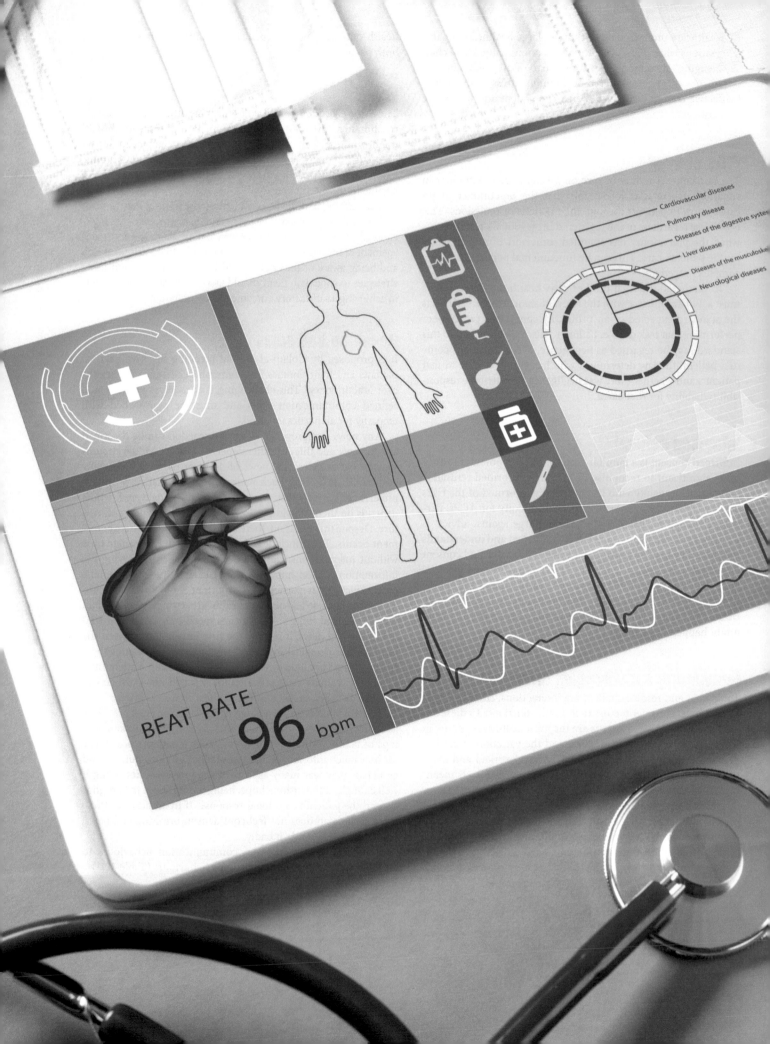

Advanced clinical interventions

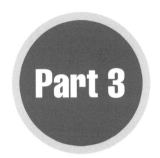

Part 3

Chapters

23 Fundamental ultrasound skills

Table 23.1 Advantages and limitations of ultrasound

Advantages	Limitiations
Portable	User must be fully trained to perform and interpret scan
Minimally invasive, painless	Interobserver variability
No ionising radiation	Operator dependent
Low cost	Limited penetration in obese patients
Comparable/superior to other forms of imaging[a]	Lesser resolution that other imaging modalities (e.g. CT, MRI)
Immediate results	Air, bowel gas and bone prevent visualisation of structures

[a] In diagnosis of specific clinical pathology.
CT, computed tomography; MRI, magnetic resonance imaging.

Table 23.2 UK ultrasound accreditation pathways

Focused	Advanced
Focused Ultrasound in Intensive Care (FUSIC)	FUSIC HD Haemodynamic Assessment
Focused Acute Medicine Ultrasound (FAMUS)	BSE Level 2 Advanced Level Echocardiography
Focused Emergency Echocardiography in Life Support (FEEL)	
BSE Level 1 Focused Echocardiography	

Figure 23.1 Ultrasound–tissue interaction

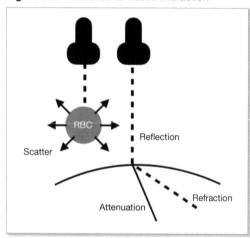

Figure 23.2 Echogenicity scale. Source: Otto[10], with permission of Elsevier

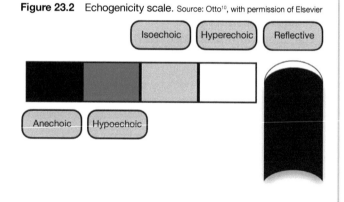

Figure 23.3 Modes of ultrasound

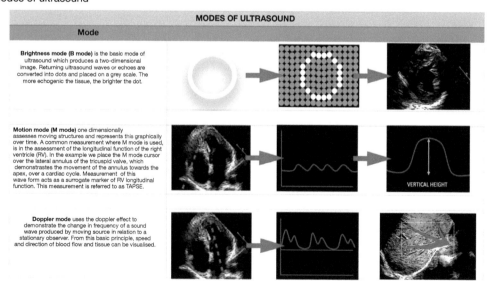

Advanced Clinical Practice at a Glance, First Edition. Edited by Barry Hill and Sadie Diamond Fox.
© 2023 John Wiley & Sons Ltd. Published 2023 by John Wiley & Sons Ltd.

Diagnostic ultrasound imaging is an invaluable tool that uses high-frequency sound waves to aid diagnosis of many conditions. Initially adopted by obstetricians,[1] it is now widely used by other medical specialties[2] as both a point-of-care assessment tool (PoCUS) and a guide for procedural interventions.

Ultrasound imaging has numerous advantages over other forms of imaging[3,4] (Table 23.1). It can be performed at the bedside so that rapid diagnosis can be made, it is lower in cost and, most importantly, it does not expose the patient to ionising radiation. Ultrasound has been found to be comparative and, in some cases, superior to other imaging modalities in the diagnosis of common acute pathologies.[5-7] There are, however. some limitations to this modality of imaging[3,4] (see Table 23.1).

Before explaining the ultrasound skills that are essential for the modern-day advanced practitioner, it is important to have a basic understanding of what ultrasound is and how it is generated to create an image that we can recognise and interpret.

Basic principles of ultrasound

Sound is a mechanical energy that travels longitudinally though an acoustic medium, in this case, human tissue. Humans can perceive audible sound up to an upper range of 20 kHz and anything above this is referred to as ultrasound.[8]

Transducer

To use ultrasound as a diagnostic tool, we first need a device that can generate sound waves and direct them into the structures we want to visualise.[9] This device is called a transducer, more commonly known as an ultrasound probe. There are different probes available for clinical use. Variations in their size, shape and operating frequency determine which probe should be used to image a particular structure.

When an electrical charge is applied to this transducer, a sound wave is created and emitted into the body. As the wave encounters various tissues and fluid media, some of it is absorbed and some is reflected back to the transducer[10] (Figure 23.1). Analysis of these reflected waves creates a two-dimensional image.

Echogenicity

Echogenicity is the tissue's ability to reflect ultrasound.[11] Human tissues possess varying echogenicity and the interface that exists between them will be represented by a different contrast (Figure 23.2). Evaluation of this information allows clinicians to differentiate between appearances of normal and pathological tissue.

Ultrasound modes

There are different modes of diagnostic ultrasound in use today.[2] Each mode provides different data that forms part of a multimodal assessment. See Figure 23.3 for a detailed explanation:

- Brightness mode (B mode)
- Motion mode (M mode)
- Doppler mode

Clinical application

Ultrasound is a tool that should complement clinical assessment and examination, rather than replace it. Most body systems can be assessed to evaluate structure and function and to detect pathology.

Brain

Ultrasound can be used to assess neurological pathology.[12] Two main techniques exist.

Optic nerve sheath diameter (ONSD) is used as a surrogate marker of intracranial pressure (ICP). The subarachnoid space lies between the optic nerve and the sheath, therefore a rise in ICP can be detected by measuring the diameter of the sheath. *Transcranial colour Doppler* (TCCD) visualises the circle of Willis and evaluates intracranial blood flow and velocity to aid diagnosis of pathology.[13]

Common pathology includes cerebral infarction, vasospasm, low cerebral perfusion pressure and increased ICP.

Airway

A more recent use of ultrasound is to evaluate the upper airway.[14] Assessment includes:

- prediction of difficulty of laryngoscopy
- correct placement of endotracheal tube and/or nasogastric tube
- presence of laryngeal oedema and subsequent prediction of postextubation stridor or likelihood of failed weaning
- aiding placement of percutaneous tracheostomy.

Heart

Ultrasound of the heart, also known as echocardiography, is carried out to assess ventricular function, evaluate haemodynamic status and identify the presence of structural heart disease or pleural/pericardial collection. Further details on this can be found in Chapter 26.

Lungs

Lung ultrasound (LUS) has become hugely popular over the last two decades due to its role in detecting pulmonary pathologies. Traditional assessment of common lung pathology (pleural effusion, alveolar consolidation, interstitial disease) using chest radiograph and auscultation is associated with poor diagnostic accuracy.[15] LUS however, is highly sensitive and specific in diagnosing these conditions, and as such can be seen as a safe alternative to conventional imaging.[15,16]

Abdomen

Outside the radiology setting, abdominal ultrasound is increasingly being used within emergency and critical care specialties.[17] It can be used to assess haemoperitoneum in trauma, biliary and urinary tract pathology, presence of intrauterine pregnancy or abdominal aortic aneurysm (AAA). Ultrasound can also be used to guide procedures such as paracentesis and urethral catheterisation.

Vascular

Obtaining intravenous (IV) access may be more difficult in some patients than others, due to tissue oedema, habitus or presence of vasculopathy.[18] Ultrasound can be used to guide placement of IV cannulas and avoid the need for repeated unsuccessful attempts, which can lead to increased patient discomfort and risk of infection or phlebitis. It is standard UK practice to use ultrasound in the placement of central venous catheters.[19]

Another role of ultrasound in the vascular system is identification of deep vein thrombosis (DVT). A simple compression test at two points on the lower limbs, femoral and popliteal veins, is highly sensitive and specific for detection of DVT.[20]

Training and governance

In the UK, there are several training programmes available to healthcare professionals (Table 23.2).[21-24] These range from basic to advanced pathways, which are comparable to training delivered to specialists in the field (i.e. cardiology, radiology). Deciding which accreditation is most suitable for the individual depends on three fundamental factors.

- Practical exposure to a range of pathology
- Support from an accredited mentor
- Minimum requirement for your area of practice

For a practitioner working in an acute specialty in which rapid assessment and diagnosis are essential, a focused level scan may be more appropriate. Conversely, if more detailed information is required, in context of a more complex presentation, i.e. structural heart disease, then a more advanced level scan is indicated.

Irrespective of the level of ultrasound scan performed, a robust governance process is required to ensure training and reporting standards are met.[25] Patient safety is vital, therefore high-quality training, dataset adherence and oversight from a local expert are key.

24 Lung ultrasound

Figure 24.1 Key ultrasound images

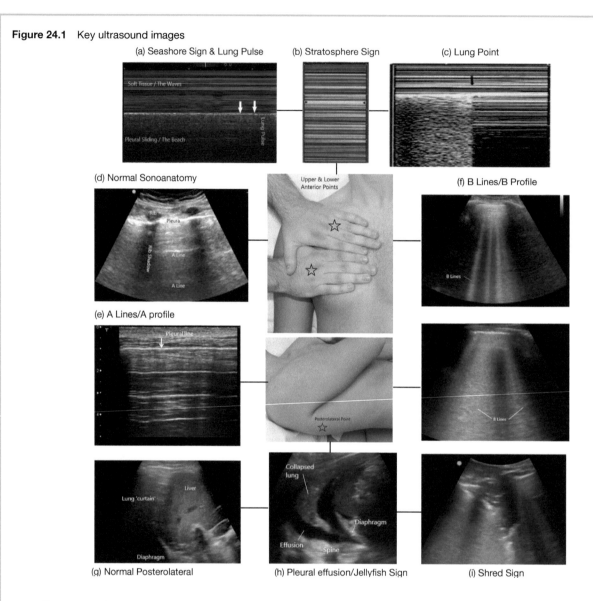

(a) Seashore Sign & Lung Pulse

(b) Stratosphere Sign

(c) Lung Point

(d) Normal Sonoanatomy

(e) A Lines/A profile

(f) B Lines/B Profile

(g) Normal Posterolateral

(h) Pleural effusion/Jellyfish Sign

(i) Shred Sign

Table 24.1 Sonographic findings of common respiratory pathologies

Pathology	Lung ultrasound findings
Pneumothorax	Absent lung sliding, absent B lines and absent lung pulse in affected area, Lung point
Pleural effusion	Varying echogenicity but often anechoic fluid above diaphragm, spine sign
Pneumonia	Focal B lines with areas of sparing, shred sign, lung hepatisation, dynamic air bronchograms. Often unilateral findings (unless bilateral pneumonia)
Chronic obstructive pulmonary disease/ asthma	A lines predominate, lung sliding may be reduced or even absent in severe cases but no lung point identified and lung pulse still present
Pulmonary oedema	B lines bilaterally, often diffuse and homogenous
Interstitial lung disease	B lines in affected zones
Acute respiratory distress syndrome (ARDS)	B lines bilaterally often heterogenous, may or may not have lung sliding, often subpleural consolidation

Advanced Clinical Practice at a Glance, First Edition. Edited by Barry Hill and Sadie Diamond Fox.
© 2023 John Wiley & Sons Ltd. Published 2023 by John Wiley & Sons Ltd.

Point-of-care lung ultrasound, when performed well, outperforms auscultation and plain chest radiographs in diagnostic accuracy, and in some instances approaches the sensitivity of CT scan. It can help to quickly differentiate the causes of respiratory failure at the bedside while avoiding the ionising radiation and risk of transfer associated with other imaging modalities. It also has an invaluable role to play in improving safety of thoracocentesis (see Chapter 28).

Probe selection and image optimisation

Although scans can be performed with linear, curvilinear or phased array probes, a curvilinear probe is generally preferred for its ability to image at appropriate depths (10–15 cm). Where closer inspection of the pleura is required, the higher frequency linear probe is preferred (or depth greatly reduced). A lung imaging preset should be chosen if available. The scan can be performed with the patient seated or supine.

Probe placement and normal sonoanatomy

Many protocols have been described, but a three-zone scan per hemithorax offers an excellent balance of speed versus diagnostic yield. With hands placed just below the clavicle with fingertips at the midline, the first point is the middle of the uppermost hand, the second the centre of the lowermost palm, and the third at the posterior axillary line at rib spaces 10–12 (Figure 24.1). The probe marker traditionally points towards the patient's head. When scanning anteriorly, this produces the classic image with soft tissue uppermost, ribs below and, deep to this, the echo-bright pleura line (Figure 24.1d). The ribs cast a shadow posteriorly, often said to look like the wings of a bat – the **bat sign**. From the posterolateral view, the liver (or spleen) is seen below an echo-bright diaphragm with the aerated lung seen as a moving curtain obscuring the diaphragm on inspiration (**curtain sign,** Figure 24.1g).

In both anterior and posterolateral views, the probe can be rotated to point the marker towards the patient's right to allow the lung to be imaged through the intercostal space, eliminating shadowing from the ribs.

Image interpretation

A lines

A lines (Figure 24.1d,e) are caused by reverberation artefacts from the pleural line and signify air below the parietal pleura. They are seen as horizontal lines extending across the screen with the distance between lines equal to the distance between probe and pleura. These are seen in normal lung tissue but also in pneumothorax.

B lines

B lines (Figure 24.1f) are thought to represent the interface between air and thickened interlobular alveolar septa and so are present in any condition affecting the interstitium. They are seen as vertical lines originating from the pleura and extending to the bottom of the ultrasound image. They obliterate A lines and move back and forth with lung sliding. Greater than three B lines in one scanning zone is considered abnormal. For B lines to be visualised, the parietal and visceral pleura must be opposed and so presence of B lines excludes pneumothorax in the zone being scanned. Unilateral B lines often represent focal infection, whereas a bilateral presentation is more likely to signify pulmonary oedema although there are other differentials (Table 24.1).

Lung sliding

In the normal lung, movement should be visualised at the pleural line, signifying an intact visceral–parietal interface. This to-and-fro movement is best seen with the high-frequency linear probe and is often described as shimmering or like marching ants. Lung sliding rules out pneumothorax at that specific scanning point. M-mode placed through the pleural line may be used where B-mode imaging is unclear – here the characteristic **seashore sign** can confirm lung sliding with pleural sliding appearing grainy (the sandy beach) with the less mobile soft tissue above the pleura represented as horizontal lines (the waves) (Figure 24.1a).

When this classic appearance is lost, and only horizontal lines remain with no 'beach', a **stratosphere sign** is said to be present representing loss of lung sliding (Figure 24.1b). Absence of lung sliding is always abnormal and should raise suspicion of a pneumothorax although other causes should be considered (see Table 24.1).

Lung pulse

Lung pulse (Figure 24.1a) represents transmission of the cardiac pulse through opposed pleura. Best seen in M-mode as vertical lines, the presence of lung pulse is useful in ruling out pneumothorax where lung sliding is absent due to alternative pathologies.

Lung point

The lung point is the transition from presence of lung sliding to absence of lung sliding and is seen where the border of normal lung and pneumothorax meet. In M-mode this can be seen as a transition from the seashore to stratosphere signs throughout respiration (Figure 24.1c). This is very specific for pneumothorax.

Pleural effusions

Pleural effusions are usually visualised in the dependent regions of the lung. The common appearance is one of anechoic fluid above the echo-bright diaphragm (Figure 24.1h). With fluid present, ultrasound is conducted more effectively, with visualisation of the spine often possible (the **spine sign**). Occasionally, fluid may appear less anechoic or include hyperechoic fibrin strands. This raises suspicion of a more complex or exudative process. Volume of effusion can be estimated and position of both lung and diaphragm marked to facilitate safe decision making for aspiration if deemed necessary.

Collapse/consolidation

Collapsed lung can often be seen 'floating' in effusion which is termed the **jellyfish sign** (Figure 24.1h). In the absence of fluid, non-aerated lung may have a similar appearance to the solid organs, particularly the liver. This is known as lung **hepatisation**. Commonly, there is also a 'shred sign' evident – discrete areas beneath the pleura with rough irregular edges bordering normal aerated lung (Figure 24.1i). There may be brighter spots within these darker areas representing air bronchograms or conversely echo-poor areas representing fluid bronchograms. These may be static or dynamic (changing with respiration).

It must be noted that consolidation deep to aerated lung is not visible and thus lung ultrasound cannot completely rule out this pathology.

Limitations

Lung ultrasound is operator dependent, and practice is needed to optimise images and interpret artefacts appropriately and thus formal accreditation with supervision from a recognised local mentor is essential. As always, findings should be incorporated into the wider comprehensive patient assessment.

25 Vascular ultrasound

Table 25.1 Risk factors for venous thromboembolism. Source: England T, Nasim A (2014) *ABC of Arterial and Venous Disease*, 3rd edn, p.51. John Wiley & Sons, Hoboken.

Acquired disorders	Inherited/congenital disorders
Malignancy	Antithrombin deficiency
Surgery, especially orthopaedic	Protein C deficiency
Presence of central venous catheter	Protein S deficiency
Trauma	Factor V Leiden mutation
Pregnancy, HRT, oral contraceptive	Prothrombin gene mutation
Prolonged immobilisation	Dysfibrinogenaemias
Dehydration	Factor VII deficiency
Age over 60	Factor XII deficiency
Obesity (BMI >30)	
Previous VTE	
Congestive cardiac/respiratory failure	
Antiphospholipid syndrome	
Myeloproliferative disorders	
Poorly controlled diabetes mellitus	
Hyperviscosity syndromes (myeloma)	
Inflammatory bowel disease	
Acute medical illness	
Behçet's disease	
Varicose veins with associated phlebitis	

Taken from: ABC of Arterial and Venous Disease : ABC of Arterial and Venous Disease (3rd Edition), edited by Tim England, and Akhtar Nasim, John Wiley & Sons, Incorporated, 2014. Page 51

BMI, body mass index; HRT, hormone replacement therapy; VTE, venous thromboembolism.

Figure 25.1 Ultrasound detection of a DVT. The probe is held lightly on the skin and advanced along the course of the vein (left). Pressure is applied every few centimetres by compressing the transducer head against the skin. The vein collapses during compression if no thrombus is present (middle) but not if a DVT is present (right). Source: England T, Nasim A (2014) *ABC of Arterial and Venous Disease*, 3rd edn, p.8. John Wiley & Sons, Hoboken.

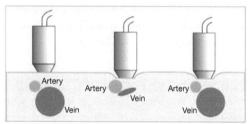

Figure 25.2 Duplex ultrasound scan demonstrating lack of flow in the common femoral vein indicating an occlusive DVT (arrow). Source: England T, Nasim A (2014) *ABC of Arterial and Venous Disease*, 3rd edn, p.51. John Wiley & Sons, Hoboken.

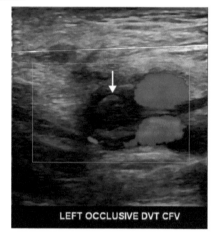

LEFT OCCLUSIVE DVT CFV

Figure 25.3 Normal duplex ultrasound scan demonstrating compression of the vein (arrow). Source: England T, Nasim A (2014) *ABC of Arterial and Venous Disease*, 3rd edn, p.52. John Wiley & Sons, Hoboken.

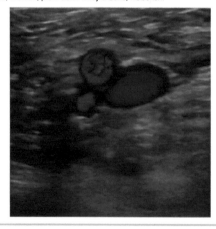 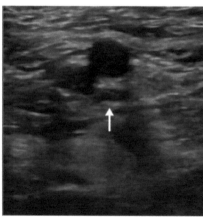

Venous thromboembolism (VTE), including pulmonary embolism (PE) and deep vein thrombosis (DVT), is a common complication of critical illness with associated morbidity and mortality; 28-day mortality rates are reported as 15% for PE and 9% for DVT.[1] Risk factors for the development of VTE are detailed in Table 25.1. These risks are further enhanced by critical care stay due to immobilisation, sepsis and invasive interventions/venous lines. Incidence of DVT varies across ICU populations, ranging from 5% to 20%[2] despite pharmacological thromboprophylaxis.

Formal departmental Doppler ultrasound is the gold standard investigation for diagnosis of DVT but can often be delayed due to the availability of trained staff to provide a portable service, with out of hours especially problematic. Point-of-care ultrasound (POCUS) allows rapid and accurate diagnosis of DVT (Figure 25.1) following a training programme (e.g. FUSIC) which has a sensitivity and specificity of 96%.[3]

Indications for use

- Unilateral extremity symptoms including:
  - Leg/arm pain
  - Tenderness
  - Swelling
  - Erythema
- Pain on calf compression during examination
- Any concern for DVT

Relative contraindications

Known DVT as there is a theoretical risk of causing dislodgement of clot leading to PE.

Sonography

Upper limb

The upper limb contains superficial veins, the basilic and cephalic, and deep veins, axillary and brachial. The cephalic vein begins at the wrist and runs up the lateral edge of the arm where it meets the axillary vein at the clavicle. The basilic vein begins on the medial aspect of the wrist and continues up the medial aspect of the arm until it joins with the brachial veins to create the axillary vein. The distal part of the axillary vein branches to create the brachial veins. The proximal axillary vein runs through the border of the axilla to the first rib where it joins the cephalic vein to become the subclavian vein. The subclavian vein then continues under the clavicle until it is joined by the internal jugular and together, they create the brachiocephalic vein which drains into the superior vena cava.

Lower limb

The lower limb contains a superficial venous system comprising the great and small saphenous veins. The deep venous system of the leg starts with the external iliac which drains into the inferior vena cava. It exits the pelvis at the inguinal ligament and becomes the common femoral vein. A short distance below the inguinal ligament, the greater saphenous joins the common femoral, which then divides into the deep femoral and superficial femoral. The deep femoral is difficult to track due to loss of acoustic window as it goes deeper into the tissues. The superficial femoral is part of the deep venous system and so any clot here is a DVT. This can be tracked down to the popliteal fossa where it becomes the popliteal vein.

Technique

To obtain images of the vasculature, a high-frequency linear probe should be utilised. The transverse plane is utilised in vascular assessment. Depth and gain should be adjusted to optimise imaging of the area of interest. Direct visualisation of echogenic clot during 2D ultrasound is the definitive method to detect DVT. Several additional techniques can be utilised to establish patency and flow of the vessels if uncertainty exists.

- Compression of the venous segment during 2D ultrasound with the probe. This confirms collapsibility of the vessel and therefore no obstruction.
- Colour ultrasound (duplex) to demonstrate flow in the vessel. Conventionally, flow towards the probe is red and away is blue (Figures 25.2 and 25.3).

When assessing peripheral vasculature, these additional methods should be employed, with caution, every 2 cm along the vessels to provide a thorough examination when excluding a DVT.

In urgent and critical care settings, a focused rapid assessment can be undertaken which should include:
- common femoral vein at inguinal ligament
- junction of common femoral and great saphenous vein
- junction of common femoral and deep femoral vein
- popliteal vein
- trifurcation of popliteal vein.

If a thrombus is identified using 2D ultrasound, no further manipulation of the vein should take place as this increases the risk of dislodging the thrombus.

DVT assessment:

Diagnostic criteria for a venous embolus do not rely solely on direct visualisation of a clot. An acute clot may be hypoechoic and therefore difficult to diagnose but as the clot ages, it will appear echogenic.[4] If intraluminal echogenic material is visualised, then compression should be limited due to the risk of dislodging the clot. Compression applied to the vein which is sufficient to deform the artery but does not cause the anterior and posterior walls to touch suggests an obstructing embolus (see Figure 25.3). Conversely, if the vein compresses completely, it is unlikely there is a DVT at this point.

Colour Doppler will allow correct identification of the vein and artery. Venous flow can be augmented by squeezing the leg distal to the scan, although caution should be advised due to the potential for clot dislodgement. If no colour flow seen or there is no increase in venous flow, this may be suggestive of occlusive thrombus. Any suspected DVT should be confirmed prior to appropriate clinical treatment.

26 Focused echocardiography

Figure 26.1 Standard patient positioning

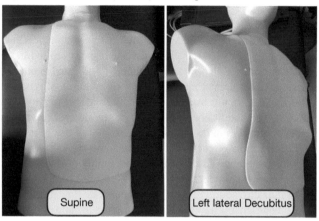

Supine

Left lateral Decubitus

Figure 26.2 The phased array probe

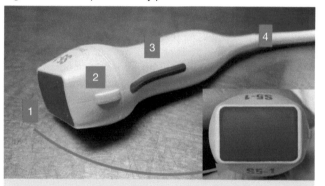

1. Footprint 2. Probe marker 3. Outer casing 4. Power cable

Table 26.1 Basic vs advanced echocardiography

	Focused	**Advanced**
Scanning mode	B mode, colour Doppler	B mode, colour, spectral and tissue Doppler
Acoustic windows	Parasternal (long and short axis) Apical four chamber Subcostal four chamber and IVC	*In addition to focused windows:* RV inflow/outflow Apical 5/3/2 chamber Suprasternal
Role in clinical practice	Rapid diagnosis in the acutely unwell patient	More comprehensive assessment of complex pathology
Associated accreditations	FUSIC Heart, FEEL, BSE Level 1	BSE Level 2, EDEC

Figure 26.3 Basic cardiac views

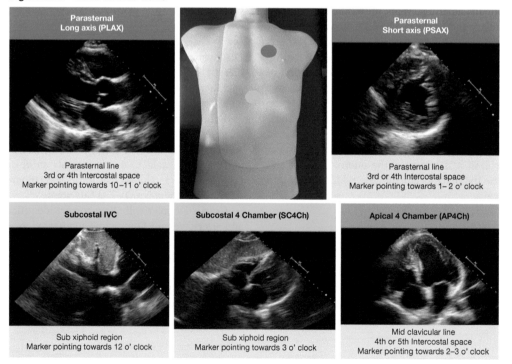

Parasternal Long axis (PLAX)
Parasternal line
3rd or 4th Intercostal space
Marker pointing towards 10–11 o' clock

Parasternal Short axis (PSAX)
Parasternal line
3rd or 4th Intercostal space
Marker pointing towards 1– 2 o' clock

Subcostal IVC
Sub xiphoid region
Marker pointing towards 12 o' clock

Subcostal 4 Chamber (SC4Ch)
Sub xiphoid region
Marker pointing towards 3 o' clock

Apical 4 Chamber (AP4Ch)
Mid clavicular line
4th or 5th Intercostal space
Marker pointing towards 2–3 o' clock

Advanced Clinical Practice at a Glance, First Edition. Edited by Barry Hill and Sadie Diamond Fox.
© 2023 John Wiley & Sons Ltd. Published 2023 by John Wiley & Sons Ltd.

The use of echocardiography within a non-cardiology setting is a rapidly expanding practice.[1] The ability to perform an ultrasound examination of the heart, at the patient's bedside, has proven to be an invaluable tool in the rapid diagnosis of many acute pathologies. Specialties such as intensive care and emergency medicine have adopted this skill, as an addition to standard clinical examination, and have integrated it within existing emergency protocols (Table 26.1).[2,3]

Within the UK there are three main focused echocardiography accreditation pathways, which are all affiliated to the British Society of Echocardiography (BSE).[2–4]

FUSIC Heart

The Intensive Care Society introduced focused intensive care echo (FICE) in 2012. Originally developed for use within critical care, it is now used across many specialties by medical, nursing and allied health professions. In 2019, FICE was rebranded as FUSIC heart, which forms one component of a larger modular accreditation pathway – focused ultrasound in intensive care (FUSIC).[2]

FEEL

The UK Resuscitation Council developed focused echocardiography in life support (FEEL) in 2013.[3] Aimed at novice practitioners, the course teaches how to integrate echocardiography into the peri-resuscitation period, to identify both causation of arrest and signs of myocardial dysfunction post return of spontaneous circulation (ROSC).

BSE Level 1

The BSE introduced level 1 echocardiography in 2018.[4] A major contributing factor to its development was the mandate of a 7-day NHS,[5] whereby access to imaging in the critically unwell should be offered within an hour of admission. Training is centred around common 'red flag' pathologies that require immediate management or referral to subspecialties.

Preparing for the examination

The optimum position for performing an echocardiogram is to have the patient in the left lateral decubitus position, ideally with the left arm raised above the head (Figure 26.1). In doing so, the heart moves closer to the chest wall and maximal distance between rib spaces is achieved to increase the *acoustic window*.[6] If the patient is too unstable to move into this position, it is possible to perform the scan supine.

Before commencing the scan, it is important to remember to attach an ECG. This will aid in identifying the correct point of the cardiac cycle at which to perform various measurements. As with any procedure, the patient's details should first be checked, and appropriate consent must be obtained.

Probe and manipulation

The probe of choice for this type of scan is the phased array (Figure 26.2). This probe operates at a lower frequency which enables deeper penetration into the thorax. To fit between narrow rib spaces, the probe surface has a small rectangular footprint. On the probe is a marker (see Figure 26.2), which is used for image orientation purposes.

The probe is manipulated in various ways to obtain a different tomographic plane or view of the heart. Broadly speaking, there are four ways in which the probe is manipulated.

Slide

The probe is moved between intercostal spaces in a sliding motion to obtain a view of the heart. The probe may also slide laterally or medially around the chest.

Rotate

To transition from a long axis plane of the heart to a short axis, the probe surface is rotated either clockwise or anticlockwise, using the probe marker as a guide. Care must be taken to ensure the surface of the probe remains within the same intercostal space when performing this manoeuvre.

Tilt

The probe is tilted on the longer edges of the probe surface. The resultant action of tilting is to 'fan' the ultrasound beam through the structures of the heart.

Rock

This is a very underutilised technique which can often be the most helpful when optimising your image. Rocking is the opposite of tilting, where the probe is 'rocked' on the shorter edges of the probe surface. Its purpose is to move the structure of interest side to side, which enables the user to centralise the image within the scan sector.

Basic views

There are five basic cardiac views that are used as part of a focused dataset. Each view corresponds to surface anatomy landmarks on the chest and a designated probe marker position, typically based on clockface landmarks (Figure 26.3).

- Parasternal long
- Parasternal short
- Apical four chamber
- Subcostal four chamber
- Inferior vena.cava (IVC)

Echocardiographic assessment

Ventricular size and function

Cardiac chamber size and degree of myocardial dysfunction are the two main parameters practitioners want to assess when performing echocardiography.[7] A dilated ventricle is often a clue that the heart is failing to 'pump' adequately, as it 'stretches' to accommodate the increased volume.[8] There are many causes of this, some of which may become clear on further echocardiographic assessment, i.e. valvular disease.[9]

Impaired myocardial contractility is prevalent in many different conditions and may be acute or chronic.[9–11] Echo examination can help identify the degree of this impairment, assess requirement for supportive therapies, i.e. inotropes, and serially assess the effectiveness of any support initiated.[8,12]

Volume-pressure overload

The left and right sides of the heart work synergistically. Therefore, any increases in pressure or volume that affect one side will deleteriously affect the other.[13] See pulmonary embolism below for further explanation.

Fluid responsiveness

Predicting fluid responsiveness with echo is a key assessment tool. Deciding whether to fluid resuscitate or de-resuscitate can aid in reversing organ dysfunction.[14] Echo features of low venous return include small ventricular end-diastolic areas, hyperdynamic function and small, collapsing inferior vena cava. Conversely, features of fluid overload include large ventricular end-diastolic areas, impaired contractility and large, non-collapsing IVC.[15]

Evidence of pericardial collection

Finally, it important to assess for evidence of pericardial collection, the volume, nature, and signs of tamponade physiology. Further explanation of this is given below.

Common pathologies

Echocardiography can aid in the diagnosis of multiple pathologies. Below are some examples of common acute presentations and their associated echocardiographic features.

Tamponade

Cardiac tamponade occurs when blood, fluid or air accumulates within the pericardial sac and creates an intrapericardial pressure that exceeds the pressures within the heart (atria and ventricle). This results in reduction of cardiac filling and, subsequently, cardiac output.[16] If left untreated, this can lead to cardiac arrest. Echocardiographic features include right atrial (RA) collapse during systole, right ventricular (RV) collapse during diastole and clear evidence of pericardial collection. It is important to note that cardiac tamponade remains a 'clinical' diagnosis.[17]

Aortic dissection

It is possible to visualise segments of the aorta using echo. Assessment includes size, presence of atheromatous plaques and evidence of intimal flap, which could signify aortic dissection. It is also important to assess for associated features of dissection, such as pericardial collection, tamponade and acute ventricular dysfunction.[18]

Pulmonary embolism (PE)

The RV is a low-pressure chamber, with thin walls. Any acute increases in pressure within the pulmonary vasculature, as seen in PE, will lead to RV dilation, dysfunction and ineffective cardiac output. Reduced cardiac output (CO) on the right will reduce filling and CO on the left, causing hypotension and, in some cases, shock leading to cardiac arrest.[19]

Sepsis-related myocardial dysfunction

During sepsis, there is increased cytokine release, mitochondrial dysfunction and tissue hypoxia, all of which can lead to acute, global myocardial dysfunction. Echo can guide decision making on fluid management and initiation of inotropic support.[20]

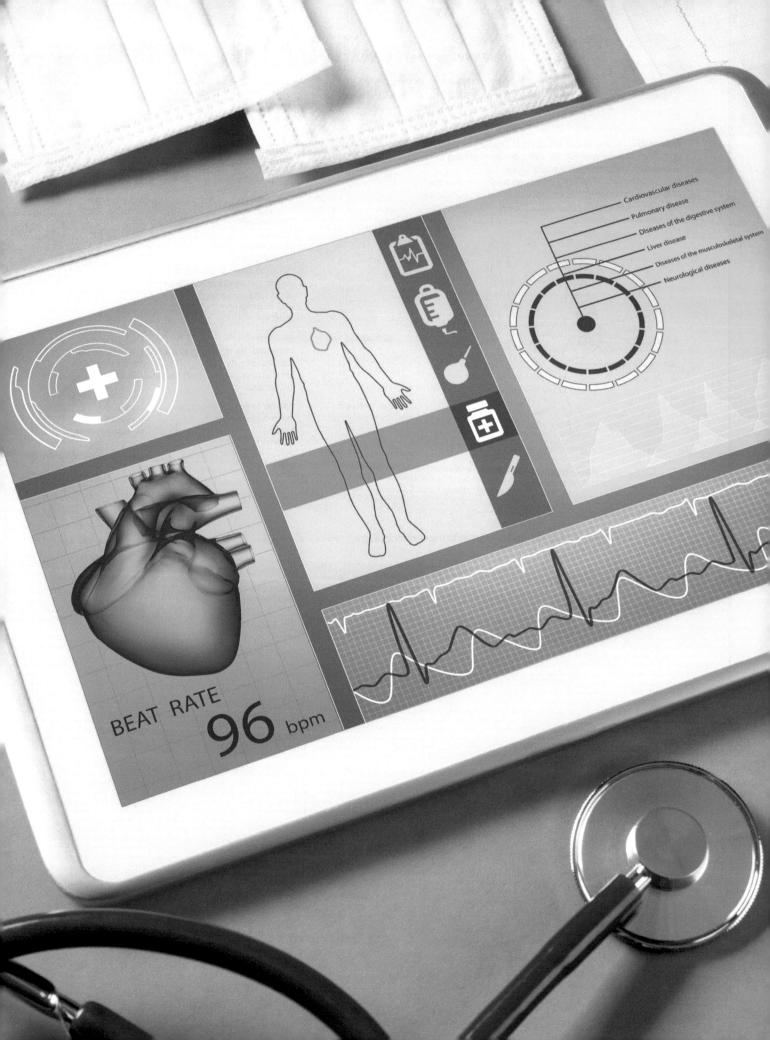

27 Central venous catheter and arterial catheter insertion

Figure 27.1 Diagram of the internal jugular vein and its divisions. The internal jugular veins are seen joining the subclavian veins to form the brachiocephalic or innominate veins. The SVC is formed by the confluence of the brachiocephalic or innominate veins. Source: Hamilton H, Bodenham A (eds) (2009) *Central Venous Catheters*, Figure 2.1, p.15. John Wiley & Sons, Hoboken.

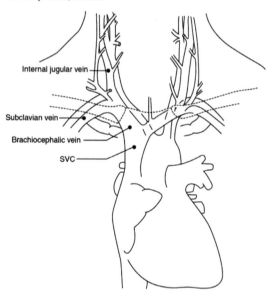

Table 27.1 Site selection

Site	Risks	Benefits
Internal jugular vein	Bleeding Pneumothorax Cardiac arrhythmia Infection Vessel thrombosis Arterial puncture Could be contraindicated in certain circumstances such as some types of cardiac surgery Risk of pneumothorax during insertion	Usually easy to insert
Subclavian vein	Bleeding Increased risk of pneumothorax Cardiac arrhythmia More challenging to insert than IJV/femoral	Cleaner site – CVC can be left in for longer period
Femoral vein	Can be more challenging to insert depending on body habitus Bleeding Higher risk of CVC-related infection	No risk of pneumothorax or cardiac arrhythmia

Figure 27.2 Central venous waveform in relation to the electrocardiogram. Source: Billington M, Stevenson M (2007) *Critical Care in Childbearing for Midwives*, Figure 10.2, p.197. Wiley-Blackwell, Chichester

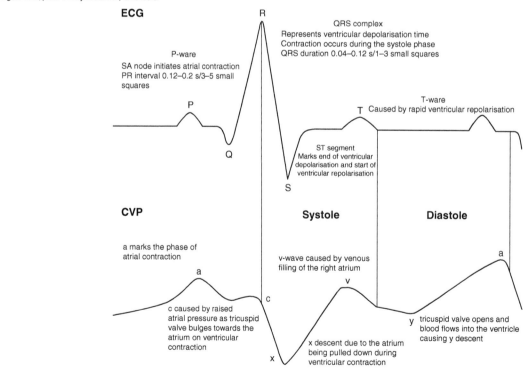

Table 27.2 Central line tip position. Source: Hamilton H, Bodenham A (eds) (2009) *Central Venous Catheters*, Table 2.1, p.25. John Wiley & Sons, Hoboken. Please see also Figure 27.3 for further explanation.

Catheter tip position	Zone in diagram	Advantages	Disadvantages
Left brachiocephalic	C	Outside pericardium	Smaller vein
		Left-sided catheters tips can be pulled back to this position	Close to junctions
			Unsuitable for long-term use, sclerosant drugs or high-volume flows
Upper SVC	B	Outside pericardium Ideal for right-sided catheters	Tip of left-sided catheters can abut SVC vein wall end on
Upper right atrium	A	Larger vessel with optimum flows (dialysis catheters)	Inside pericardium
			Arrhythmias or tricuspid valve damage can occur if catheter migrates inwards
		Tip position suitable for all routes of access	Risk of tamponade if perforation occurs

Reproduced with permission from *British Journal of Anaesthesia* (Stonelake and Bodenham 2006).

Figure 27.3 Stylised diagram of heart and great veins, and areas where catheter tips may lie (angles between veins may be more acute in vivo). See Table 27.1 for further explanation. Source: Hamilton H, Bodenham A (eds) (2009) *Central Venous Catheters*. John Wiley & Sons, Hoboken.

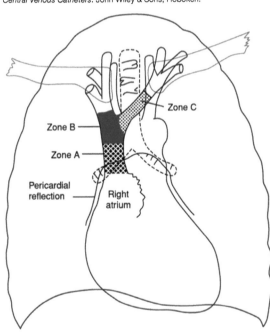

Figure 27.4 Modified Allen test. (a) With the patient's arm flexed at the elbow and the fist tightly clenched, the operator should occlude both ulnar and radial arteries simultaneously. (b) The fist is subsequently unclenched, and the palm should appear white. The compression is then released from the ulnar artery while maintaining pressure over the radial artery. (c) Once the compression is released, the color should return to the palm, usually within 10 seconds. The test is repeated on the same hand while releasing the radial artery first and continuing to compress the ulnar artery if evaluation of radial collateral blood flow is required.[1] Source: Dougherty L (2015) *Royal Marsden Manual of Clinical Nursing Procedures*, 9th edn, Figure 10.7, p.528. John Wiley & Sons, Hoboken.

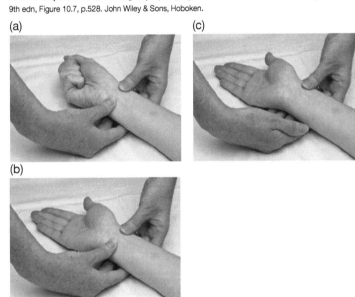

Figure 27.5 Arterial waveform. Source: Al-Aamri I, Derzi S, Moore A et al (2017) Reliability of pressure waveform analysis to determine correct epidural needle placement in labouring women. *Anaesthesia*, **72**, 840–844.

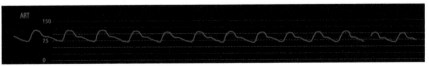

Central venous catheter insertion

Central venous access refers to lines placed into the large veins of the neck, chest or groin. To measure central venous pressure, the tip must lie within the thoracic cavity and preferably in the superior vena cava. Central venous access is a frequently performed invasive procedure which carries a significant risk of morbidity and even mortality.

Indications

- Monitoring of central venous pressure (CVP)
- Infusion of medications which are irritant to smaller veins
- Insertion of pacing wires
- Insertion of pulmonary artery catheter (PAC)
- Renal replacement therapy
- Parenteral feeding
- Emergency venous access
- Fluid resuscitation

Contraindications

- Uncorrected coagulopathy
- Thrombocytopenia
- Skin infection at the site of access
- Recent surgery to other nearby structures such as carotid endarterectomy

Anatomy

Internal jugular vein (IJV)

The IJV (Figure 27.1) runs from the jugular foramen to the sternal margin of the clavicle. At this point it terminates by joining the subclavian vein (SCV) to form the brachiocephalic vein. The IJV is surrounded by the carotid sheath which also contains the carotid artery and the vagus nerve. When the vein forms, it initially lies superficially in the anterior triangle of the neck and overlies the internal carotid artery. As it descends, it moves to lie lateral to the artery.

Subclavian vein (SCV)

The SCV is a continuation of the axillary vein. It begins at the outer border of the first rib and ends at the medial border of scalenus anterior, where it joins the internal jugular vein to form the brachiocephalic vein behind the sternoclavicular joint.

Femoral vein

The femoral vein is the continuation of the popliteal vein and ends medial to the artery at the inguinal ligament where it becomes the external iliac vein. The femoral artery, vein and nerve lie within the femoral triangle, arranged from lateral to medial: nerve, artery, vein. The artery can easily be palpated on a patient, and the vein lies 2 cm medial to the pulsation.

Site selection

The anatomy of these areas is complex and the risk of damaging nearby structures is significant. The choice of site depends on a combination of factors which are summarised in Table 27.1.

Step-by-step guide

1 Inform the patient and gain consent.
2 Assess the insertion site visually and with ultrasound to ensure the site is suitable for central venous access.
3 Prepare the environment and patient, ensuring you have adequate access to the insertion site.
4 Set up your trolley and prepare the central venous catheter.
5 Ensure that a pressurised monitoring system is set up.
6 Complete a team brief and Local Safety Standard for Invasive Procedures (LocSSIPs) as per local policy.
7 Don a surgical hat and mask.
8 Scrub and then don a sterile surgical gown and sterile gloves.
9 Clean the area with antiseptic (2% chlorhexidine in 70% isopropyl alcohol is recommended) and drape the area.
10 Cover the ultrasound probe with a sterile cover.
11 Using ultrasound guidance, infiltrate local anaesthetic (e.g. 1% lidocaine) into the insertion site area.
12 With the ultrasound, identify where the vein is largest and most lateral to the artery.
13 Insert the introducer needle attached to the syringe just proximal to the probe and whilst aspirating the syringe, watch the screen. The needle will appear as a bright white, echo-dense, spot which you can angle towards the vein until it deforms the wall of the vein as it pierces it.
14 Once blood is aspirated, keep the needle still and detach the syringe.
15 Insert the guidewire through the introducer needle (the guidewire should pass freely). During insertion of the guidewire, observe the ECG. If the guidewire passes too far and touches the endocardium, atrial or ventricular ectopics can be observed. If this occurs pull back the wire.
16 Once the guidewire has been inserted to an appropriate length, remove the needle.
17 Use the ultrasound to confirm the guidewire is within the vein by visualisng the wire, vein and artery.
18 Use the scalpel to make a small nick in the skin around the insertion site.
19 Pass the dilator over the guidewire and dilate the skin and subcutaneous tissue, keeping hold of the guidewire.
20 Remove the dilator whilst holding sterile gauze over the site.
21 Place the central line over the wire and into the vein.
22 Use a syringe with saline to ensure you can aspirate and flush all ports.
23 Secure the line as per local guidelines.
24 Confirm appropriate catheter tip position via:
    - transducing the distal port of the CVC and analysing the central venous pressure waveform in relation to the electrocardiogram (Figure 27.2)
    - chest X-ray (Table 27.2, Figure 27.3).[xsublist]

Arterial catheter insertion

Arterial lines are commonly used within the critical care setting and allow a beat-to-beat display of a patient's blood pressure. In addition, they allow arterial blood sampling without the need for repeated arterial punctures.

Indications

- Inotropic or vasopressor support
- Frequent arterial blood sampling
- Cardiac output monitoring

Contraindications

- Ischaemic limb where arterial catheter is being placed
- Infection/wound at insertion site
- Fistula on same side as insertion site

Anatomy

The radial artery tends to be the most common insertion site for arterial catheters. The radial artery (Figure 27.4) is superficial and lies between the tendons of the brachioradialis and flexor carpi radialis. The tissues that are supplied with blood by the radial artery are also supplied by the ulnar artery which reduces the risk of ischaemic damage. Arterial catheters can also be placed in the brachial, dorsalis pedal and femoral arteries.

Step-by-step guide

1 Explain the procedure to the patient and gain consent if appropriate.
2 Identify the insertion site by palpating the pulse or using ultrasound.
3 Ensure that a pressurised transducer system has been set up.
4 Perform modified Allen test (if intending to place catheter in radial artery) (see Figure 27.4).
5 Prepare the equipment required.
6 Position the patient with the wrist dorsiflexed.
7 Complete a team brief or Local Safety Standards for Invasive Procedures (LocSSIPs).
8 Don sterile gloves.
9 Clean the area with antiseptic (2% chlorhexidine in 70% isopropyl alcohol is recommended).
10 Palpate the artery and infiltrate subcutaneous local anaesthetic (0.5–1 mL 1% lidocaine).
11 Whilst palpating the artery, puncture the skin with the needle at a 30–40° angle.
12 Advance the needle until a flashback of blood is seen.
13 Insert the guidewire to an appropriate length.
14 Remove the needle.
15 Place the arterial catheter over the guidewire.
16 Remove the guidewire.
17 Connect the pressurised transducer system and ensure you see an arterial wave form on the monitor (Figure 27.5).
18 Suture/secure the arterial catheter as per local policy.
19 Dress the catheter and insertion site with an appropriate dressing.

28 Pleural procedures

Table 28.1 Pleural pathologies & suggested first line management to support pleural procedures

Condition	Essential investigations	Potential interventions	Referral considerations
Tension pneumothorax	Peri/cardiac arrest use physical examination +/− CXR	In an emergency use needle decompression followed by chest drain	ED Resus & hospital-based care
Pneumothorax (primary or secondary)	CXR, +/− HRCT, FBC, Coag screen, UE	Conservative longitudinal observation	Respiratory for consideration of possible underlying congenital factors or ambulatory management of chest drain
		If symptomatic consider aspiration +/− chest drain	May require referral for surgical intervention
Pyothorax/empyema	CXR, +/− HRCT, PocTUS, Pleural fluid: MC&S, pleural fluid PH, Septic screen BBV screen FBC, Coag, UE	Inpatient chest drain +/− intrapleural lytic agents, IVAB therapy	Respiratory for hospital based care
			If severe refer to thoracic surgeons for urgent decortication
		Consider treatment alongside lifestyle factors i.e. risk of self-discharge with chest drain device	
Haemothorax (may be related to trauma or malignancy)	PocTUS, CXR, +/− HRCT, Blood tests: FBC, UEs, Coag, Group & Save. Pleural fluid cell count & MC&S, pleural fluid cytology	Consider chest drain	Surgical care with onward referral to thoracic surgeons if active bleeding
		Review active antiplatelet or anticoagulation therapy	
		If associated with rib fracture, provide analgesia	
		Monitor for sepsis	
Chylothorax mostly related to neoplasm or injury	CXR, +/− HRCT, PocTUS pleural fluid cholesterol	Pleural aspiration	Consider referral to thoracic surgeons for VATs if suspected related to trauma/injury
		Modification of underlying pathophysiology e.g diet	
Bilateral pleural effusion	Treat underlying cause e.g. cardiac failure". "Consider blood tests to investigate immunological causes	Attempt to treat systemic cause first	Refer for specialist management of underlying condition, e.g. renal or rheumatology
		Palliation with indwelling pleural catheter may be possible in terminal stages	
Unilateral pleural effusion important to exclude malignancy	PocTUS +/− CT Thorax Abdomen/Pelvis + contrast FBC, UEs, LFT, Coag, CRP	Pleural aspiration especially when malignancy is suspected	Referral to respiratory team for investigation
Multiple causation including infection (parapneumonic)	Pleural fluid cytology MC&S, TB, Glu, Protein, LDH		
		If the cause is likely to be reversible, e.g. infective or related to medications, consider holding to await therapeutic effects of treatment	Consider referral for medical thoracoscopy or VATs in cases of probable primary malignancy of the pleura
		In known cases of malignancy more definitive palliation may be undertaken with chest drain +/− pleurodesis or an indwelling pleural catheter	

Advanced Clinical Practice at a Glance, First Edition. Edited by Barry Hill and Sadie Diamond Fox.
© 2023 John Wiley & Sons Ltd. Published 2023 by John Wiley & Sons Ltd.

Figure 28.1 The pleural space and movement of pleural fluid under normal circumstances. Source: Adapted from Ferreiro L, Toubes ME, San José M et al. (2020) Advances in pleural effusion diagnostics. *Expert Review of Respiratory Medicine*, **14**(1), 51–66, with permission from Taylor & Francis.

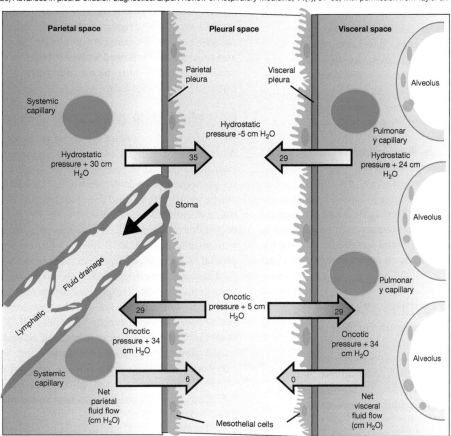

Figure 28.2 Triangle of safety for chest drain insertion.
Source: Reproduced with kind permission from Oxford Medical Education.

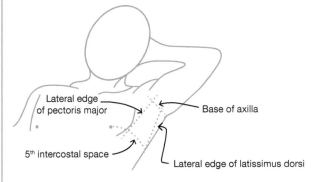

Table 28.2 Light's criteria. Source: Based on Light RW, Erozan YS, Ball WC Jr (1973) Cells in pleural fluid. Their value in differential diagnosis. *Archives of Internal Medicine*, 132(6), 854–860.

	Transudate	Exudate
Pleural:serum protein	<0.5	≥0.5
Pleural:serum LDH	<0.6	≥0.6
Pleural fluid LDH	<2/3 upper limit of normal	>2/3 upper limit of normal
Main causes		• Malignancy
		• Bacterial/viral pneumonia
	• Heart failure	• Tuberculosis
	• Cirrhosis	• Pulmonary embolism
	• Nephrotic syndrome	• Pancreatitis
	• Pulmonary embolism	• Esophageal rupture
		• Collagen vascular disease
		• Chylothorax/mothorax

Table 28.3 Diagnostic accuracy of Light's criteria for diagnosing transudative vs exudative pleural effusion. Source: Based on Light RW, MacGregor MI, Luchsinger PC et al. (1972) Pleural effusions: the diagnostic separation of transudates and exudates. *Annals of Internal Medicine*, 77, 507–513.

	Sensitivity (%)	Specificity (%)
Light's criteria (1 or more of the following)	98	83
Pleural fluid protein/serum protein >0.5	86	84
Pleural fluid LDH/serum LDH >0.6	90	82
Pleural fluid LDH >2/3 serum LDH upper limit of normal	82	89

Clinical skills in pleural procedures are relevant in the diagnosis and treatment of patients with intrapleural collections. These collections are categorised according to their composition (e.g. air–pneumothorax and blood–haemothorax) and are attributable to various conditions related to, but not exclusively: idiopathic, malignancy, infection, trauma or a pulmonary manifestation of a concurrent disease process (e.g. rheumatoid). Conditions such as primary spontaneous pneumothorax or haemothorax related to trauma may be managed initially by emergency services. However, guidelines recommend onward referral of most pleural conditions to respiratory review[1,2] (Table 28.1).

Supported by point-of-care thoracic ultrasound (PocTUS) skills, practitioners in relevant specialties can, with training and following a period of supervised practice, become skilled in undertaking various pleural procedures to autonomously manage the patient from presentation to diagnosis and treatment.[3] The three most common procedures required of practitioners to be discussed here are diagnostic pleural aspiration, therapeutic pleural aspiration and the placement of an intercostal chest drain (ICD).

Understanding the pleural space

Within the pleural space (Figure 28.1), there is normally approximately 0.25 mL/kg of pleural fluid. This allows opposing surfaces of the lung to 'glide' across each other during breathing and holds the lungs to the chest wall during inspiration. The pressure within this space is normally negative. Homeostasis is maintained by equal production of pleural fluid from the capillary bed in the parietal interstitium with equal drainage from the lymphatic system. When large volumes of fluid or air collect in the space, this creates positive pressure, often resulting in lung collapse and decreased lung volume. Ultimately, this may result in breathlessness and dyspnoea with symptoms associated with the weight of fluid affecting diaphragmatic movement. In previously healthy patients, large collections of air and fluid can be accommodated with little change to physiological observations. Massive air leak can, however, rapidly result in tension in the space and circulatory collapse with resulting cardiac arrest requiring emergency intervention.

Diagnostic pleural aspiration

A large-volume syringe (50–60 mL) and green needle can be used to actively aspirate pleural fluid for diagnostic purposes in small-volume collections. This procedure may limit the volume of fluid for cytology.

Therapeutic pleural aspiration

A specific thoracocentesis kit may be used to syphon up to 1.5 L[4] of pleural fluid or air from the pleural space to relieve symptoms in large-volume collections. Pleural fluid obtained during therapeutic aspiration can also be sent for investigation.

Intercostal chest drain (surgical and Seldinger)

This refers to a tube inserted and sutured in the pleural space as a temporary or semi-permanent drain using either blunt dissection for large surgical/Argyle type chest drains or Seldinger techniques for smaller gauge drains (12–18 FG), including semi-permanent indwelling pleural catheters (IPC) used in palliation. The tube will either have a one-way valve (IPC) or be connected to an underwater seal drainage bottle or flutter device to create a one-way valve. The type and gauge of drain are related to the mechanism of injury and viscosity of fluid.

Local Standards for Safe Invasive Procedures (LocSSIPs)

Pleural procedures incur risks for patients and as such, except in extreme emergency, require written consent and must adhere to LocSSIPS. LocSSIPs take care to ensure the correct patient, site and processes are followed with care taken to avoid anticoagulation medications and blood dyscrasia associated with an increased risk of bleeding.

Complications of pleural procedures

PocTUS is used to ensure the safest position for pleural procedures, to avoid iatrogenic injury. It is mandatory for pleural effusion and can assist in pneumothorax. It must be done as part of the procedure and remote marking is not advised. Operator consideration regarding fluid depth and skin to fluid depth is essential in deciding where to place the device. PocTUS in the hands of a skilled operator is used to demonstrate other findings to help with diagnosis, such as B lines, indicating interstitial fluid, or pleural nodularity and thickening related to malignancy.

The safe triangle (Figure 28.2) should be used where possible for chest drain insertion. The point of device insertion is just above the inferior rib of the intercostal space to best avoid the neurovascular bundle normally found directly behind each rib. This reduces any risk of serious injury to vascular structures and subsequent bleeding.

All pleural procedures are undertaken with strict aseptic non-touch technique with the use of good skin preparation, sterile US gel, sterile gown, gloves and equipment to reduce infection. Introduction of infection in the pleural space is difficult to treat and can be fatal.

Effect of pleural procedures

Pleural aspiration or chest drains act as a valve to allow excess fluid/air to syphon and pressures to potentially normalise, allowing the lung to reinflate. During active/rapid drainage, the operator should stay with the patient to monitor for adverse signs and symptoms related to lung re-expansion (e.g. pulmonary oedema, cough) and loss of hydrostatic pressure (e.g. vasovagal collapse). If the lung is unable to reinflate due to chronic pleural thickening or malignancy, severe chest pain may be experienced as other structures are pulled to equalise intrathoracic pressure. Postprocedure CXR in this case may demonstrate a 'unexpandable/trapped lung' with hydropneumothorax.

In very frail patients, towards end of life, pleural aspiration can directly result in death and careful consideration of any temporising palliative effect of aspiration should be carefully weighed against this and other anticipatory medications. Young patients with a healthy pleura may experience significant pleurisy once the lung has reinflated following ICD insertion so an effective analgesia regime is essential.

It is important to hand over the care plan of chest drainage to the nursing team and ensure that the patient is adequately observed with recording of physiological observations.[5] Saline flushes should be prescribed and administered to ensure chest tube patency in smaller guage drains (12Fg-18Fg) via a three way tap. Any adverse events related to chest drain insertion or care should be recorded with oversight across the organisation.

Investigations

Sampling of pleural fluid and subsequent laboratory analysis may aid diagnosis. Diagnostic algorithms may be used to determine the aetiology of the effusion and subsequent treatment (Tables 28.2 and 28.3). It is important to consider that Malignancy related to unilateral pleural effusion is common, with an estimated 50 000 new cases each year[6] and should be investigated by a specialist respiratory team.

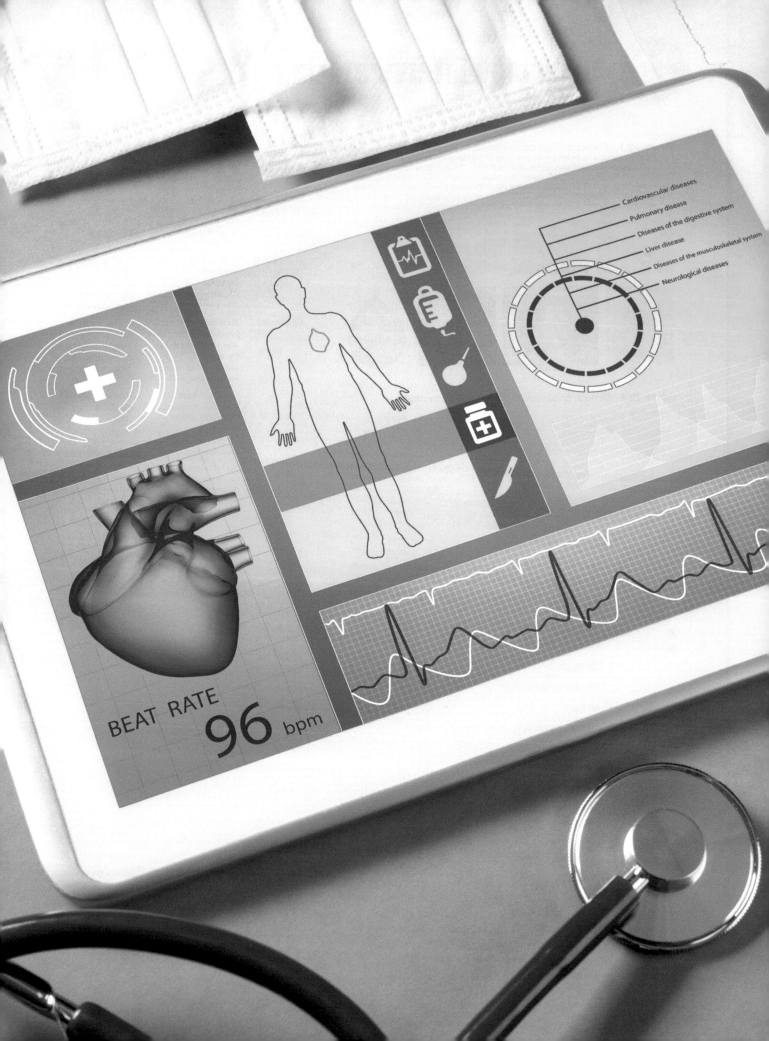

29 Radiology interpretation

Figure 29.1 Radiation dose comparisons. Source: Society of Radiographers (2019) Communicating Radiation Benefit and Risk Information to Individuals Under the Ionising Radiation (Medical Exposure) Regulations (IRMER). Source: Steve Hopson / Wikimedia commons / CC BY- SA 2.5; Quintin Soloviev / Wikimedia commons / CC BY- SA 4.0; Quadell / Wikimedia commons / CC BY- SA 3.0; Augustus Binu / Wikimedia commons / CC BY- SA 3.0; Mikael Häggström / Wikimedia commons / CC0 1.0 Universal; Glitzy queen00 / Wikimedia commons / Public domain; Mikael Häggström / Wikimedia commons / CC0 1.0 Universal

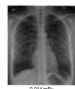
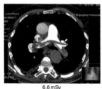
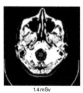

0.014 mSv   6.6 mSv   1.4 mSv

Figure 29.2 General principles of plain X-ray interpretation

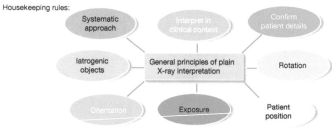

Table 29.1 Comparison of imaging modalities

Imaging modality	Pros	Cons
Plain radiography	Inexpensive Accessible/portable Quick Good first-line imaging option	Radiation exposure 2D images – layers of anatomy difficult to interpret
Fluoroscopy	Inexpensive Accessible Dynamic Allows simultaneous intervention	High radiation exposure Dependent on patient mobility and compliance
Ultrasound	Relatively inexpensive No radiation exposure Accessible/portable Dynamic Allows simultaneous intervention	Image quality is operator dependent Image interpretation more difficult
CT	Good contrast between structures High anatomical definition 3D images Fast scans possible	High radiation exposure Cost
MRI	No radiation exposure Good soft tissue differentiation Multiplanar Can be functional	Cost Long scan time Patient compliance required Complex interpretation Implant patients contraindicated

Table 29.2 Radiation doses by modality

Examination	Typical dose (mSV)	Equivalent period of natural background radiation for context
XR limbs or joints	<0.01	<1.5 days
XR teeth	<0.01	<1.5 days
XR PA chest	0.014	3 days
XR cervical spine	0.08	2 weeks
XR hip	0.3	7 weeks
XR thoracic spine, abdomen, pelvis	0.7	4 months
XR lumbar spine	1.3	7 months
CT head scan	1.4	1 year
CT thorax	6.6	3.6 years
CT abdomen or pelvis	10	4.5 years

Plain radiographs

Plain X-rays provide information about bone, joint and soft tissue structures. They have a number of advantages over cross-sectional imaging techniques such as computed tomography (CT), magnetic resonance imaging (MRI) and ultrasound (US), but they also present certain limitations. These are summarised in Table 29.1 to aid decision making. Despite their limitations, plain films are valuable in providing a preliminary overview of anatomy and pathophysiology, guiding further, more focused imaging and informing ongoing medical management.

Advanced Clinical Practice at a Glance, First Edition. Edited by Barry Hill and Sadie Diamond Fox.
© 2023 John Wiley & Sons Ltd. Published 2023 by John Wiley & Sons Ltd.

Radiology referrals

- Observe IRMER regulations (see below).
- Fill in request form accurately; it is a legal document!
- Include correct patient ID, mode of transport to radiology department, IV or oxygen attachments, patient mobility.
- Highlight risks, allergies and implants. Include renal function if referring for contrast studies.
- Correct referrer details including bleep/extension number.
- Accurate and relevant past medical history and presenting condition to justify the request and radiation exposure (see Table 29.2 and Figure 29.1 for radiation dosage examples), ensure efficient use of resources and enable the development of an informed report.
- Consider the clinical question you are asking. Imaging should confirm or exclude your question, not provide the answer.
- If unsure as to the most appropriate imaging modality, ask the radiographers/consultant radiologist for advice. Know your patient and be prepared to present the case succinctly.
- Use your institution's i-Refer resource link to the Royal College of Radiologists referral guidelines.

Further reading: www.rcr.ac.uk/clinical-radiology/being-consultant/rcr-referral-guidelines/about-irefer

IRMER

The Ionising Radiation Medical Exposure Regulations (2000) govern the safe and effective use of ionising radiation, ensuring patient exposure is both rationalised and minimised, that the benefits outweigh the risks and the lowest dose possible is used. They outline the responsibilities of the duty holders who include employer, referrer, clinician and operator, all of whom must complete certified IRMER training. As non-medical referrers, advanced practitioners must ensure that they comply with national and local competencies and remain up to date on the advanced practice register held by the employer. Further reading: www.cqc.org.uk/guidance-providers/ionising-radiation/ionising-radiation-medical-exposure-regulations-irmer

Plain X-ray

The three main types of plain imaging are chest, abdominal and musculoskeletal radiographs. By adopting a systemic approach when interpreting these images, the practitioner ensures a comprehensive evaluation which may identify or rule out certain pathologies, inform the medical management or justify the need for further investigations including cross-sectional or continuous imaging such as fluoroscopy.

CXR interpretation: RIPE ABCDEFGH

A structured approach to chest X-ray interpretation is essential. Figure 29.2 summarises the fundamental considerations underpinning the interpretation of any radiograph. Taking these principles into account at the beginning of the radiographic appraisal minimises misinterpretation due to technical aspects and enables more balanced, contextual interpretation. The following may be useful.

- **R**otation – the medial aspect of each clavicle should be equidistant from the spinous processes. Spinous processes should also be vertically orientated against the vertebral bodies.
- **I**nspiration – the 5–6 anterior ribs, lung apices, both costophrenic angles and the lateral rib edges should be visible.
- **P**rojection – note if the film is anteroposterior (AP) or posteroanterior (PA).
- **E**xposure – the left hemidiaphragm should be visible to the spine and the vertebrae should be visible behind the heart.
- **A**irway – (trachea, bronchi, carina) deviation, obstruction, ETT, tracheostomy.
- **B**ones – alignment, bony contours, fracture, lesions.
- **C**ardiac + aorta – heart size/borders, aortic contours, deviation, valves, pacemaker.
- **D**iaphragm – position, costophrenic/cardiophrenic angles, adjacent organs, density above/below.
- **E**ffusions/pleura – pneumothorax, haemothorax, empyema, thickening, lesions.
- **F**ields (lung) – lung markings, symmetry, density, masses, anatomical borders, deviation silhouette sign.
- **G**astric bubble – present or not.
- **H**ilar + mediastinum – mediastinal contours, symmetry, density, size, position, lymphadenopathy.

Don't forget to also review soft tissues for abnormalities; identify lines, nasogastric tubes, etc.

Musculoskeletal (MSK) X-ray interpretation

Plain radiographs can reveal a wide range of bony, cartilaginous and joint pathology, but soft tissue or synovial abnormalities may not be visualised and CT may be required.

Radiographs produce a two-dimensional image which may not show certain pathologies in a different plane – consider imaging multiple views.

The following mnemonic may be used.

- **A**lignment – joint space, dislocation/subluxation
- **B**ones – cortex, contours, texture (trabecular pattern), fracture, bony fragments, arthropathy
- **C**artilage – joint space narrowing, contours, osteophytes, calcification
- **S**oft tissue – disruption, effusion, swelling, foreign bodies, calcification

Abdominal X-ray (AXR) interpretation

AXR is only useful for abnormal gases, masses, bones and stones. It involves a relatively high dose of radiation, so the practitioner should consider the value of AXR versus abdominal US or CT scan. AXR may be useful as part of an acute abdominal series (AP supine, PA erect, chest radiograph to evaluate free gas).

When interpreting an AXR, consideration should be given to the following.

- *Bowel:* diameter (small bowel <3 cm, large bowel <6 cm, caecum <9 cm = '3/6/9 rule'), mass, obstruction, gas patterns, free air.
- *Organs/soft tissue:* lung bases, liver, gallbladder, stomach, psoas muscles, kidneys, spleen, bladder – contours, size, intraparenchymal air, calcifications, masses.
- *Bones:* lower ribs, lumbar vertebrae, sacrum, coccyx, pelvis, proximal femurs – fracture, deformity, focal lesions, degenerative changes, joint disease.

Cross-sectional imaging

Cross-sectional imaging includes advanced imaging techniques that have the ability to image the body in cross-section.

- *Computed tomography (CT):* the high contrast and excellent spatial resolution enable differentiation of soft tissue structures which are similar in attenuation, and the ability to detect subtle changes in these.
- *Magnetic resonance imaging (MRI):* extremely high resolution and high contrast allow images to be reconstructed in multiple planes, and the detection of subtle or early pathological change.
- *Ultrasonography (US):* although unable to reveal the anatomical detail of the above techniques, US allows for evaluation of moving structures in real time, is easily utilised at point of care, involves no radiation exposure and can be used to guide invasive procedures or allow Doppler examination of vessels.

Fluoroscopy

Offers the same high-resolution, real-time images as USS, but the soft tissue contrast is less than that achieved with US, making it difficult to differentiate between structures or identify effusions. Also, it is not portable and relies on ionising radiation.

30 The advanced practitioner's role in organ donation and transplantation

Figure 30.1 (a) DBD donor optimisation care bundle 1. (b) DBD donor optimisation care bundle 2

NHS Blood and Transplant — Donation after Diagnosis of Death using Neurological Criteria (NC)
Donor Optimisation Care Bundle

Name.................... DOB.................... MRN....................

Patient Name .... DOB .... MRN .... Weight .... Height ....

IMMEDIATELY AFTER DIAGNOSIS OF DEATH

- Perform lung recruitment manoeuvre.
- Set tidal volume to 4-8mls/kg (ideal body weight).
- Set optimum PEEP (5 to 10cm H2O).
- Add vasopressin (0.48 to 4U/hr), where vasopressors are required. Wean noradrenaline.

Time of death.................... Signed.................... Name.................... GMC....................

WITHIN 1 HOUR OF CONSENT/AUTHORISATION

- Administer methylprednisolone (15mg/kg, maximum 1G).
- Request an ECG.
- Request an echocardiogram.
- Request a CXR – post recruitment manoeuvre.

Time completed.................... Signed.................... Name.................... GMC....................

WITHIN 4 HOURS OF CONSENT/AUTHORISATION

- ECG report complete.
- Echocardiogram report complete.
- CXR report complete.
- Site cardiac output monitoring, if able.

Time completed.................... Signed.................... Name.................... GMC....................

DRUGS

- Vasopressin 20 units in 50mls 5% dextrose; rate 1.2 to 10mls/hour.
- DDAVP 1 TO 4mcg IV.
- Methylprednisolone 15mg/kg (max 1G).

CONTINUOUSLY

- Ensure ongoing lung protective strategy.
- Nurse 30-45 degrees head up.
- Continue physiotherapy including suctioning.

- Review intravascular fluid status and correct hypovolaemia.
- Wean noradrenaline as able.
- Treat DI with DDAVP.

- Continue NG feed, as directed by SNOD.
- Monitor blood glucose and treat as per unit protocol.
- Monitor serum sodium concentration.

- Continue use of mechanical thromboprophylaxis.
- Ensure prophylactic low molecular weight heparin use.

- Continue hourly observations.
- Maintain normothermia.
- Stop all unnecessary medications.
- If not already present, insert a central line (right sided IJ or SC is preferable).

- Other tests or therapies may be indicated. SNOD to direct.

GOALS

PaO2 ≥ 10 kPa	U.O. 0.5 – 2 mls/kg/hr
PaCO2 5 – 6.5 kPa	Na < 150 mmol/L
pH >7.25	Glucose 4 – 10 mmol/L
MAP 60-80 mmHg	Temp 36 – 37.5 °C

NHS Blood and Transplant — Donation after Diagnosis of Death using Neurological Criteria (NC)
Donor Optimisation Care Bundle

Name.................... DOB.................... MRN....................

Patient Name .... DOB .... MRN .... Weight .... Height ....

	Start	+1hr	+2hr	+4hr	+6hr	+8hr	+10hr	+12hr	+14hr	+16hr	+18hr
PaO2 ≥ 10 kPa (FiO2 < 0.4 as able)											
PaCO2 5 – 6.5 kPa (or higher as long as pH >7.25)											
MAP 60 – 80 mmHg											
Cardiac index > 2.1 l/min/m² (if applicable)											
Urine output 0.5 – 2 mls/kg/hr											
Temperature 36 – 37.5 °C											
Blood glucose 4 – 10 mmol/L											
Signature											
Surname											
Date											
Time											

PLEASE RECORD ACTUAL VALUES

Table 30.1 Additional resources concerning organ donation and transplantation

Donor identification and referral	www.odt.nhs.uk/deceased-donation/best-practice-guidance/donor-identification-and-referral/
Consent and authorisation	www.odt.nhs.uk/deceased-donation/best-practice-guidance/consent-and-authorisation/
Donation after brainstem death	www.odt.nhs.uk/deceased-donation/best-practice-guidance/donation-after-brainstem-death/
Diagnosing death using neurological criteria	www.odt.nhs.uk/deceased-donation/best-practice-guidance/donation-after-brainstem-death/diagnosing-death-using-neurological-criteria/
Donation after circulatory death	www.odt.nhs.uk/deceased-donation/best-practice-guidance/donation-after-circulatory-death/
Donor optimisation	www.odt.nhs.uk/deceased-donation/best-practice-guidance/donor-optimisation/
Clinical calculations relating to organ transplantation	www.odt.nhs.uk/transplantation/tools-policies-and-guidance/calculators/
Policies and guidance relating to organ transplantation	www.odt.nhs.uk/transplantation/tools-policies-and-guidance/policies-and-guidance/

Advanced Clinical Practice at a Glance, First Edition. Edited by Barry Hill and Sadie Diamond Fox.
© 2023 John Wiley & Sons Ltd. Published 2023 by John Wiley & Sons Ltd.

Advanced practitioners (APs) play an important role in supporting organ and tissue donation. Each potential donor is precious, saving and improving lives through transplantation.

Types of donation

In the UK, once a decision has been made to withdraw life-sustaining treatment (a decision separate from any organ donation decision), donation can occur in two ways: following death by neurological criteria (DBD) or following planned withdrawal of life-sustaining treatment and circulatory death. Commonly, in both cases, patients are receiving invasive ventilation and possibly other supportive treatments, such as vasopressor therapy, so that once withdrawn, asystole is expected imminently.

In donation after circulatory death (DCD), the potential donor will be palliated within, or close to, the retrieval operating theatre, and subsequently diagnosed dead using typical cardiorespiratory criteria following a period of 5 minutes witnessed cardiorespiratory arrest.[1] The Maastricht classification of Donation after Circulatory Death states that APs may diagnose these deaths in accordance with local policies and procedures following suitable approved training.[2]

The clinical observations of the patient and the timing of asystole influence the outcome of a DCD donation, death usually occurring within 3 hours of extubation.

Diagnosing death by neurological criteria ('brainstem death testing')

Defined as the irreversible loss of capacity for consciousness, combined with irreversible loss of the capacity to breathe and therefore irreversible cessation of the integrative function of the brainstem.[3] Strict 'red flag' preconditions are required to make this diagnosis using the Faculty of Intensive Care Medicine (FICM) approved national form.[4] Preconditions include identifying a cause for the patient's coma, excluding reversible and non-neurological causes and ensuring the patient's physiological stability during testing. Brainstem function is tested by assessment of associated cranial nerves (see Figure 31.1, page 84). The tests are performed twice, by two senior General Medical Council (GMC) registered doctors; one must be a consultant and neither of them can be part of the transplant team. The completion time for the first set of tests denotes the time of death to be registered.

The AP can be expected to support stabilisation and optimisation in preparation for testing and have an awareness that the preconditions are met. Following testing, lung re-recruitment and restoration of physiological optimisation are essential until the patient's end-of-life decisions have been clarified and agreed with their family.

Role of the specialist nurse for organ donation (SN-OD)

The SN-OD is a specialist nurse whose role is to verify suitability to donate, discuss decisions around donation, co-ordinate the teams involved and organise the donation process. They provide expertise in bereavement support for the donor family during and after donation. The discussion and decision to withdraw life-sustaining treatment must be consultant led but the donation discussion is typically led by the SN-OD.

Although some potential donors may be referred in the emergency department, most donations occur in the critical care unit. Early notification to, and working collaboratively with, the SN-OD ensures sensitive, safe, effective and efficient preparation and optimisation of any potential donor and their family. It is considered best practice in the UK that the SN-OD is notified of any plan to test for neurological death or when planning treatment withdrawal, attending to support the clinical team and patient's family.[5] APs can assist in the SN-OD's predonation assessment by ordering investigations and gathering medical information about the potential organ donor.

Optimisation of the potential organ donor

In both DBD and DCD, once a decision to donate has been established, in the period prior to the donation operation in collaboration with the SN-OD, the AP should help with physiological optimisation in an effort to improve the success outcome of any organs transplanted. In DBD, NHS Blood and Transplant Services advocates use of its 'optimisation care bundle'.

Optimisation focuses on improving the perfusion of organs intended for donation and limiting periods of instability. Maintenance of adequate perfusion and oxygenation whilst avoiding excessive doses of vasoconstricting medicines is essential. Electrolyte and fluid balance must be monitored and corrected, along with maintenance of thromboembolic prophylaxis to prevent microvascular emboli. Hormone replacement should be administered to patients following a neurological death, replacing those no longer secreted from the pituitary axis (typically methylprednisolone, desmopressin and vasopressin). Successful optimisation can support up to nine transplants and the management of the potential donor should remain a clinical focus of the AP (Figure 30.1).

UK law and ethics

The rights of the unconscious patient are protected by the Mental Capacity Act.[6] The MCA uses the term 'best interests' when determining what should happen to the patient who lacks capacity to make decisions. Where end-of-life decisions are being taken, in law, organ donation is now, or is about to be, supported in each UK jurisdiction under a 'deemed' consent arrangement. Each jurisdiction has slightly different qualifying conditions, but in essence, an adult patient's written or verbal decision to donate or not is regarded as a lawful decision. Where no decision is registered, with qualified exceptions, adult patients are assumed to support organ donation. Family discussions are then constructed to verify, respect and support that decision. The SN-OD provides expertise in the lawful execution of these complex conversations and will do so by planning collaboratively with the consultant and bedside nurse as per national guidance.[5] If the family raises the subject of organ donation, the AP should notify the SN-OD for further advice, ensuring the family's expectations are met and accurate information is given.

Tissue donation

Where solid organ donation is not suitable, tissue donation may be considered. Corneas and heart valves are consistently in high demand with skin, bone, cartilage and tendons offering transformational life changes. The acceptance criteria are more stringent than for organ donation. However, as retrieval may be undertaken up to 48 hours after death, the assessment process can be performed after the patient has died, following a referral to the National Referral Centre. The AP should be aware of this option and their local notification procedure along with basic knowledge of the process to facilitate positive discussions with families (Table 30.1). The patient does not need to have died in the critical care setting to be a tissue donor.

31 Verification of death

Figure 31.1 Criteria for the diagnosis of death.
Source: Gardiner D, Shemie S, Manara A, Opdam H (2012) International perspective on the diagnosis of death. *British Journal of Anaesthesia*, **108**(suppl 1), i14–28, with permission of Elsevier

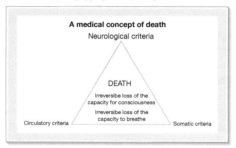

A medical concept of death
Neurological criteria

DEATH
Irreversible loss of the capacity for consciousness
Irreversible loss of the capacity to breathe

Circulatory criteria   Somatic criteria

Table 31.1 Recognition of life extinct

Signs unequivocally associated with death
Rigor mortis
Hemicorporectomy
Decapitation
Massive cranial or truncal injury
Incineration of more than 95% of the body surface
Hypostasis
Decompostition

Table 31.2 Documented criteria for the diagnosis of death following cardiorespiratory arrest

Criteria	
Preconditions	Identification of the patient Irreversible and simultaneous apnoea, loss of circulation and unconsciousness No indication to commence or continue CPR
Diagnosis	Minimum observation period of five minutes Absence of central pulse on palpation and heart sounds on auscultation Absence of respiratory effort Following minimum observation period: • absence of papillary reaction to light • absence of corneal reflex • absence of motor response to supraorbital pressure
Documentation	Date and time at which the criteria are fulfilled Additional information including persons present (family, friends, nursing staff) Concerns regarding death Name, signature, grade and registering body membership number, contact telephone number

Figure 31.2 Tests for the absence of brainstem function

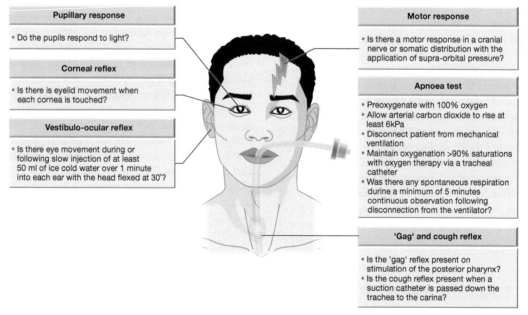

Pupillary response
• Do the pupils respond to light?

Corneal reflex
• Is there is eyelid movement when each cornea is touched?

Vestibulo-ocular reflex
• Is there eye movement during or following slow injection of at least 50 ml of ice cold water over 1 minute into each ear with the head flexed at 30°?

Motor response
• Is there a motor response in a cranial nerve or somatic distribution with the application of supra-orbital pressure?

Apnoea test
• Preoxygenate with 100% oxygen
• Allow arterial carbon dioxide to rise at least 6kPa
• Disconnect patient from mechanical ventilation
• Maintain oxygenation >90% saturations with oxygen therapy via a tracheal catheter
• Was there any spontaneous respiration durine a minimum of 5 minutes continuous observation following disconnection from the ventilator?

'Gag' and cough reflex
• Is the 'gag' reflex present on stimulation of the posterior pharynx?
• Is the cough reflex present when a suction catheter is passed down the trachea to the carina?

Ancillary investigations
• Useful where neurological examinations not possible, primary metabolic or pharmacological derangement cannot be ruled out, high cervical cord injury, uncertainty in spontaneous or reflex movements
• Clinical - Absent doll's eye response (not in cervical spine injury)
      - Atropine 3 mg does not increase heart rate (more than 3%)
• Neurophysiological - EEG
               - Evoked potentials
• Radiological - CT angiography
         - Transcranial doppler

Diagnosis of death

In the United Kingdom in 2019, over 600 000 deaths were registered, with a significant increase of 14.5% in England and Wales in 2020, partially due to the coronavirus pandemic.[1] Death results in the irreversible loss of characteristics which are essential and necessary to a living human person's existence, defined as the irreversible loss of the capacity for consciousness, in conjunction with the irreversible loss of the capacity to breathe.[2]

Recent guidance[3] regarding care after death advocates that death is dealt with:

- according to the law and coroner requirements with specific criteria for coroner investigation and notifiable infectious diseases, ensuring the health and safety of others[4,5]
- in a timely and sensitive approach
- by respecting the privacy, dignity, spiritual, religious and cultural needs and wishes of the patient and their key contacts or family members, where practicable and within legal obligations.

Legal aspects

Certification of death requires completion of the Medical Certificate of the Cause of Death (MCCD), in accordance with The Births and Deaths Registration Act 1953,[6] by a registered and General Medical Council (GMC) licensed medical practitioner.

Diagnosis of death is the process of confirming that death has occurred. Terminology is varied, including confirmation of death by registered medical practitioners, recognition of life extinct by ambulance clinicians, and verification of death by registered nurses.[2,3,7]

There is clear societal and professional demand for a timely and reliable means of diagnosing and certifying death. Diagnosis should occur within 1 hour or 4 hours of death, in the hospital or community respectively.[8,9] Any competent registered medical practitioner or healthcare professional (HCP) may diagnose death within the scope of their practice.[2,10,11] However, the coronavirus pandemic has led to the development of remote verification of expected death out of hospital guidance, wherein care workers, family or friends may complete this process, if appropriate, with the general practitioner via video consultation.[12]

Diagnosis of death guidance and practice

In the UK, there was a dearth of guidance and standard criteria regarding the diagnosis of death, prior to the publication of the Code of Practice.[2] Traditional teaching and advice produced by professional organisations were variable, leading to conflicting practice and uncertainty concerning the correct approach.

The unifying medical concept of death encompasses three sets of criteria, the most appropriate of which is used, depending upon the circumstances in which the diagnosis of death is required. They include somatic criteria, circulatory criteria and neurological criteria (Figure 31.1).

Somatic criteria tend to be applied within the community setting where death may have occurred hours or days prior, with signs present that negate the need for clinical examination (Table 31.1).

Diagnosis of death using circulatory criteria confirms irreversible and simultaneous apnoea, loss of circulation and unconsciousness, as a result of cardiorespiratory arrest. Essential criteria to be met prior to diagnosis of death include full and extensive reversal of contributing causes, and one of the following:

- criteria for not attempting cardiopulmonary resuscitation (CPR) have been met
- recognition of failed CPR
- withdrawal of life-sustaining treatment, as this is of no further benefit to the patient, not in their best interests to continue or is the patient's wishes, as indicated via an advanced directive to refuse treatment.

The minimum period of observation for diagnosing death varies from 2 to 20 minutes, with a standard of 5 minutes in the UK. Irreversible cardiorespiratory arrest is confirmed by apnoea, the absence of central pulse on palpation and heart sounds on auscultation, and is sufficient for diagnosis in primary care. Electrocardiography, intra-arterial pressure monitoring or echocardiography may corroborate this within the hospital setting. Spontaneous return of respiratory or cardiac function requires a subsequent 5-minute observation period from the point of cardiorespiratory arrest. The absence of pupillary reaction to light, corneal reflex and supraorbital pressure motor response is consequently confirmed. The time at which diagnosis occurs, through fulfilment of these criteria, is the documented time of death (Table 31.2).

Organ donation is inextricably linked to the diagnosis of death. Donation after circulatory death (DCD) is the retrieval of organs for transplantation, following the diagnosis of death, according to circulatory criteria. In this context, diagnosis is time-critical, minimising warm ischaemia time and increasing the likelihood of successful transplantation. It should be managed sensitively, with respect, maintaining public confidence. DCD occurs within the critical care setting and following changes in the law, leading to the 'opt-out system' in the UK, increasing donor numbers are projected over the next 10 years. Advanced critical care practitioners may be trained to provide this vital service, with support from clinical leads for organ donation and intensive care clinical leads, under local governance, in order to facilitate all DCD opportunities.[13]

National professional guidance supports the diagnosis of death by neurological criteria for patients with evidence of irreversible brain damage, of known aetiology, wherein mechanical ventilation maintains cardiorespiratory activity, regardless of organ donation.[14] This should take place within the critical care environment and must be conducted by two qualified doctors, competent in brainstem testing and interpretation, one being a consultant and both registered with the GMC for more than 5 years, with testing performed on two occasions.[2] Essential components include fulfilment of precondition criteria, exclusion of reversible conditions criteria, in addition to the demonstration of apnoea, loss of consciousness and brainstem activity (Figure 31.2). There are both short and long forms for the diagnosis of death using neurological criteria, as well as supplementary guidance for patients receiving extracorporeal membrane oxygenation (ECMO).[15–17] National procedures for identifying potential donors for donation after brain death (DBD) should be followed, with notification of the specialist nurse for organ donation[18,19] (SNOD).

Training and Competence

Registered medical practitioners, nurses and HCPs are trained in the diagnosis of death via e-learning modules and simulation courses under local governance structures. Individuals are assessed with various competency assessment tools, including directly observed practical skills. Doctors specialising in critical care medicine are trained and assessed in diagnosis of death using circulatory and neurological criteria as part of the Intensive Care Medicine High Level Learning Outcomes curriculum.[20]

32 Home-based care, crisis response and rehabilitation

Figure 32.1 Home-based care

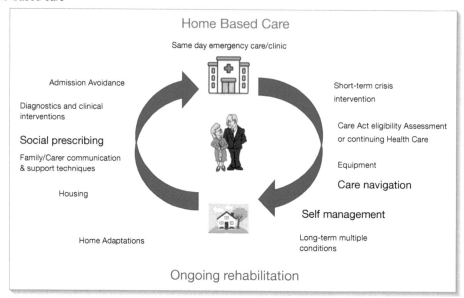

Home Based Care

Same day emergency care/clinic

Admission Avoidance

Diagnostics and clinical interventions

Social prescribing

Family/Carer communication & support techniques

Housing

Home Adaptations

Short-term crisis intervention

Care Act eligibility Assessment or continuing Health Care

Equipment

Care navigation

Self management

Long-term multiple conditions

Ongoing rehabilitation

Figure 32.2 The advanced clinical practitioner's role in managing long-term conditions, as part of the multidisciplinary team

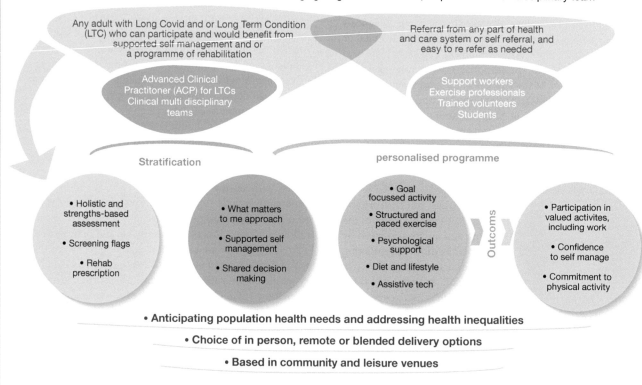

Any adult with Long Covid and or Long Term Condition (LTC) who can participate and would benefit from supported self management and or a programme of rehabilitation

Referral from any part of health and care system or self referral, and easy to re refer as needed

Advanced Clinical Practitoner (ACP) for LTCs Clinical multi disciplinary teams

Support workers
Exercise professionals
Trained volunteers
Students

Stratification

personalised programme

- Holistic and strengths-based assessment
- Screening flags
- Rehab prescription

- What matters to me approach
- Supported self management
- Shared decision making

- Goal focussed activity
- Structured and paced exercise
- Psychological support
- Diet and lifestyle
- Assistive tech

Outcomes

- Participation in valued activites, including work
- Confidence to self manage
- Commitment to physical activity

- **Anticipating population health needs and addressing health inequalities**

- **Choice of in person, remote or blended delivery options**

- **Based in community and leisure venues**

Advanced Clinical Practice at a Glance, First Edition. Edited by Barry Hill and Sadie Diamond Fox.
© 2023 John Wiley & Sons Ltd. Published 2023 by John Wiley & Sons Ltd.

Improving Outcomes

There is growing evidence that care closer to home has better outcomes for patients. Indeed, admission to hospital can cause significant and irreversible harm for some, due to hospital-acquired deconditioning (HAD). Hospital-acquired infections (HAI) increase the risk of delirium and iatrogenic complications and harm. Delivering care at home brings significant advantages, with a reduction in deconditioning, fewer HAIs and the possibility of maintaining social interactions, but also a number of challenges. Access to specialist services and high-tech diagnostics such as X-rays and CT scans may be harder, and there may be complex environmental challenges to delivering care. Care at home is popular with patients as they feel more confident in their own environment, and are able to continue with their usual social, psychological and environmental supports (Figure 32.1).

The COVID-19 pandemic has accelerated the development of home-based care teams with government initiatives to incentivise using them. Services have been developed which offer a crisis response to a significant decompensation or change in function. The crisis response team responds with an advanced level of diagnostic skill and interventions to ensure safe and effective care at home. Some services are lead by consultant geriatricians, others by GP extensivists or consultant practitioners from a variety of clinical backgrounds. Most services are multidisciplinary in nature with a balanced skill set and range of capabilities, from support workers to advanced practitioners.

Skills and knowledge

Advanced practitioners working in these settings need all the skills and knowledge of acute medicine in order to assess, diagnose and deliver appropriate interventions within the prescribed ceilings their team is able to offer. These vary from team to team. Some offer home-based intravenous (IV) antibiotics and infusions while others use ambulatory clinics with closer patient observation for IV infusions, but undertake point-of-care diagnostics and interventions. Current policy is facilitating further development and investment in these hospital-at-home teams.

Identification of a crisis may come from GPs, ambulance services, either on the road or at the call centre, or other community-based colleagues who are concerned over deterioration in both health and social care. This integration of systems is critical for efficiency and to avoid unnecessary duplication of assessments and interventions. Integrated care systems deliver better patient satisfaction and perceived quality of care, but there is no evidence for lower costs.

An advanced practitioner in this setting needs to be flexible in their approach, as they may face a crisis from many precipitators, both intrinsic and extrinsic, such as falls, infections, deterioration or exacerbation in any long-term condition, including mental health crises. They need to follow treatment guidelines for acute interventions and long-term conditions, and have clinical decision-making skills to support adaptations to guidelines for person-centred care.

The use of digital technology is an important part of supporting people to stay well at home. This may include remote monitoring of complex physiological parameters via telehealth, such as pulse oximetry services used during COVID-19, and telecare using specialist alert devices for falls, and mobility to support people who are at high risk of falling or may have a cognitive impairment.

Once the crisis has been averted, there must be an appropriate response to support onward anticipatory care planning, rehabilitation and engagement with social prescribing, to proactively support ageing well in the community. The advanced practitioner needs to have skills in supporting rehabilitation to maintain or regain functional abilities.

Rehabilitation

Rehabilitation is described as 'a process aiming to restore personal autonomy in those aspects of daily living considered most relevant by patients or service users and their family carers'. Rehabilitation aims to assist people who have disabilities to recover, improve or limit further decline in their physical, mental and social skills. Rehabilitation is key to every episode of care. It maximises mental and physical health, independence and occupation.

Rehabilitation is relevant at any stage in the lifecourse, but is often most efficacious after a crisis or functional decline, such as a stroke, fall or significant injury. Rehabilitation forms the backbone for management of those with long-term conditions.

It is increasingly acknowledged that effective rehabilitation delivers better outcomes and improved quality of life and has the potential to reduce health inequalities and make significant cost savings across the health and care system. Rehabilitation for community-dwelling older people reduces nursing home admissions, falls and acute hospital admissions, but there is scant evidence for reduction in deaths.

Prehabilitation prior to invasive or disabling treatments, such as chemotherapy or surgery, maximises fitness and results in better recovery outcomes and a reduction in hospital length of stay.

Rehabilitation is delivered in a variety of settings, including hospital, home, gym or clinic. The advanced practitioner delivering rehabilitation is able to undertake diagnostic assessments and implement appropriate rehabilitation interventions depending on the person-centred goals of the patient. The highly skilled clinician is able to tailor their interventions to the individual needs of the person. The clinician will facilitate the person to self-manage their own care. The advanced practitioner sets management plans to be supported by other staff within the MDT, with oversight of the trajectories and realistic achievement of goals set (Figure 32.2).

Specialist rehabilitation is offered for neurological conditions, cardiac and pulmonary rehabilitation, as well as long COVID. There are specific NICE guidelines for cardiac rehabilitation,[1] stroke rehabilitation[2] and pulmonary conditions,[3] which advanced practitioners use to develop systems and services to meet the needs of their patient cohorts.

Home-based care is a growing area of specialism for advanced practitioners to work in, providing a variety of models, across the spectrum of patient needs, from acute crisis interventions to longer term rehabilitation.

33 Frailty

Figure 33.1 A pictorial demonstration of how frailty can impact upon recovery from a relatively 'minor' insult

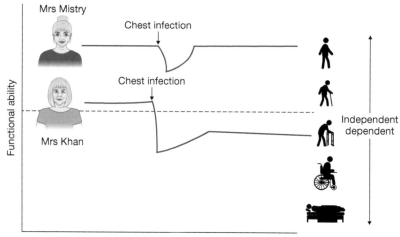

Mrs Mistry

Chest infection

Chest infection

Functional ability

Mrs Khan

Time

Independent
dependent

Mrs Mistry is a fit 85-year-old.
PMH-OA Knees-Right TKR 2 years ago,
HTN, T2DM,
SH-Drives, plays 9 holes of golf twice a
week, self caring.

Mrs Khan is a mildly frail 85-year-old.
PMH- OA Knees, HTN, T2DM, CKD III,
Breast Cancer 10 years ago.
SH-Walks with a stick, 2 falls in 6
months, has microwave meals as too
tired to cook, struggling to stand from
her chair.

Table 33.1 Models of frailty

Phenotype model[1]	Cumulative model[2]
1. Unintentional weight loss of ≥5% of body weight or 10lbs in last year 2. Self-reported exhaustion (some/most of the time) 3. Low physical activity level 4. Slowness (in the slowest 20% to walk 15 feet) 5. Weakness (grip strength in lowest 20%) or sarcopenia Score: 0 = robust 1 or 2 of above = pre-frail 3 or more of above present = frail	1. Deficits accumulate with age. 2. 92 aspects of health were measured 3. The more of these 92 aspects in which an individual has a deficit, the greater the degree of frailty 4. Add up all the deficits, then divide them by the total number of deficits that were considered (e.g. 92) to arrive at a frailty index 5. The higher the frailty index, the more frail someone is

Table 33.2 How to identify frailty: the five frailty syndromes[4]

Falls, e.g. legs gave way, 'found on floor'

Immobility, e.g. sudden deterioration in mobility, unable to get out of the chair/off the toilet – 'off legs'

Delirium, e.g. new onset of confusion or sudden worsening of existing confusion in someone with dementia

Incontinence, e.g. new onset or worsening of urine or faecal incontinence

Susceptible to medication side-effects, e.g. confusion with stronger analgesics, constipation with antimuscarinics

Figure 33.2 Screening tools recommended by the British Geriatric Society

Step 1- Suspect Frailty	**Step 2- Screen Frailty**	**Step 3- Assessment**
Patient presents with/reports one of 5 frailty syndromes or you have other reasons to suspect frailty	-PRISMA 7 -Gait speed over 4 metres -Timed Up And Go Test (TUGT)	If screening indicates frailty is likely perform a Comprehensive Geriatric Assessment (CGA)

PRISMA 7

1. Are you more than 85 years?
2. Male?
3. In general do you have any health problems that require you to limit your activities?
4. Do you need someone to help you on a regular basis?
5. In general do you have any health problems that require you to stay at home?
6. In case of need can you count on someone close to you?
7. Do you regularly use stick, walker or wheelchair to get about?
Score of > 3 = potential frailty and need for further assessment.

TUGT

Taking more than ten seconds to get up from a chair, walk three meters, turn around and sit down = potential frailty and need for further assessment.

Gait Speed

Taking more than five seconds to cover four metres = potential frailty and need for further assessment.

Advanced Clinical Practice at a Glance, First Edition. Edited by Barry Hill and Sadie Diamond Fox.
© 2023 John Wiley & Sons Ltd. Published 2023 by John Wiley & Sons Ltd.

What is frailty?

Someone living with frailty has a biological syndrome with significant cumulative decline in multiple physiological systems. Instead of being able to 'shrug off' seemingly minor events such as a fall or chest infection, a person with frailty will find that these events significantly affect their ability to function and that it is increasingly difficult to return to their prior level of function (Figure 33.1). Consequently, they are more likely to require increased help with their activities of daily living, be admitted to a nursing home and die than those with a similar health condition or those of a similar age who are not frail. It is widely acknowledged that there are two models of frailty: phenotype[1] and cumulative[2] (Table 33.1).

Who has frailty?

Frailty is more common the older you are and is more prevalent amongst women than men. Although figures differ, it is estimated that 25–50% of those aged 85 and over have a degree of frailty.[1,3] It is important to bear in mind that although frailty is more common the older you get, it is not something that automatically occurs when you reach a particular age. There are many robust older adults living without frailty, who are working, competing in triathlons and caring for grandchildren.

How to identify frailty

Step 1 Suspect frailty

Screening for frailty should ideally be performed every time an older person sees a health or social care professional, but it is particularly important when a patient presents with or reports that they have one of the five frailty syndromes (Table 33.2).

Step 2 Screen for frailty

There are a variety of tools that can be used to screen for frailty. Screening tools recommended by the British Geriatric Society,[4,5] such as gait speed, TUGT and PRISMA 7 (Figure 33.2), follow the phenotype model of frailty. If the screening tool indicates the likelihood of frailty, further detailed assessment by a healthcare professional should occur. There may be other reasons for slow gait speed, for example pain, that could have resulted in the person being erroneously flagged as frail. This is particularly important if someone is acutely unwell when it is highly likely that their gait speed will be impaired.

The cumulative deficit model has given rise to the generation of various tools, such as the Clinical Frailty Scale (CFS), electronic frailty index (eFI) and hospital frailty risk score. The eFI is used in primary care to identify frailty using 36 deficits. A hospital-based version, the Hospital Frailty Risk Score, will shortly be rolled out across the UK. Although not what it was original designed for, the

CFS is widely recommended as an emergency department frailty screening tool. The CFS should be completed based on the individual's baseline state; that is, how they were 2 weeks prior to admission. Therefore, if someone has delirium, getting a detailed reliable collateral history is crucial when completing the CFS.

Step 3 Comprehensive geriatric assessment (CGA)

Following screening, if someone is believed to have frailty then a CGA should be used to formally diagnose frailty. A CGA is a multidimensional holistic assessment of an individual's needs that is performed to devise a patient-centred problem list and develop a patient-lead intervention plan. A CGA should be completed for everyone who is believed to have frailty and should ideally be performed in a proactive manner when the patient is not acutely unwell. It should be co-ordinated by a designated healthcare professional who enables the multidisciplinary team, the patient and their family/carers (if the patient wishes) to contribute to it.

When someone is experiencing an acute deterioration in their health requiring admission to hospital, it may be challenging to undertake a CGA and is not the ideal time to do it. However, research has shown that inpatients who receive a CGA on admission to hospital are more likely to be alive and to return home, so it is something that we should all strive to undertake.[6]

Why is it important to recognise frailty?

We know that those with frailty will be more likely to fall, be admitted to hospital, require assistance with activities of daily living, die and when experiencing an illness or stressor be more likely to experience delirium and have a prolonged and more uncertain recovery period. Identifying frailty, and indeed pre-frailty, means that interventions can be planned to identify and address the issues contributing to it potentially resulting in a reduction in the severity of frailty following medical intervention or lifestyle changes. Additionally, diagnosing frailty should prompt healthcare professionals to establish what matters most to the individual in their care and to keep their wishes at the centre of all decisions. It should also prompt healthcare professionals to carefully consider the risks (including the risk of worsening the degree of frailty) against the intended benefit of any proposed intervention.

Unfortunately, it is more common that the severity of frailty will worsen over time, rather than improve. Having an awareness of this can help individuals (and those closest to them) make decisions about their future.

How do I find out more?

A free e-learning package is available via e-Learning for Healthcare for those wishing to develop their knowledge further: www.e-lfh.org.uk/programmes/frailty/

34 Advanced practitioner-led inter- and intrahospital transfer

Box 34.1 MINT mnemonic entails considerations for personnel, equipment and transportations methods/modes
Source: Mowplass et al.[13] with permission of the American Thoracic Society.

M	**Medical**	• Doctor • Advanced practitioner • Grade required (consultant/registrar/advanced practitioner/trainee advanced practitioner)
I	**Instrumentation**	• Transfer bag – preferably set out in ABCDE approach • Alternative oxygen delivery means (bag-valve mask or a Mapleson circuit) • Oxygen cylinders (calculate requirements) • Advanced airway (endotracheal tube/tracheostomy/surgical airway kit) • Suction • Invasive and non-invasive ventilator • Monitors (ECG, NiBP, arterial, CVP, capnography, SpO_2, BG, temperature) • Defibrillator (with externally pacing) • Syringe drivers with a spare device • Additional device batteries • Drugs (both maintenance and emergency) • Fluids (crystalloids including hypertonic saline or mannitol; colloids including blood products)
N	**Nursing**	• Nurse (ITU, ED, CCOR, CCU)? • Operating department practitioner (ODP)? • Paramedic?
T	**Transportation**	• Certified bed/trolley for transfer • Patient transport service • Blue light double-crewed ambulance (paramedic +/- emergency care assistant or a technician) • Air Ambulance (including land ambulance transfer at base and destination)? • Expected journey time?

Box 34.2 Generic oxygen calculation for invasive ventilated patients

For an invasive ventilated patient transfer for a calculated 60-minute journey, the oxygen requirement equation is as follows.

• $2 \times$ transport time in minutes $\times$ [(minute volume $\times FiO_2$) + ventilator driving gas]
• Ventilator driving gas can be 0.5 L/min – please check manufacturer's instructions for use
• A minute volume of 6 L/min at an FiO_2 of 0.6 for a 60-minute transfer O_2 required:
  – 2×60 (mins) $\times$ [(6 x 0.6) + 0.5] = 120 mins $\times$ 4.1 l/min
  – 492 litres

Box 34.3 A–E approach and considerations pretransfer Source: Mowplass et al.[13] with permission of the American Thoracic Society.

A	**Airway**
	(with C spine)
		• Is the patient self-ventilating or invasively ventilated?
		• Is the endotracheal/tracheostomy secure and patent?
		  • Migration (what level is the endotracheal at the lips?)
		  • Cuff inflation pressure (is there a leak)?
		• Does the patient require immobilisation, with a vacuum mattress, scoop stretcher or long spine board equivalent, cervical collar and/or head blocks and tape?

B	**Breathing** (with ventilation)	• Breathing assessment including auscultation and a chest X-ray • Chest drains below the level of the heart and secured? Not pulling and ensure they are swinging, draining or bubbling • What is the ventilation mode (BiPAP, SIMV, PS, CPAP) is the patient including settings (RR, tidal/minute volume, FiO_2)? • Ventilator tubing secured? • Is there CO_2 capnography? • Has there been a blood gas within the last 15 minutes before departure whilst on the transport ventilator? • Does the blood gas show adequate oxygenation/ventilation (if not, can this be optimised?) • What are the calculated oxygen requirements?

Advanced Clinical Practice at a Glance, First Edition. Edited by Barry Hill and Sadie Diamond Fox.
© 2023 John Wiley & Sons Ltd. Published 2023 by John Wiley & Sons Ltd.

Box 34.3 (Continued)

C	Circulation (with haemorrhage control)	• Cardiovascular assessment including inotropic support (which inotrope, strength, rate and mcg/kg/min?)
		• What are the calculated infusion requirements?
		• Are there any haemorrhage concerns?
		  • Does any coagulopathy need to be reversed?
		  • Does the patient require blood products for transfer?
		• All monitoring leads (ECG, invasive/non-invasive BP, SpO_2) are running centrally along the patient and will not cause skin damage
		  • Are they on and all working?
		• All IV, CVC and arterial lines secure and accessible from the patient's right-hand side
		  • At least two IVs accessible?
		• Have all non-essential infusions been detached?
		• Are there IV bolus fluids attached?
		• Urinary catheter is running centrally down the patient?

D	Disability (with neurological control)	• Neurological assessment including pupils, blood glucose and noting any seizure activity • Is the patient 15–30° head up? • ETT ties appropriate if suspected raised intracranial pressure • Has secondary neurological injury prevention been considered? • Is the patient adequately sedated? • Are muscle relaxants required? • Are anticonvulsants required?
E	Exposure (with temperature regulation)	• Are there any patient temperature concerns? • Does the patient require active or passive warming or cooling? • Have all attempts at minimising pressure damage been considered? • Have all wounds been dressed? • Is the patient secured to the stretcher and stretcher secured to the ambulance?

Box 34.4 Transferring team considerations Source: Mowplass et al.[13] with permission of the American Thoracic Society.

P	Phone	• Is it a personal mobile? • Is it charged and do you need a charging cable?
E	Enquiry number and name	• Do you have the receiving unit's phone number and the name of the receiving consultant? • Do you have your consultant's phone number in case of emergency and requiring advice/help en route?
R	Revenue	• Has the transfer team got money in case of an emergency or a return taxi is required?
S	Safe clothing	• Has everyone got high-visibility clothing? • Are there sufficient gloves, aprons, eye protection for personal protection? COVID PPE? • Warm clothing?
O	Organised route	• What is the route? • Is there a back-up route in case of obstruction? • Do you have the correct hospital site?
N	Nutrition	• Is there food and water for the transfer team (if a prolonged transfer)?
A	A-Z map	• Is there one? • If using GPS, do you have the correct postcode?
L	Lift home	• Is the ambulance bringing the team home? • Proposed method of returning to base location? • What if the ambulance gets redirected on the way back?

Facilitating safe patient transfer is an important aspect of the advanced practitioner (AP) role. This may be to another location within the same facility (intrahospital) or to a different hospital (interhospital). This chapter provides an overview for the AP involved in transfers.

Since the establishment of the first intensive care unit (ICU) in the 1950s, demand has grown exponentially.[1] When demand exceeds supply, or when centralised specialised care is required, interhospital transfer of the critically ill patient becomes necessary.[1–3] Numbers are believed to be increasing because of supply–demand imbalances.[1,3] Interhospital transfer is often time-critical, although some patients require transfer for specialist treatment in less time-sensitive situations. It is a high-risk care episode for potentially unstable patients.[3,4] The goal of interhospital transfer should be maintenance of high-quality care[1] while moving the patient to an appropriate location in an expedient and safe manner.[5] This occurs following initial resuscitation and stabilisation.[3] Despite this, patients may be in a dynamic and often precarious condition yet transfer carries risks and exposes them to different potential harms and instability.[5] While the reasons for intrahospital transfer are different, many of the potential risks are common to all transfers. Therefore, clinicians should approach all transfers with the same degree of rigour.

The transfer of patients illustrates Murphy's Law: 'If anything can go wrong it will'. Since the late 1970s, safety concerns have led to several studies into the risks of transferring critically ill patients.[1] Published studies conclude that serious adverse events (AEs) occur, with rates reported between 12.5% and 62%.[6,7] Over 91% of these are preventable.[7] This is regardless of the transport modality used or clinicians involved[1] and this data has not changed over time.[7] Avoidable AEs occur[8] and the AP requires an appreciation of the potential risks and complications that can occur throughout transfer.

Patient stabilisation and preparation for transfer

Preparing a patient for transfer, either inter- or intrahospital, can be daunting and demanding for multiple reasons.[7] In most clinical situations, the patient should have received initial resuscitation and physiological optimisation prior to transfer. However, in some truly time-critical situations, critical interventions (e.g. airway management) are performed initially, while less complex resuscitation (e.g. volume resuscitation or osmotherapy) is continued during the transfer. Achieving relative stability/stable physiology should be carefully balanced with the urgency of the transfer and should be guided by senior clinicians and a 'scoop and run' approach may be required if it is time-critical. Therefore, optimisation may be required en route.[9]

Patient safety is paramount. Pretransfer preparation must be meticulous; several mnemonics have been developed and provide useful frameworks. A useful preparation is a mnemonic of 'MINT' which considers transfer personnel, equipment and transportation modes/methods (Box 34.1),[1] not forgetting adequate analgesia, sedation and antiemetics. The transferring team must be self-sufficient and not reliant on the ambulance clinicians for equipment. It is imperative that the volumes of oxygen and drugs available are sufficient for the entire journey, bearing in mind the potential for delays. This applies particularly to oxygen and drugs which are doubled for the journey time, or a minimum of 60 minutes.[3,4] For ventilated patients, the oxygen equation is outlined in Box 34.2. The ABCDE approach is the gold standard in assessing a patient pretransfer (Box 34.3).[3] 'PERSONAL' is a mnemonic that can be used to plan personnel and equipment requirements for transfer (Box 34.4).[10]

Finally, the team should consider actions to be taken in the event of unexpected AEs, including vehicle failure, failure of ventilator/pumps/monitor/oxygen, deterioration/cardiac arrest, or dislodged airway, and always have a dedicated intravenous access labelled for emergency drugs.[3,10]

During and after transfer

The goal during inter- and intrahospital transfer is the continuation of high-quality care while preventing deterioration and untoward AEs. Factors associated with reduced incidents are teamwork, patient assessment, equipment and interpersonal skills.[1]

Dynamic risk assessment must be carried out prior to and during transfer and should consider the patient's condition, specific risks, likelihood of deterioration, potential for additional intervention required en route and duration of transfer.[3]

Use of checklists reduces physiological derangement and AEs[11] and can minimise AEs.[12] Checklists are key to detecting underlying factors and improving safety during transfer[13] and this should be undertaken immediately before transfer. Failure of equipment is the most common AE during transfer.[14] Therefore, standardised equipment and transfer bags are recommended. Specifically designed critical care transfer trolleys should be used. Patients' pressure areas must be protected and tubes, lines and drains should be secured, with oxygen cylinders safely stowed.[3] All equipment must be stowed below the patient.[1] APs must be familiar with switching to the trolley or vehicle's oxygen and electricity supplies and how to safely secure on/to the trolley.

Minimum standards of monitoring in the ICU ventilated patient must include end-tidal carbon dioxide, invasive blood pressure (non-invasive blood pressure is unreliable on transfer), three-lead electrocardiogram, oxygen saturations and temperature.[9] Ventilation settings, airway pressures and drug infusions, including boluses given en route, must be recorded. If adequate stabilisation and preparation for transfer has been undertaken, there should be minimal need to perform interventions en route. Clinician safety is also paramount so clinicians should be in a secure seat, with seatbelt, throughout the transfer. If intervention is required, the vehicle should stop in a safe location.[3]

Communication is key for a successful transfer. This includes providing relatives with contact numbers of the receiving unit, visiting times and directions.[1,4] Handover at the receiving unit is a crucial point in ensuring the quality of the transfer. After the patient is safely transferred into the bedspace and monitoring, ventilation and infusions are in situ, both teams focus on a structured verbal handover to medical and nursing staff simultaneously.[5]

Governance

Governance surrounding transfer is key to identifying and minimising AEs that may lead to patient or team harm. Hospitals should nominate a lead with responsibility for guidelines, AP training, competencies, certified transfer equipment and audit. This individual should report to the trust critical care delivery group/governance meeting and network transfer forums.[3]

In AP-led transfers, varying approaches have been considered through guidance documents to minimise untoward AEs.[3,9,15–17] These include consultant-led triage; a logbook of all transfers; indemnity to undertake this role; and mandating training.[3,8,9,14–17] Conversely no clear guidelines exist for methods to train an AP for transfer.[1,6] Guidance states that training should be a blended education approach to achieve transfer competencies with lectures, supervised transfers and simulation training,[17,18] with continuous professional development after initial training.

Conclusion

This chapter has provided an overview of AP transfers which occur within and between hospitals. All transfers carry potential risks to patients and clinicians. Meticulous planning and preparation is required to promote safety, and several mnemonics provide effective frameworks for this. Patients should be adequately resuscitated prior to transfer, taking the urgency of the transfer into consideration. The chapter outlines the importance of following clear governance frameworks and receiving comprehensive training.

This chapter will help to ensure that patients undergoing inter- or intrahospital transfer are cared for by a vigilant process.

Independent prescribing

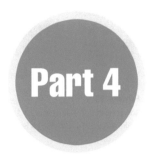
Part 4

Chapters

35 Principles of pharmacology

Figure 35.1 Types of targets for drug action (RICE).
Source: Nuttall D, Rutt-Howard J (2011) *The Textbook of Non-Medical Prescribing*, Figure 5.2, p.171. John Wiley & Sons, Hoboken.

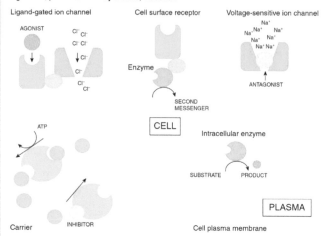

Figure 35.2 Routes of drug absorption.
Source: Nuttall D, Rutt-Howard J (2019) *The Textbook of Non-Medical Prescribing*, Figure 5.1, p.155. John Wiley & Sons, Hoboken.

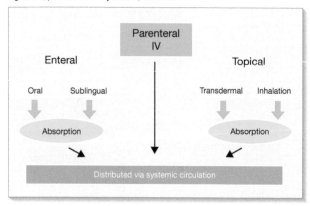

Figure 35.3 Therapeutic index. Schematic diagram of the dose–response relationship for the desired effect (dose–therapeutic response) and for an undesired adverse effect. The therapeutic index is the extent of displacement of the two curves within the normal dose range.
Source: McKay GA, Reid JL, Walters MR (2011) *Clinical Pharmacology and Therapeutics*, John Wiley & Sons, Hoboken.

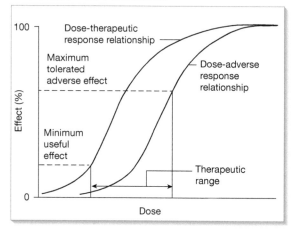

Table 35.1 Factors affecting speed and extent of absorption of non-parenteral medications

Factor	Remarks
Age of the body	Variability in absorption between neonates, children and the elderly
Physiological problems	Malabsorption, gut motility, blood flow and perfusion
Route of administration	Drugs that need to cross membranes will take longer to show an effect
Interactions	Drug–drug, drug–food
Chemical nature of the drug	Lipid solubility (lipid-soluble drugs are absorbed across the lipid cell membrane more easily), acid–base relationship of the drug and the body (acid drugs are absorbed more quickly in an acid environment, alkaline drugs are absorbed more quickly in an alkaline environment)

Table 35.2 Terms used to describe lipid and water solubility

Terms describing lipid solubility	Terms describing water solubility
Lipophilic	Hydrophilic
Non-polar	Polar
Unionised	Ionised
Uncharged	Charged
Hydrophobic	Lipophobic

Table 35.3 Hydrolysis

The drug reacts with water. The chemical bond within the drug is broken and two compounds are formed. Simultaneously, the water molecule splits in two, a hydrogen molecule transfers to one of these new compounds and a hydroxide molecule transfers to the other. This increases the drug's water solubility

Table 35.4 Drugs that commonly induce or inhibit CYP450 enzymes

Enzyme inhibitors Increase rate of drug metabolism CASA SICKFACES.COM	Enzyme inducers Decrease rate of drug metabolism SCRAPS GPS
Cranberry juice Allopurinol SSRI Amiodarone Sodium valproate Isoniazid Cimetidine Ketoconazole Fluconazole Alcohol (acute) Chloramphenicol Erythromycin Sulfonamides Ciprofloxacin/ clarithromycin Omeprazole Metronidazole	Sulphonylurea Carbamazepine Rifampicin Alcohol (chronic) Phenytoin St John's wort Griseofulvin Phenobarbitone Smoking

Table 35.5 First-order and zero-order kinetics

First-order kinetics	The higher the concentration in the plasma, the quicker a drug is cleared
Zero-order kinetics	A constant amount of the drug is eliminated; the rate is dependent on time Quite rare. Notable examples are alcohol, phenytoin, salicylates, omeprazole and fluoxetine

Pharmacology is the study of pharmacodynamics, the effect of a drug on the body, and pharmacokinetics, what the body does to the drug and how it moves the drug through itself.

Pharmacodynamics

The drug has four main targets where it can exert its effect: receptors, ion channels, carrier molecules and enzymes (RICE) (Figure 35.1). Drugs will act as agonists (bind to a receptor and cause the same biological response) or as antagonists (bind to a receptor and block the biological response). To bind, a drug must have affinity for that receptor. The likelihood of the bound drug causing an effect is called *efficacy*. A potent drug will cause effect at low concentrations.

Pharmacokinetics (ADME)

Absorption

Drugs can be administered in a variety of ways (Figure 35.2). Absorption of a drug refers to it crossing cell membranes from the site of administration into the plasma. Bioavailability is the amount of drug reaching the plasma that can be distributed around the body. IV medications are already available to the plasma so have 100% bioavailability, whereas some drugs need to be secondarily absorbed into a target area (i.e. across the blood–brain barrier). Bioavailability does not equal efficacy; a drug in the bloodstream does not mean it is more effective. Bioavailability is the relationship between the amount available and the amount administered. The speed and extent of absorption of non-parenteral medications will depend on numerous factors (Table 35.1).

Distribution

The drug is moved to its target site of action by the bloodstream. Distribution may be within body compartments such as intracellular fluids, fat, interstitial fluid, blood plasma or transcellular fluid. Many drugs bind to plasma proteins to be transported; plasma proteins are a transport system, not a drug target, and this binding will not induce a physiological response. Only the unbound drug will be able to exert a pharmacological effect; as the unbound drug is absorbed into the tissue, plasma proteins will release more of the bound drug.

Distribution will be affected by illnesses causing hypoalbuminaemia, which can lead to higher concentrations and consequently a greater effect of the free drug. Competition for the same plasma-binding site between two drugs may increase the unbound concentration of the less competitive drug. Lipid solubility will affect distribution; lipophilic drugs will distribute more readily into fat whereas hydrophilic drugs will concentrate more into the bloodstream (Table 35.2).

Metabolism

Metabolism changes the drug from one form to another, either by enzymatically converting an active drug into an inactive form or by converting an inactive prodrug to an active metabolite form. Lipid-soluble drugs need to be metabolised to increase their water solubility and enable better excretion by the kidneys. This principally happens in the liver but can happen the blood plasma, gut wall and lungs.

Drug metabolism has two phases and drugs will be metabolised in one, or both of these phases.

- *Phase 1* – oxidation, reduction and hydrolysis; makes the drug more water soluble, does not automatically make the drug inactive, enables better excretion by the kidneys (Table 35.3).
- *Phase 2* – conjugation; joining with a polar chemical group, usually glucuronic acid, mostly makes the drug inactive and allows the metabolites to be secreted into bile or excreted by the kidneys.

The most important enzyme system in drug metabolism is the cytochrome P450 (CYP450) system, predominantly used in oxidation and reduction that takes place in phase 1 metabolism. CYP450 may be affected by a person's genetics or by drugs that inhibit or induce this enzyme (Table 35.4). First-pass metabolism refers to drugs that are metabolised before they reach the bloodstream; this is extremely variable and decreases with disease or age, and these drugs should be administered by an alternative route.

Drug clearance involves metabolism and excretion and is the rate at which the drug is removed from the body. Drug clearance may be affected by decreased liver or renal blood flow that occurs with older age, or diseases that affect either of these organs, or their perfusion. In liver or renal impairment, reduced drug doses may be needed to prevent drug accumulation. Drug half-life is the time it takes for the plasma concentration of a drug to be halved (Table 35.5).

The therapeutic index refers to drug concentrations in the body that are high enough to be effective but not so high that they are toxic. Some drugs have a narrow therapeutic window; concentrations in the plasma need regular monitoring, and drug doses may need adjusting to maintain plasma concentrations within this window (Figure 35.3).

Excretion

Drugs are excreted by the kidneys in urine, and by the biliary system in faeces. Drug excretion can be affected by age, disease or reduced blood flow to hepatobiliary or renal systems, urine pH, urine flow or drug interactions.

Some renal excretion of free, unbound drugs will occur through glomerular filtration but drugs bound to plasma and drugs with large molecules are unable to enter the glomerular capsule. Certain drugs are excreted by secretion into carrier systems in the proximal convoluted tubule. Effecient carrier systems work against a concentration gradient and the kidneys use different carriers for acids and bases, although this is competitively inhibited. Drugs may be reabsorbed via passive diffusion; drugs that are lipophilic are easily reabsorbed, hydrophilic drugs cannot easily cross membranes so stay in the renal tubule.

Biliary excretion occurs when conjugated metabolites are actively secreted into bile by carrier systems. The biliary system conveys drugs to the small intestine for excretion in the faeces. Enterohepatic recycling occurs when conjugated drugs are hydrolysed by bacteria in the intestine, releasing the free drug which is reabsorbed into the blood.

36 Non-pharmacological and pharmacological interventions

Figure 36.1 Neural circuit of gate control of pain. In the top panel, the non-nociceptive, large-diameter sensory fiber (orange) is more active than the nociceptive small-diameter fiber (blue), therefore the input to the inhibitory interneuron (red) is net positive. The inhibitory interneuron provides presynaptic inhibition to both the nociceptive and non-nociceptive neurons, reducing the excitation of the transmission cells. In the bottom panel, an open 'gate' (free-flowing information from afferents to the transmission cells) is pictured. This occurs when there is more activity in the nociceptive small-diameter fibers (blue) than the non-nociceptive large-diameter fibers (orange). In this situation, the inhibitory interneuron is silenced, which relieves inhibition of the transmission cells. This 'open gate' allows for transmission cells to be excited, and thus pain to be sensed.
Source: John Tuthill / Wikimedia Commons / PD CC BY SA 4.0

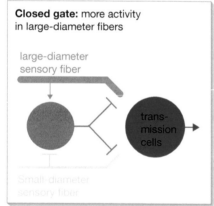

Closed gate: more activity in large-diameter fibers

large-diameter sensory fiber

trans-mission cells

Small-diameter sensory fiber

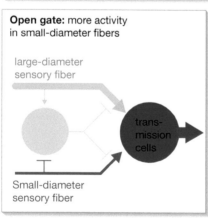

Open gate: more activity in small-diameter fibers

large-diameter sensory fiber

trans-mission cells

Small-diameter sensory fiber

Figure 36.2 The effect of pharmacological and non-pharmacological pain management. Interventions along the nociceptive pain pathway where each type of intervention exerts its mechanism of action to relieve pain. Source: Manworren RC (2015) Multimodal pain management and the future of a personalized medicine approach to pain. *AORN Journal*, **101**, 307–318, with permission of Elsevier

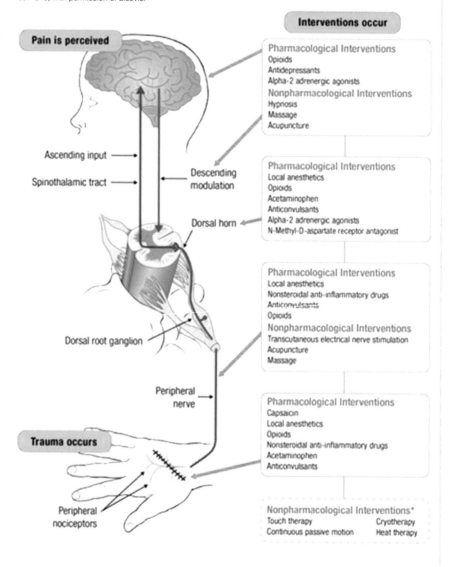

Pain is perceived

Ascending input

Spinothalamic tract

Descending modulation

Dorsal horn

Dorsal root ganglion

Peripheral nerve

Trauma occurs

Peripheral nociceptors

Interventions occur

Pharmacological Interventions
Opioids
Antidepressants
Alpha-2 adrenergic agonists
Nonpharmacological Interventions
Hypnosis
Massage
Acupuncture

Pharmacological Interventions
Local anesthetics
Opioids
Acetaminophen
Anticonvulsants
Alpha-2 adrenergic agonists
N-Methyl-D-aspartate receptor antagonist

Pharmacological Interventions
Local anesthetics
Nonsteroidal anti-inflammatory drugs
Anticonvulsants
Opioids
Nonpharmacological Interventions
Transcutaneous electrical nerve stimulation
Acupuncture
Massage

Pharmacological Interventions
Capsaicin
Local anesthetics
Opioids
Nonsteroidal anti-inflammatory drugs
Acetaminophen
Anticonvulsants

Nonpharmacological Interventions*
Touch therapy   Cryotherapy
Continuous passive motion   Heat therapy

When discussing patient care, it can be all too easy to reach for the medicines cupboard when the patient requires an intervention. This section will explore the options and considerations for both pharmacological and non-pharmacological interventions.

Splinting

Broken bones can cause extreme discomfort and patients often require large amounts of analgesia. The movement of the broken aspect is usually the largest source of pain, greater than the injury itself. Reducing the ability for the broken aspect to move can therefore reduce both the pain and the need for pharmacology.

Simply placing the patient into a sling, splint or traction device and reducing movement can reduce the amount of pharmacology required to manage the patient's distress.

Psychology, physiology and pharmacology

Distraction can be a useful technique for managing issues such as pain, with the magnitude of distraction inversely correlated with the level of pain. Enabling patients to focus away from the initial insult may reduce the need for pharmacology.

The gate theory of pain (Figure 36.1) encompasses the perception of pain and is subdivided into sensory-discriminative, motivational-affective and cognitive-evaluative aspects. A commonly used example of the gate theory is using cold temperatures to modulate pain as the cold temperatures are said to stimulate afferent nerve fibres and thus inhibit transmission of pain to the second-order neurons. This also provides a theoretical basis for the modulation of pain by touch (i.e. stroke or rub) by inhibiting the signals at the level of the dorsal horn.

Utilising non-pharmacological interventions can improve the patient experience and their psychological welfare.

Altered pharmacokinetics

Pharmacology can be affected by non-pharmacological factors which should be considered when prescribing.

Consider the hydration status of the patient. If the patient is dehydrated, their circulating volume may be depleted and therefore the concentration of any drug may be increased but also the distribution and metabolism may be unpredictable.

Nutritional status may affect pharmacology. If the patient is protein depleted, the risk of increased unbound drug is greater.

There may be an increased risk of toxic drug levels from standard dosing regimes.

Multimodal approach (Figure 36.2)

Utilising more than one method of analgesia can have increased acute and chronic benefits, especially when considering the use of regional and local anaesthetics. Systemic analgesia may be required to gain immediate control of a situation but lower level analgesics may be utilised as a stop-gap before local/regional techniques can be used. A good example of this might be a Colles fracture where a drug such as Entonox* or Penthrox* can provide rapid analgesia before a haematoma block can be administered to provide longer lasting and more effective analgesia.

Distraction techniques

Distraction can be useful in managing not only anxiety but pain in a range of patients. It is typically utilised most often in children but may be used elsewhere. There is evidence to suggest both physiological reduction and self-reported reduction in pain when using distraction techniques, which can include video games, movies and parental involvement for children.

Home remedies

Non-prescription or over-the-counter medication may interfere with the medicines you wish to administer. Often, patients may not consider these as medications and may not list them during clinical examination and history taking. Care facilities such as residential homes should have processes in place to monitor non-prescription medications and alert a prescriber. Not eliciting these medications can result in unexpected and potentially serious consequences to the patient. A good example is St John's wort which is a popular herbal remedy taken by patients for a range of health conditions; however, it has been shown to significantly induce enzymes, including CYP450 substrates. This can affect various medications including antidepressants and immunosuppressants along with a range of cardiac and other medication.

Health promotion

Clinical interactions can be a useful time to identify health and lifestyle factors that may affect the patient's physical and mental health. Clinicians should be aware of the Making Every Contact Count initiative.[1]

37 Shared decision making

Table 37.1 The two-stage test and five statutory principles of the Mental Capacity Act (2005)

Two-stage test
1. Does the patient have an impairment of the mind or brain?
2. Does that impairment mean they are unable to make specific decisions?

Principles
1   A presumption of **capacity**
2   Individuals should be supported to make their **own decisions**. All steps must be taken to aid this
3   An **unwise decision** is not a reason to class the patient as being unable to make a decision if it is an informed decision
4   Decisions should be made in **their best interest** by the multidisciplinary teams
5   **Least restrictive options** to their rights and freedoms.

Figure 37.1 Choose Wisely UK advocated questions (BRAN) to aid the decision-making process

1. What are the Benefits
2. What are the Risk
3. What are the Alternatives
4. What if I do Nothing

Table 37.2 'Ask 3 Questions' advocated by the Health Foundation Campaign

1. What are my options?
2. What are the possible benefits and risks of these options?
3. What help do I need to make my decision?

Advanced Clinical Practice at a Glance, First Edition. Edited by Barry Hill and Sadie Diamond Fox.
© 2023 John Wiley & Sons Ltd. Published 2023 by John Wiley & Sons Ltd.

In this chapter we will look at the partnership that should be created with service users and their families/carers. We will consider the relationship of capacity and consent in the decision-making process. The goal of communication is gaining mutually agreed decisions. Finally, we will discuss the role of reflection and self-awareness that support us as independent prescribers in the decision-making process.

Mental capacity, informed consent and prescribing decisions

Before we embark on any decision-making process, we need to be clear on the prescriber's role in ensuring consent and capacity during a consultation. If these aspects are not present, a shared partnership cannot be created. Ascertaining *capacity* and ensuring we provide clear communication to enable informed *consent* are integral parts of the prescribing process. As per principle 1 of the Mental Capacity Act (MCA) (2005), we can make an assumption of capacity in our patients but we must be confident in them having it. Capacity is a fluid concept and someone who has lacked capacity in the past does not necessary lack capacity now. Without capacity, we cannot be sure that despite best information giving, our patients are making an informed decision and thus consenting to treatment.

Capacity is assessed by the two-stage tests set out in the MCA (Table 37.1). Does the patient have an impairment and does that impairment inhibit them from making specific decisions? Remember that capacity is fluid and someone not having capacity in one instance does not mean they will lack it in another.

The MCA principle 2 focuses on the individual being supported to make their own decisions. In 2019 the Act returned to Parliament for a key amendment which was concerned largely with changes to the previously named Deprivation of Liberties (DOLs) which following this change in legislation is now Liberty Protection Safeguards. The shift is more about supporting and protecting rather than explaining why freedoms are being deprived.

Prescribers need to encourage and support service users to participate in the decision-making process. Even when we consider capacity, and at times the need to act in the best interest of others (principle 4), we recognise that best practice is treatment in the least restrictive form. Remember, an unwise decision is not an incorrect decision as long as it has been based on the most appropriate information. This is further discussed under the reflection heading.

More detailed information about capacity and the advanced practitioner can be found in Chapter 11 of this book. Table 37.1 demonstrates the key considerations.

Creating a partnership

Competency 3 of the Royal Pharmaceutical Society Prescribing Competency Framework focuses on the core skills a prescriber needs to demonstrate in practice when reaching a shared decision. It highlights the need for a partnership to be created that allows open and honest transfer of information. Respect the patient's choices regarding treatment. Ensure we address adherence in a non-judgemental way. Ensure we build a rapport that encourages appropriate prescribing and that a prescription will not always be supplied. Finish consultations with a check that patients/carers understand what has been discussed and thus we have reached a satisfactory outcome.

As independent prescribers, we should utilise *consultation models* to ensure we complete a thorough care episode and do not miss opportunities. Using different models for different scenarios can be useful. Consultation models are discussed in detail in Chapter 7 of this publication.

Ensure you use clear communication that is jargon free and pitched at the level of the individual you are talking with. Understanding of information can be checked throughout and again at the end to maintain key messages. Techniques such as 'chunk check' are recommended to assist in understanding but also a mixture of techniques including non-verbal, digital, written, etc. can be utilised.

Finally, consider the environment where the consultation is taking place. All parties need to feel able to ask questions without fear of judgement. This can be challenging in some places. Signposting to support mechanisms for patients can be helpful. Charities such as Choose Wisely UK and Health Foundation Campaign promote healthcare providers and service users making better decisions together. Choose Wisely is a global initiative improving conversations to focus on what is important to both. It highlights the negative impacts of the overuse of medications and harmful effects of unnecessary investigations. It suggests using the BRAN questions to support patients to get the best out of consultations and reach a shared decision that matters to them (Figure 37.1). The Health Foundation Campaign's 'Ask 3 Questions' also gives three simple questions patients and carers can use (Table 37.2).

Reflection and self-growth to facilitate a better understanding

In order to create a dialogue that is open and honest, we must be aware of our own judgements and inherent bias. Regardless of our professional background, we as independent prescribers are encouraged to reflect as part of the prescribing process. Knowing our own boundaries and staying within our scope of practice are essential for safe prescribing. However, without reflection, how can we both identify these boundaries and also look to develop?

Through the process of reflection and considering the decisions of others, we can start to unpick the rationale behind them. Decisions that patients make may not be in alignment with our own. But if you have adequately supported the patient and given the rationale and reasons behind why their decisions might have associated risk, then that is all you can do. At times, it will be hard to accept this but as practitioners we must. By looking at the process and reflecting, you can develop your consultation strategy and strengthen your communication so that you will know you did all you could. You may also see things from the perspective of others and come to realise it was not that unwise a decision after all.

This process aligns with the Royal Pharmaceutical Society Prescribing Competency Framework – Competency 7.1 Prescribe Safely, Competency 8.4 Prescribe Professionally and Competency 9.1 Improve Prescribing Practice. It is also key that we reflect on the practice of others to ensure our patients' interests remain at the forefront of what we do. The overarching remit is about making better decisions together for the good of all.

38 Prescribing practice and patient education

Figure 38.1 The dimensions of health. Source: Adapted from Leach RM (2014) *Fundamentals of Health Promotion for Nurses*, Figure 1.1, p.6. John Wiley & Sons, Hoboken

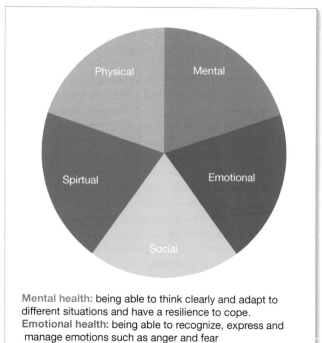

Mental health: being able to think clearly and adapt to different situations and have a resilience to cope.
Emotional health: being able to recognize, express and manage emotions such as anger and fear
Social health: being able to form and maintain relationships.
having energy and vitality and feeling well.
Spiritual health: being able to be at peace with oneself and find calm.

Figure 38.3 Methods of education delivery

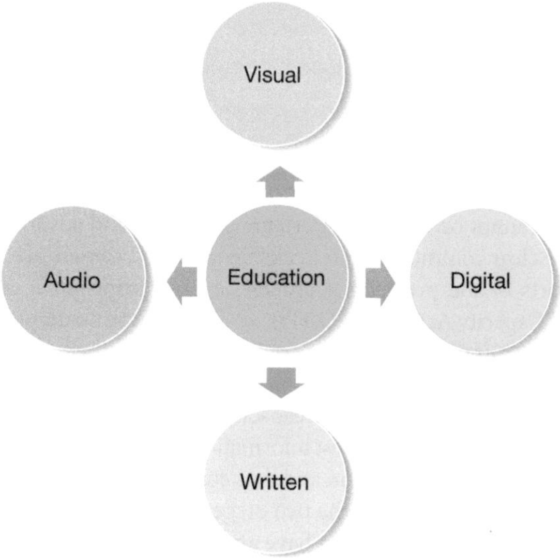

Visual — Education — Digital — Audio — Written

Figure 38.2 The influences that potentially threaten, promote or protect health. Source: Browne GR et al. (2015)/John Wiley & Sons

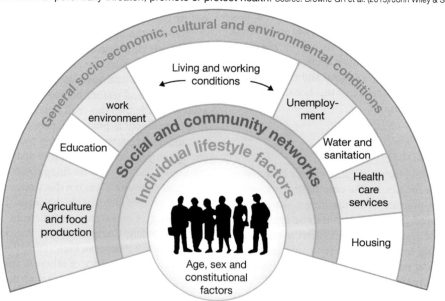

Advanced Clinical Practice at a Glance, First Edition. Edited by Barry Hill and Sadie Diamond Fox.
© 2023 John Wiley & Sons Ltd. Published 2023 by John Wiley & Sons Ltd.

This chapter will highlight the opportunities independent prescribers have in patient education. It will address the key messages to get across and how as advanced practitioners we are integral to health and well-being. Our role as independent prescribers covers both actively promoting health to reduce the necessity of medicines in some cases and how health beliefs link with adherence of treatment to benefit patient outcomes.

Education

This is multifactorial in terms of prescribing. We are educating patients on the conditions that we diagnose and the role of medication for these. This is to ensure we have concordance with treatment, informed consent to taking the medications we offer them and also to ensure they will adhere to the treatment plan.

As advanced practitioners, we are in a unique position to support wider public health agendas. We are ideally placed to educate in relation to health promotion and to introduce and support the concept of well-being. Also to highlight health inequalities and tackle these head on.

All health professionals have multiple interactions daily with members of the public and as prescribers we are able to monitor the health state of others. Our consultations provide a holistic picture of the individuals we see. This means we can consider health much more broadly and introduce risk screening tools in our daily practice. As a prescriber, it is important to build a rapport with the patient and ensure they feel comfortable to disclose and engage. This requires strong communication skills and expertise at handling sensitive conversations.

Patient education should consider the following aspects.
- Taking advantage of education technology where appropriate (websites, apps, etc.).
- Knowledge level and health beliefs.
- Attitude toward change.
- Determine the individual's learning style.
- Stimulate the individual's interest.
- Consider the individual's strengths and limitations.
- Include the individual's wider social network in healthcare management (family, friends, etc.).
- An appreciation of the dimension of health (Figure 38.1).
- The influences that threaten, promote or protect health (Figure 38.2).
Remember we are looking to bring about changes by influencing these behaviours, in the hope that this will improve or maintain health. First, the person must want to change and also be able to see the benefits that will accompany change.

Behaviour change

It is important to address patient expectations when looking at health behaviour change, helping them set achievable goals and suggesting ways for them to track their progress. Barriers to learning must be identified and addressed. Also, patients need to believe they have the necessary skills to achieve change.

Practitioners need to have the knowledge to support this process so a strong understanding of behaviour models is essential, along with the ability to translate them into practice. You must be able to relate the national health agenda to the person in front of you. Engage them and empower then to make the changes necessary for a healthier lifestyle.

Case study – Suzanne

Suzanne is in her early 20s. She presents at A&E after a fall with a swollen right ankle. Her worry is that it is broken. On taking a full history, you discover that she has a 5-year history of smoking three packs of cigarettes a week. She also consumes 16–20 units of alcohol, mostly on Friday and Saturday night. Her BMI is 29. She has a sedentary job at a desk in an office. She shares a flat with two friends. Suzanne also reports three hospital admissions with exacerbation of her asthma in the last year. Her parents are still alive. Her mother is in good health but her father had a heart attack 6 months ago. After examination and X-ray, you are able to reassure Suzanne that her ankle has no fracture. It will take a few days to settle down. Simple analgesia is discussed and Suzanne is happy to take what she has at home.

There are a lot of opportunities to challenge health behaviour here. Immediate concerns are listed below.
- Smoking with asthma
- Alcohol intake
- Weight and diet
Now take a moment to consider the wider factors that might affect Suzanne's health – environment, mental health, finances, etc. Some factors are out of our individual control (see Figure 38.2). However, working in partnership with local agencies and national initiatives will ensure you have access to a wider pool of resources to signpost your patients on to.

Social prescribing

So what can we do on a more local level to support the above discussed case? First, we need to address Suzanne's health beliefs. We can discuss the link of decreased life expectancy with asthma exacerbations and the link between smoking and poor asthma control. Does she see the link between her BMI and risk factors for heart disease, especially in view of recent family history? She may be more open to change after her father's myocardial infarction. She has a sedentary job so are there ways to build daily exercise in?

As independent prescribers, our role is wider than medication. Social prescribing could be really helpful here. Social prescribing is a way of putting patients in touch with local agencies that can help improve their health, social welfare and well-being. Document clearly in her records that the conversation has taken place. Recommend GP follow-up

Addressing these issues is linked to the knowledge of the prescribers. You will need knowledge of activities that help individuals but also understanding of the wider factors that allow individuals to engage with these activities. Making Every Contact Count (MECC) is a Health Education England initiative using local providers to support people with making positive changes to their mental and physical health. It partners with multiple agencies at all levels to support providers in this. Some of its key priorities are smoking, alcohol, weight and mental health. The use of risk stratification tools to help explain to patients the impact of their lifestyle can be helpful.

Materials

Having an understanding of the way people learn will help us to support them. Patient education can be delivered in a variety of formats (Figure 38.3). The Patient Education Materials Assessment Tool (PEMAT)[1] is a validated tool to assess the understandability and actionability of print and audiovisual patient education materials. The following definitions are utilised within the tool.
- *Understandability*: patient education materials are *understandable* when consumers of diverse backgrounds and varying levels of health literacy can process and explain key messages.
- *Actionability*: patient education materials are *actionable* when consumers of diverse backgrounds and varying levels of health literacy can identify what they can do based on the information presented.
The PEMAT was designed to be completed by healthcare professionals who design and provide high-quality educational materials to patients or consumers.

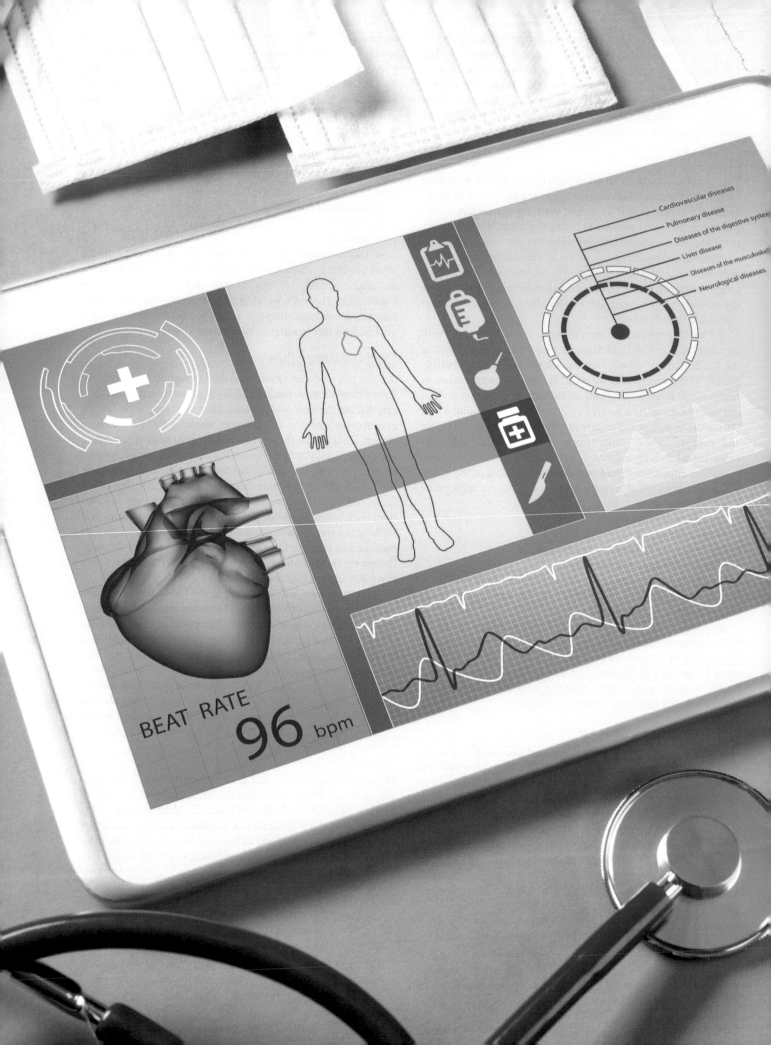

Advanced clinical practice leadership and management

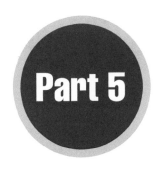

Part 5

Chapters

Leadership in healthcare settings

Table 39.1 Examples of attributes of effective healthcare leadership in teams and organisations

Authenticity and transparency

Emotional intelligence and compassion

Accountability and integrity

Role modelling and living values

Inspiring a vision and shared purpose

Positive inclusion and diversity

Facilitation of and flourishing in others

Motivational and inspiring

Quality and safety focused

Person, citizen and patient centric

Clarity of team and organisational objectives

Connectivity and collaboration

Table 39.2 Examples of consequences of effective healthcare leadership in teams and organisations

Positive workplace culture

Effective teams

Person-centred, safe, effective, compassionate care

Positive patient experience and satisfaction

Staff engagement and satisfaction

Workforce retention and development

Connected and trusting relationships

Robust safety and learning cultures

Innovation and continuous improvement

Capability and talent management

Purpose alignment throughout organisation

Empowering leadership at all workforce levels

Improved productivity

Collaboration and connectivity across systems

Advanced Clinical Practice at a Glance, First Edition. Edited by Barry Hill and Sadie Diamond Fox.
© 2023 John Wiley & Sons Ltd. Published 2023 by John Wiley & Sons Ltd.

Over the years there have been many approaches and strategies for healthcare leadership. However, for the NHS, healthcare leadership was brought sharply into focus in 2013 following the shocking findings of the public inquiry led by Sir Robert Francis into the failings of care at Mid Staffordshire NHS Foundation Trust between 2005 and 2008. The report highlighted a leadership culture that focused more on the trust's business than its patients' care, and became a catalyst for an invigoration of studies and reports identifying that healthcare leadership must be more patient and person centred in healthcare settings of the future.[1]

Subsequently in 2009, the Care Quality Commission (CQC) was introduced as a combined monitoring body for standards in health and social care and continues to assess leadership in healthcare settings as one of its five key quality standards. These CQC reports show us that organisations that have outstanding reports demonstrate leadership which enables high-quality care with a focus on learning, innovation and patient experience.[2]

In recognition of the value of leadership in healthcare, the NHS Leadership Academy was formed in 2012 with the aim of delivering inclusive and system-wide approaches to grow healthcare leaders through a variety of professional development programmes. The academy's Healthcare Leadership Model is an evidence-based approach comprising nine leadership dimensions which identifies both individual leadership behaviours and areas for leadership development.[3]

Leadership in healthcare settings

Leadership in healthcare is widely recognised as a complex process with multiple dimensions, behaviours, styles and approaches, and remains difficult to precisely define.[4] Leadership has been described as accepting responsibility to create conditions that enable others to achieve shared purposes,[5] as well as the art of influencing human behaviour to guide others towards a specific goal in such a manner as to evoke dedication, motivation, trust, respect and co-operation.[6]

The challenge for healthcare leadership is to avoid disconnect between healthcare staff and those leading the organisation in order to maintain a patient-focused safety culture that is innovative and influences productivity.[7] This can be realised by organisations which demonstrate attributes of effective leadership, including clear objectives at all levels, inspiring shared visions, engaging with staff and focusing on effective team working (Table 39.1). Thus, effective leadership is the most influential factor required to not only create an impact on developing positive work-based cultures that deliver safe and effective care[5] (Table 39.2) but also to nurture leadership by all and inspire the next generation of healthcare leaders.[8]

Approaches to leadership in healthcare settings

With increased discussion on leadership approaches in healthcare settings, a move away from historical heroic styles has emerged with a validated shift towards those leadership approaches that encourage collaboration, working across professional and organisational boundaries.[5,6] These include the following leadership approaches.

Collective leadership

Collective leadership involves an approach in which there is leadership contribution from all levels of the team, service or organisation. Shared leadership, rather than hierarchical dominance, is a key feature, enabling environments where everyone acts together to achieve high-quality organisational goals. In healthcare settings, collective leadership is not only reliant on the leadership skills of individual leaders, but requires a strategic mindset change within organisations with dedication and commitment to create a direction and enhance sustainability. This involves distribution of leadership to enable those with expertise to share the responsibility and thus, when successful, can create consistent professional leadership that is continually improving and provides high-quality compassionate care.[9,10]

Compassionate leadership

Compassionate leadership requires inclusive behaviours that are attentive, understanding, empathising and helpful to those being led. A focus on 'including all' is essential to meet the nature of compassion. Understanding that healthcare professionals have compassion as a core value within practice is crucial for organisations, as staff will expect this same compassion from their organisation's culture and leadership. Therefore, when compassion is not aligned between healthcare staff and organisational culture, staff satisfaction and motivation are affected. This has been recently demonstrated during the COVID-19 pandemic when effective teams were more likely to thrive in compassionate leadership cultures.

Compassionate leadership, however, should not be misunderstood as being a soft touch approach, as it involves courageous conversations that provide clear and honest feedback to challenge negative or disruptive behaviours.[10,11]

Transformational leadership

Identified as an important aspect of clinical leadership in order to influence workplace culture, transformational leadership has been endorsed as a healthcare leadership approach for its collection of motivational leadership behaviours. These behaviours include role modelling, inspiring shared visions and enabling others with the ability to transform people, teams or organisation through motivational and visionary leadership. Transformational leadership is recognised for transforming the workplace and safety culture through staff engagement and satisfaction.[5,12]

Systems leadership

Systems leadership represents an emerging shift away from individual organisations, with independent or silo working, to whole-systems thinking with a series of interconnected and interdependent organisations or health economies. Aimed at overcoming structural and process barriers, systems leadership enables partnerships across organisational boundaries with a focus on integrating health economies that meet the needs of their citizens within services. Enabling collaboration and connectivity, whole-systems leadership can influence large-scale changes and quality outcomes across local, regional or national systems.[8,13]

Opportunities for advanced practice

Within clinical practice, advanced practitioners have the opportunity to apply and demonstrate the core attributes of leadership whether that be via clinical leadership within the workplace or influencing strategic priorities across the healthcare system. Importantly, ensuring development of all four pillars of advanced practice will realise the value and impact of this multiprofessional workforce in delivering the healthcare needs of the future.

40 Leadership and management theories

Figure 40.1 Leadership and management traits.

Leadership	Management
• Inspires others (often described as inspirational) • Demonstrates honesty and integrity in their role • Communicates a vision effectively • Able to articulate a strategic view • Leads by example • Demonstrates informed decision making and can justify decisions • Compassionate leadership style • Displays confidence in their own ability and the ability of their team • The desire to create a learning culture • Takes responsibility for challenging decisions and the outcome • Visionary	• Understands and designs good processes • Able to execute a vision or plan • Able to effectively direct (teams, resources, plans) • Accomplished in Process Management: establish work rules, processes, standards and operating procedures • Team and people focused • Coaching skills • Productive and results orientated • Demonstrates emotional resilience

Figure 40.2 Major management theories.

Lewin's 3 Stage Change Model Kurt Lewin 1947	1. **Unfreezing**: Identifying & preparing the team to accept that change is necessary. Developing a compelling reason for change. Challenging beliefs, values, attitudes and behaviours. Stakeholder involvement important for success. Listen, manage & understand concerns. 2. **Change**: Personal transitions take place. Team members begin to resolve their uncertainty about this issue & look for ways to achieve outcomes. Lots of communication is key. Describe benefits of the change. Be able to describe how change will affect everyone. Empower the team 3. **Refreeze**: Teams will have embraced the new way of working. The change becomes embedded. It has become the new normal. Teams feel confident with the change and it is sustained. Feedback, and ongoing support and training are crucial.
Kotter's 8 Step Change Model John Kotter 1995	1. Create Urgency 2. Form a powerful coalition 3. Create a vision for change 4. Communicate the vision 5. Remove obstacles 6. Create short term wins 7. Build on the change 8. Anchor the change in organisational culture

Figure 40.3 Major leadership theories.

Timeline	Theory	Main Authors	Concepts
1840s	Great Man Theories	Historian: Thomas Carlyle	Thought that natural leaders were born with the required leadership characteristics rather than had the ability to learn these
1930s	Trait Theory	Francis Galton	Leaders can be inherited or acquired through training in leadership traits
1940s	Behavioural approaches	Rensis Likert	Believed particular leadership traits can be learned, emphasis on the behaviour of the leader. Development of leadership styles we know today
1960s	Contingent/Situational	Fred Fiedler	Believed leaders have fixed styles, so different leaders are contingent on the situation. Developed least preferred co-worker (LPC) scale to discover whether a leader was task or relationship orientated Based on leadership in particular situations; need to assess the situation & leadership style required.
1990s onwards	Transactional	Max Weber & Bernard Bass	Focus on leadership as a cost-benefit exchange
	Transformational	James MacGregor Burns	Focuses on a leadership style that inspires others and is inspirational
	Collaborative	Hank Rubin	Focuses on team members leading and supporting each other
	Servant	Robert Greenleaf Ken Blanchard & Mark Miller	Leaders who support their team members & seek to serve people first
	Inclusive	Jennifer Brown Mahzarin R. Banaji	Focuses on a person centred approach, and empowers team members to become leaders
2010 onwards	NHS Leadership Model (2013)	NHS Leadership Academy, Open University & Hay Group	NHS Values based evidenced based approach to effective leadership 9 dimensions: • Inspiring shared purpose • Leading with care • Evaluating information • Connecting services • Sharing the vision • Engaging the team • Holding to account • Developing accountability • Influencing for results
	Compassionate Leadership	Michael West	Four Key Elements • **Attending**: visibility of leaders • **Understanding**: listening with fascination • **Empathising**: really understanding the issue or problem or concern • **Helping**: what needs to happen to address this Leaders need a clear vision, alignment of clear goals at every level, and commitment, leadership that is authentic, open & honest, with humility, curious, optimistic, appreciative & compassionate.

Advanced Clinical Practice at a Glance, First Edition. Edited by Barry Hill and Sadie Diamond Fox.
© 2023 John Wiley & Sons Ltd. Published 2023 by John Wiley & Sons Ltd.

As an advanced clinical practitioner (ACP), understanding the major approaches to leadership and management theories will help you to develop your skills in this pillar of advanced practice as well as understand what may be driving others' behaviours and performance. Leading and managing teams, contributing to positive safety cultures, leading projects and implementing changes as well as influencing system change successfully as part of your ACP role mean you will be utilising leadership and management tools and theory, whether consciously or unconsciously.

While leadership and management approaches and characteristics tend to overlap, it can be helpful to remember that a *leadership approach* tends to refer to the ability to influence a team and share a vision while a *management approach* refers to someone who manages by monitoring and controlling performance, in order to maintain order and stability (Figure 40.1). Learning from history is important and there are many examples in the NHS where leadership of teams was inadequate and catastrophically failed to meet the needs of patients, their families and staff – Mid Staffordshire, Winterbourne View and Morecombe Bay come to mind. This is why understanding leadership and management theories and learning to become an effective leader are so important and incumbent on clinicians.

Management theory

Figure 40.2 gives an overview of the major management theories. These can be thought of as a set of general rules or concepts which have been designed from a specific perspective, e.g. sciences or psychology.

Change management theory

As an ACP, you will be involved in leading change rather than managing performance. This theoretical approach provides guidance for successful implementation, embedding and evaluation of change. Lewin's Model of Change and Kotter's Model of Change are two commonly adopted approaches (see Figure 40.2).

Leadership theory

Figure 41.3 gives an overview of key leadership theories. The theories commonly seen in the NHS are transactional, transformational, compassionate and the health leadership model.

Transactional leadership

This approach tends to be used by managers. It focuses on motivating and directing followers through appealing to an issue they feel strongly about; an example of this could be seen in the relationship of the sports coach and player. The power attributed to transactional leaders comes from their formal authority through the organisational culture and their use of reward and punishment. It is seen as a more authoritarian approach. A more responsive leadership approach is used through one of four methods

- *Contingent rewards*: an approach which rewards a team for achieving tasks.
- *Active management by exception*: an approach in which the leader adopts a style of managing by 'reporting by exception'. This is seen as an effective project management approach, with the assumption that everything is going to plan, using a project plan to address any goals or deadlines that are not being met, with RAG (red, amber, green) ratings in the project plan.
- *Passive management by exception*: missed deadlines and goals are not actively managed but only addressed once they affect other aspects of a team or project.

- *Lassez-faire*: while this approach is not viewed favourably by many in healthcare, there is a school of thought which believes it is a more positive approach associated with an attitude of trust and reliance on team members. Leaders avoid micromanagement and strong guidance. This is thought to encourage team members to develop their own leadership skills but there are associated risks in situations where strong direction may be required, such as in a resuscitation situation.

Transformational leadership

This differs from a transactional style in that the leader takes a more motivational approach to leadership. The mainstay of this approach involves encouraging, inspiring and motivating a team. It is seen as an ideal approach to take when an organisation is going through significant change. Transformational leaders are generally seen as energetic, enthusiastic and passionate who create a vision and inspire others to share their goal. Examples of transformational leaders include Steve Jobs and Bill Gates.

Compassionate leadership

Michael West believes that compassionate leadership enhances the intrinsic motivation of staff and reinforces their fundamental altruism. It helps promote a culture of learning, where risk taking is seen as acceptable within safe boundaries, and it is accepted that not all innovation will be successful. This approach promotes staff psychological safety and in turn the team feel able to raise safety concerns, as well as feeling empowered to develop and implement new and different ways to solve problems in a system, while accepting that not everything will be successful. This approach results in collaborative and co-operative working in teams with increased staff cohesion, optimism and well-being.

There are four core elements which underpin this approach.
- Being present
- Understanding staff distress
- Ability to empathise
- Motivation to intervene and make a difference

Health leadership model

Developed by the NHS Leadership Academy, this comprises 9 elements (see Figure 40.3). It is an evidence-based research model which highlights the importance of clarifying the behaviours expected of leaders working within the NHS that reflects:
- the values of the NHS
- what is known about effective leadership
- patients' views of leadership in the NHS.

Three core themes were developed from the evidence-based approach.

1 Providing and justifying a clear sense of purpose and contribution which embraces behaviours and skills in leaders to promote an explicit focus on the needs and experiences of service users.
2 The motivation of teams to work effectively, including the ability to work collaboratively with other organisations and occupations and construct a positive team emotional climate.
3 Focus on improved system performance, by encouraging service improvement.

This leadership approach synthesises a variety of approaches to provide a toolkit for best practice in leadership within the NHS.

Conclusion

This chapter has provided an overview of the main leadership and management theories that ACPs may incorporate into their professional practice, at both a systems and an organisation level.

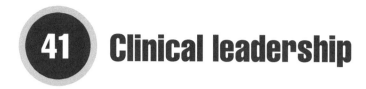

41 Clinical leadership

Table 41.1 Attributes of a clinical leader

Role model	Resilient	Demonstrate courage
Effective communication skills	Supportive	Self-awareness
Inspirational	Current	Compassionate
Transparent	Technologically comfortable	Kind
Honest	Adaptable to change	Innovative
Skilled	Responsible	Driven
Confident	Visionary	Emotional intelligence
Committed	Capable of building strong relationships	Discipline
Enthusiastic	Open-minded	Invested
Consistent	Clinically competent	Willingness to try
Intuitive		Integrity

Figure 41.1 Leadership capabilities of advanced practice (adapted from https://onlinelibrary.wiley.com/doi/full/10.1002/nop2.150)

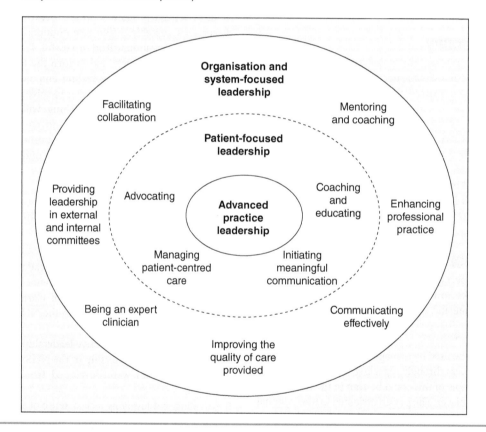

Healthcare services are facing unprecedented challenges: a global health pandemic, ageing population, limited funding and a workforce crisis. Strong clinical leadership is vital in ensuring high-quality, safe, compassionate, inclusive and cost-effective care. Effective clinical leadership delivered throughout an organisation, from the board of directors to patient-facing clinicians, is influential in shaping culture and improving care. As identified in the NHS Long Term Plan, priority must be given to developing the next generation of clinical leaders. The focus has shifted from the traditional role of trained managers to promoting and engaging clinicians to take formal and informal roles in strategic leadership. This is echoed in the publication of *Clinical Leadership – A Framework For Action* which outlines the importance of widening opportunity for all clinicians to be given access to leadership roles. The vision is to drive quality care and innovation, with patient experience and safety remaining the common goals. This shared leadership allows clinicians to use their expertise and experience to contribute to improving organisational performance.

What is clinical leadership?

Clinical leadership refers to anyone with a clinical background in a leadership role. Their leadership style is founded on clinical expertise, enabling them to identify, influence and drive care and innovation to improve patient safety and outcomes. Clinical leadership can be delivered in both a formal leadership role, as part of a clinical management team, or informally in everyday work by undertaking additional roles and responsibilities. It is integral to both maintaining a standard of care and driving transformational change to improve services, patient and population outcomes. By recognising that clinicians are central to shaping services and driving change, organisations can empower and support all members of staff to reach their full potential. Individually, the clinician adopts their leadership role as part of their clinical identity and professional responsibility, motivating them to deliver efficient, good quality safe care.

Clinical leadership vs management

It is important to understand the difference between clinical leadership and management because an organisation cannot function without both. Managers focus on the task in hand, directing individuals within an already structured team or through policy and procedure. Clinical leaders drive change by creating a vision, setting direction and developing relationships with key stakeholders, inspiring engagement from the team.

What makes a good clinical leader?

Through the evolution of the current healthcare structure, it is recognised that clinical leadership cannot be the responsibility of one professional body of clinicians. Instead, it is a shared concept, with everyone identified as having the potential to develop into a leadership role. Shared leadership is achieved by focusing on developing the collective, not just individuals. Whilst there are personal attributes that highlight an individual's potential to progress (Table 41.1), core skills like change management can be learned through competency frameworks and internal and external courses. To provide opportunities for everyone, the organisation must commit to investing in mentorship, education and development programmes. This will enable an enhanced opportunity to build advanced practice capabilities (see figure 41.1).

Personal attributes

Effective clinical leaders are those who demonstrate personal attributes including, but not limited to, self-awareness, integrity, confidence, positivity, approachability, consistency and emotional maturity. They understand their strengths and weaknesses, and manage their behaviour depending on both the situation and the behaviours of their team and organisation. This is essential to meet the needs of the team and service users and will positively impact on overall engagement, reinforcing a focus on care and service delivery.

Clinical competence

In addition to personal attributes, clinical competence is key in leading a team successfully. Clinical leaders who understand the clinical environment and possess the skills to maintain a high level of safe care can cultivate an environment of clinical safety, enabling the workforce to identify necessary areas of change. Effective communication, empowering the team to raise concerns, promoting well-being, self-care and embedding a supportive culture are key in ensuring a healthy workforce, which will then improve focus, service delivery and patient experience.

Organisational structure

To promote and value clinical leadership, organisations must be open to change and support the development of clinical leaders. They will in turn drive change, both within the clinical area and more globally, to improve overall experience and promote excellent clinical practice, efficiency and outcomes for patients. Clinicians should be both supported and encouraged to undertake leadership programmes and empowered to apply their own leadership styles and their own judgement in clinical scenarios.

Introducing leadership opportunities and mentorship at every level emphasises the value of collective clinical leadership. For collective leadership to be successful, the organisational culture must be clear about its vision, values and expectation. It must also promote cross-boundary working to inspire and encourage clinicians to work as a team towards a common goal, rather than solely on their individual achievements. Financial investment is required to secure the future leadership team and demonstrate a commitment from the organisation to the clinical team in driving change.

Clinical leadership within advanced practice

In the current structure, advanced practitioners are often overlooked for formal leadership roles because they predominantly work in clinical settings. However, they provide leadership at the forefront of patient care and lead change. They often work in complex situations, applying clinical expertise and decision making in unpredictable settings.

As with all clinicians, advanced practitioners should be encouraged and supported to develop their clinical leadership skills. This includes encouraging enrolment in leadership development programmes and being supported to recognise transferable skills from everyday practice which can be applied to more formalised clinical leadership roles. NHS England offers a range of programmes and resources to aid budding advanced practice leaders in discovering their full potential: www.leadershipacademy.nhs.uk/.

Advanced practitioners play a vital role in patient safety, service delivery and research, and should be both recognised and valued for their potential contribution to clinical leadership in informal and formal settings.

Conclusion

- Clinical leadership plays a vital part in an organisation's overall performance, improving service delivery and patient safety.
- Clinical leadership is a driving force in shaping the future of healthcare systems and should be embraced.
- Healthcare organisations must commit to investing in the education and development of future clinical leaders at all career levels.
- Clinicians need to be open and comfortable with the process of adaptive change.
- Clinical leadership cannot succeed without the engagement of a team.

42 Educational leadership

Figure 42.1 The leadership capabilities of advanced practitioners. Source: Lamb et al.[2]/John Wiley & Sons.

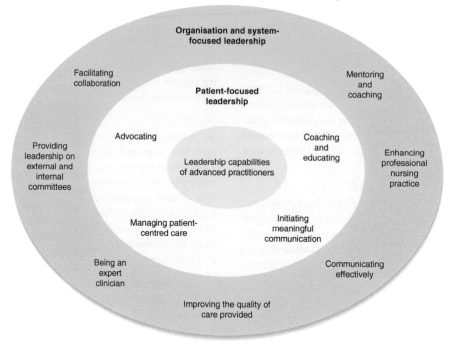

Table 42.1 Patient-focused leadership capability domains and capabilities. Source: Adapted from Lamb et al.[2]/John Wiley & Sons.

Domain and definition	Capabilities
1. Managing patient-centred care: using clinical expertise in combination with advanced nursing knowledge to provide appropriate, high-quality, patient-centred care to patients and families	1.1 Providing clinical expertise in a specialty area – having specialised clinical expertise that is refined to meet the unique needs of the population they serve
	1.2 Leading teams – taking on a leading role within the healthcare team
	1.3 Promoting goal-oriented care – focusing on achieving the healthiest outcomes for patients and families
	1.4 Using system-level knowledge – understanding how the healthcare system operates, who and what is involved at different levels and moving patients through the system was described by all participants as necessary for creating a seamless care experience for patients
2. Coaching and educating – fostering trusting relationships and capitalising on teachable moments. The two capabilities of this domain are:	2.1 Facilitating independence and autonomy – capitalising on opportunities to educate patients and families about disease processes, medications and new therapies
	2.2 Listening and explaining – taking the time to listen to patients and clearly explain a diagnosis or a new treatment is crucial for patient acquisition of skills for self-management
3. Advocating – being a patient advocate	3.1 Being a strong voice, negotiating an their behalf – representing and voicing patient and family needs at different forums and assisting patients and families to feel safe and that the system is meeting their needs
4. Initiating meaningful communication – communicating with patients regardless of circumstances	4.1 Addressing the uncomfortable topics – initiating and addressing the more challenging topics and the tough conversations is perceived to positively affect patients and families, because they are able to talk about uncomfortable and difficult elements of their care

Advanced Clinical Practice at a Glance, First Edition. Edited by Barry Hill and Sadie Diamond Fox.
© 2023 John Wiley & Sons Ltd. Published 2023 by John Wiley & Sons Ltd.

As healthcare organisations are rapidly changing to meet the needs of the population they serve, those within the service need to be able to adapt to and steer this change based on their knowledge of the system and recognition of the quality improvements required.[1] Leadership is a crucial part of the ACP role, with multiple themes and capability domains having been identified in previous studies[2] (Figure 42.1, Tables 42.1). There are clear links between organisational awareness and commitment to commissioning education that bring clear benefits to patient care.

Organisational level

The advanced clinical practitioner's (ACP) educational role at the organisational level is to play a part in ascertaining the learning needs of the organisation, to lead on quality improvement projects and to involve key stakeholders in a spirit of co-production to benefit patients and provide high-quality care. This will involve collaboration across professions and other agencies, as well as engagement with the wider community to build relationships and support workforce transformation. A key focus will be on the development and evaluation of training programmes across the organisation to develop the workforce to meet the population's needs. As such, ACPs need to lead on and contribute to clarification of the organisation's strategic objectives, allocation of resources and training aligned to these organisational goals.

Teamwork

It has long been recognised that effective multiprofessional teamworking improves both patient outcome and satisfaction of team members and much of the ACP role should focus on team cohesion, motivation and development. The ACP is also a role model for others by recognising their development needs and ensuring the development of a solid skill mix to meet the needs of diverse population whilst also enabling team members to support each other and work towards maximising their potential.

This is achieved through development of learning activities, supervision and assessment. The focus is not just on competency development but also on creating a supportive learning culture where staff can be open and honest, and engage in peer review and critical reflection. Whilst the ACP will create educational packages, and map against competency requirements, a key focus is on workforce development to ensure a highly skilled, knowledgeable workforce that can engage in complex decision making to ensure the needs of the population are met and to develop succession plans for the future workforce.

Advanced clinical practitioners thus require continued development in their own roles so that they can provide this coaching, mentorship, peer review and support of others and maintain both their strategic influence and guidance of workforce development. This is both an individual and employer responsibility.

Individual level

The requirement for educational development was recognised in the Department of Health proposals to reform professional regulation in 2017. These included the development of standards for higher levels of practice. The resultant standards set out in the Multi-Professional Framework for Advanced Clinical Practice in England[1] advocated for ACPs to be educated to Master's level. There has been little research specifically addressing the educational preparation of ACPs, but the variety of roles and remits makes a generic education programme challenging and highlights the importance of flexibility as the key to success. The Multi-Professional Framework for Advanced Clinical Practice in England[1] requires the ACP to consistently demonstrate skills of critical reflection on one's own practice, both professionally and personally, and supporting others to reflect on their practice.

Distributive leadership and education

There has been a recent shift toward leadership styles that acknowledge the unique and differing influences that healthcare professionals, particularly within ACP roles, have upon the leadership style that educators must adopt. Effective leadership is becoming increasingly recognised as paramount to the delivery of high standards of education, research and clinical practice. As such, an emerging leadership style within healthcare settings is that of distributive leadership through a 'consortium approach'.

Distributive leadership encompasses multiple parties (e.g. higher education institutes, Health Education England, healthcare professionals), there is more than one designated leader, ideas are shared, democratic principles are promoted and there is a fully collaborative approach. DL can help to maximise mutual mentoring capacity to establish a sustainable teaching and learning community of practice.

Case study – Demonstrating Educational leadership

Lorna Malcolm works as clinical team lead for a community palliative care team. As a physiotherapist, Lorna has played a leading role in advancing rehabilitative palliative care practice.

Bedside education

Lorna's main education role is through bedside education, championing a rehabilitative approach to care throughout the hospice and through continued professional development of herself and her staff team.

Formal evidence-based teaching

Lorna, as a senior team member, plays a part in the strategic development of education in line with the organisational goals. She also regularly leads and teaches study days run out of the hospice. Her teaching is informed by her practice, her own research into patient experiences of group exercise classes in a hospice setting, and continued peer review evaluation of her teaching by those who attend.

Presentations and publications

Inspiring learning outside her own institution, Lorna has presented her work at conferences such as the European Association of Palliative Care and written a chapter in Wiley's *Palliative Care Nursing at a Glance* textbook. Conference attendance, presentations and publications widen access to networks of diverse disciplines informing individual and team practice.

43 Research leadership

Table 43.1 Key research leadership competencies for advanced clinical practitioners

- *Technical proficiency* – necessary to evaluate, generate and implement evidence.
- *Capacity building* – vital to sustain and grow the critical mass of ACPs engaged with and leading research.
- *Research situational awareness* – demonstrating a critical gaze about practice at individual, organisational and professional levels.
- *Social consciousness* – embracing a person-centred approach to practice which uses research to advocate for solutions to societal challenges.

Table 43.2 Leadership Skills

Leadership skills	Advanced leadership skills
Performing a SWOT analysis of yourself and healthcare organisation	Intercultural leadership
Conflict resolution and management	Transformational leadership
Providing constructive feedback	Effective delegation
Defining and communicating innovative vision	Empowerment of patients and service users
Motivating people	Empowerment of colleagues at all levels
Situational leadership	Change management & negotiating
Effective communication	Awareness and ethical utilisation of finances and spending
Complex project management of multiple projects	Effective and transparent notes and administration

Figure 43.1 Plan Do Study Act (PDSA) cycle.
Source: [9]/Gov.UK/Public Domain (OGL)

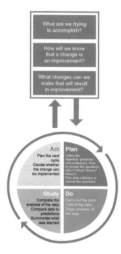

Advanced Clinical Practice at a Glance, First Edition. Edited by Barry Hill and Sadie Diamond Fox.
© 2023 John Wiley & Sons Ltd. Published 2023 by John Wiley & Sons Ltd.

The Health Education England Advanced Clinical Practitioner (ACP) framework emphasises expectations of research leadership which go far beyond the demonstration of adequate technical research skills (i.e. the necessary knowledge to appraise evidence, conduct research studies, analyse data, author publications, etc.), to demand a critical gaze which continuously examines individual, organisational and collective practice (Table 43.1).

This mandate to review and refine clinical practice in an iterative manner should not be taken, obviously, as a limitation for other nursing professionals or any other members of the interdisciplinary team to engage in research, but for ACPs to recognise the emphasis placed on them to shape and influence systems and services through research and the research agenda. In such sense, it would not be so much about one's own evidence-based practice, but the promotion of collective practice which is underpinned by evidence.

Further, this critical perspective should not just encourage an up-to-date practice, defining the boundaries of what is known or how practice should be enacted, for example in relation to models of care or emerging competencies. ACPs aiming to be proficient in research leadership competencies should also embrace how to stop ineffective and wasteful practices, for example by championing Choosing Wisely perspectives.[1]

Advanced clinical practitioners often report uncertainty and insecurity about their ever-growing and frequently changing scope of practice and spheres of influence. Even with those restraints, or precisely because of the fluidity of the role, ACPs are ideally positioned to span boundary, intersecting different professional disciplines, pivoting on the various levels of expertise held by different roles (i.e. from specialists to consultants), influencing care settings (i.e. primary or secondary) and supporting practice networks (i.e. clinical and academic, and even industry). They can act as 'knowledge brokers', promoting opportunities and accepting a responsibility to nurture structures which facilitate and promote their own research as well as the research of others.

Advanced clinical practitioners may harness the current policy and political environment regarding clinical academic roles and embed their research leadership efforts in lobbying and advocacy messages, acting in synergy with other professionals at different levels of practice and stages in the clinical and academic journey to underpine claims for far-reaching consideration of ACP roles.

Advanced clinical practitioner research leadership is vital to induce a ripple effect which could sustain a critical mass of ACP researchers who would then continue generating evidence about not only their own practice but the ACP role in general. This evidence would help mitigate the uncertainties mentioned, if not about the ACP role itself, then about areas such as the implementation, evaluation, growth and optimal scope of practice of ACPs. If these gaps are addressed, then it is likely that the adoption of advanced clinical roles in other healthcare systems would be galvanised and expanded. In essence, it would be the responsibility of ACPs to consider what evidence is required to enable more similar and innovative posts to be funded, demonstrating clinical, professional and social impact.

Embracing social responsibilities within research leadership

The idea that research leadership of ACPs should include social and societal perspectives may be counterintuitive, such seems to be the importance attributed to the 'clinical' label in their title. For this reason, it may be tempting to consider research mainly from a clinical, bedside, biology and pathology angle. However, a person-centred approach to clinical practice should ensure that determinants at all levels which influence and shape the health and well-being of patients are considered, with ACPs attuned to the interventions and solutions needed to address societal challenges.

This societal perspective of research leadership is coupled with a need to demonstrate social skills in research, among them communication, engagement, influencing and negotiating to advocate for the diffusion, implementation and adoption of research findings, as the HEE framework clearly stresses when it mentions 'alerting appropriate individuals and organisations' of the gaps in the evidence base. This alerting could also be interpreted as an opportunity to engage with and steer professional and scientific organisations so they recognise the evidence and gaps, contributing to the determination of practice.

Combining the influencing and communication skills held by ACPs, their participation in professional societies and the mandate to disseminate and promote research findings suggests a clear pathway for ACPs to get involved in shaping health and social care policies so that they are based in evidence. This involvement of ACPs in policy by providing their research expertise and highlighting existing evidence may also help to further reduce the variations in expectations, poor role recognition among citizens and the different professions feeding into ACP roles, and from a global perspective, the alignment of roles in the UK with innovative thought and evidence currents worldwide.

Impact – an unexplored domain of research leadership in advanced clinical practice

A final area where ACPs ought to demonstrate research leadership is impact. Whilst there seems to be little doubt of the clinical benefits for patients, organisations and health and social care services once ACP roles are implemented, debates about their impact often do not take into account education and particularly research activity. Additionally, proposals to balance clinical and research time for ACPs portray research as an opportunity cost of clinical time (i.e. research is costed using the estimated value of clinical work which could have been carried out instead) or appreciate the value of research in terms of funding income generated for the organisation or savings from reduced organisational costs incurred,[2] without reflecting upon the benefits of mentorship, supporting and encouraging future ACP leaders.

Conclusion

In summary, excellence in research leadership for ACPs encompasses much more than conducting research, affording wider and richer opportunities and responsibilities for professionals in advanced roles.

44 Improving quality of care

Table 44.1 Principles of quality improvement

Quality principle	Description in relation to quality improvement
Safety	Avoidance of harm through identification and management of risk to people from healthcare that is intended to help them
Person-centred	Provision of care that is focused on the needs, values and choices of the individual, including enabling codesign of care with service users, families, carers and colleagues
Effectivity	Use of evidence to provide care that has an intended and expected beneficial effect
Efficiency	Aimed at producing maximum beneficial effect with minimum wasted expense or effort. This requires improvements to be timely and sustainable, with judicious use of resources to achieve the desired outcome
Equity	To ensure personal characteristics (e.g. age, gender, ethnicity, socioeconomic status) do not unfairly affect the quality of care received

Figure 44.1 Outline of the quality improvement process. Source: ⁹/Gov.UK/ Public Domain (OGL)

1. Start out	2. Define and scope	3. Measure and understand	4. Design and plan	5. Pilot and implement	6. Sustain and share

Table 44.2 Root cause analysis tools

Tool	When to use it
Affinity diagram	To brainstorm ideas and/or group them into themes
Cause and effect (fishbone) diagram	To visually summarise the findings of the affinity diagram
'5 Whys'	To identify why issues are happening by developing a questioning attitude to problems
Data check sheet	To gather and store data in a structured format
Pareto analysis	To identify the major causes of a problem needing improving
Histogram	To show continuous data and highlight where or when problems happen to help focus improvement interventions
Scatter diagram	To illustrate the relationship and the association between two variables which may be correlated (or not)
Questionnaire and survey	To gain feedback on the service delivered from the patient and family perspective
Quantitative analysis (i.e. audit, service analysis)	To evaluate the service against national standards and measure results after implementing interventions and over time
Identify frustrating problems	To illustrate, discuss and solve problems within the work environment

Table 44.3 Mapping process tools

Tool	When to use it
Conventional process mapping	Before making any service changes to help gain better understanding of how a whole-patient pathway works
Value stream mapping	To understand the steps in the patient journey and patient experience. Often undertaken during rapid improvement events when key stakeholders use a dedicated block of time to make improvements happen
Spaghetti diagram	To assess time wasted through unnecessary movement through a ward, clinic, department or whole hospital. Helps to identify how to save time by visualising unnecessary movement of products, staff or patients
Mapping the last 10 patients	To demonstrate what is really happening to patients along their journey. It may expose differences in practice or workload, which can cause unhelpful variation and unnecessary delays, and compromise safe care
Process template	When undertaking a conventional process map or value stream map to identify the bottlenecks/constraints in the patient journey
Tracer study	To understand the flow of information that supports clinical care processes. Use this tool in addition to conventional process mapping to give a more detailed picture of what happens in real time within information processes and flow
Sort and share	To focus on how the working environment affects services; this is a useful tool as it helps to identify where changes need to be made in addition to helping staff to create and maintain a safer environment for patients, staff and visitors

Advanced Clinical Practice at a Glance, First Edition. Edited by Barry Hill and Sadie Diamond Fox.
© 2023 John Wiley & Sons Ltd. Published 2023 by John Wiley & Sons Ltd.

What is quality improvement in healthcare and why is it important?

The King's Fund and the Health Foundation[1] note that:

'Now, more than ever, local and national NHS leaders need to focus on improving quality and delivering better-value care. All NHS organisations should be focused on continually improving quality of care for people using their services. This includes improving the safety, effectiveness and experience of care'.

Whilst their report was completed in 2017 and much has changed in that time (including a global pandemic), there has been a continued commitment to improving quality of care.[2]

In agreed definitions of advanced clinical practice, quality improvement is a key feature.[3-5] This includes an expectation that ACPs use their knowledge, skills and experience to engage with complex decision making, using the autonomy afforded by their role to enable 'innovative solutions to enhance people's experience and improve outcomes'. ACPs are expected to 'lead new practice and service redesign solutions in response to feedback, evaluation and need, working across boundaries' to 'continually develop practice in response to changing population health need, engaging in horizon scanning for future developments'.[3]

Quality improvement is multifaceted, and whilst quality may mean different things to different people at different times, there is a set of principles that underpin quality improvement (Table 44.1). These are echoed in the standards expected of ACPs as registered healthcare professionals through their regulatory bodies.[6,7]

Stakeholders and assessing feasibility

In order for a quality improvement project to be successful, consideration must be given to both the needs of and possible impact (positive or negative) on those affected by the project. We should not underestimate the powerful contribution that can be made by patients, families, carers and colleagues in shaping the project to ensure it achieves its goals. Determining who the key stakeholders are should occur at an early stage, before specific aims, actions and outcome measures are planned, to ensure they are fit for purpose.

Use of SCOT analysis to collect the perspectives of stakeholders on the Strengths, Challenges, Opportunities and Threats to the project can be helpful in shaping initial planning and assessing the feasibility of a project. Stakeholder analysis can also be used to identify persons who can be engaged to facilitate the project and those who may need persuasion to prevent blockages or obstructions to the project's progress.[8]

Feedback should be actively sought from stakeholders, with the default position being that they are involved in the design and production of the project. Through engagement with stakeholders, the resources that will be needed to successfully deliver the project can be identified. Resource consideration is not just ensuring that sufficient funding is in place, but also working out what facilities, access arrangements, people and information may be needed.

A communications plan or matrix should be developed to capture who needs to know what, and when, about the project. This will help to keep the project on track and ensure people remain on board with the proposed changes. Responsibility charting can be used alongside the communications plan and updated as the project is developed to ensure everyone involved is clear about their role and responsibilities in delivering the quality improvement.[8]

Problem identification and models for improvement

The six steps of the quality improvement process can be found in Figure 44.1. This starts with identifying the scope of the project. Define what will be included/excluded by answering the questions 'What? When? Where? Who?'. This will promote clarity and ensure each member is working in the same direction.[9]

A root cause analysis of the problem is paramount as the project should focus on the cause, rather than the effect of the problem. Initial quantitative or qualitative analysis will help to capture and evaluate relevant data.[8] Specific tools can support development of understanding by gaining insight into the causes of the problem, before making interventions or changes based on assumptions (Table 44.2). This prevents mistaken conclusions and ensures problem solving is factual and evidence based.[10]

Improbable causes should be removed through general agreement and the verified causes should be ordered in terms of priority.[11] If a project is large and complex, the team may focus on issues which will have the biggest impact within the resources available (time, funding, staff, expertise). Through this process, the project objectives can be agreed and established; these will be the focal points for the 'design and plan' stage. It is important in this stage to identify all the tasks and activities that need to be delivered. During this process, the use of SMART goals and GANTT charts can help in identification of actions and timelines.[8]

When implementing changes, it is advisable to pilot the intervention on a small scale first before wider implementation. Using the Plan, Do, Study, Act (PDSA) cycle enables testing interventions and learning in a structured framework (see Chapter 43, Figure 43.1).[8]

Quality improvement methods

In deciding which methods to use, it is important to know what needs to be tested, what should be achieved, and how outcomes will be measured.[12,13] Process mapping allows visual representation of the different steps of the journey and overall picture (Table 44.3). This enables teams to understand the project, engage effectively in their part of the process, and identify any points of inefficiency and duplication. Tracking the project through a process map can highlight how well the project is developing and offers the opportunity to reflect on issues that may arise and address them where needed.[14]

Process mapping should connect with measuring the project's actual performance to evaluate the real impact of decisions and actions taken.[15] The Statistical Process Control tool can support data analysis of the outcomes previously defined in the 'design and plan' stage.[8,9] Indicator measurements should be recorded and analysed throughout the project delivery and beyond to ensure that the changes implemented are beneficial.

Regardless of the outcome, dissemination of the results of the project should form part of the communications plan. Mistakes should be highlighted to avoid them being repeated by others, and examples of effective practice should be shared widely to act as a beneficial learning experience.[15]

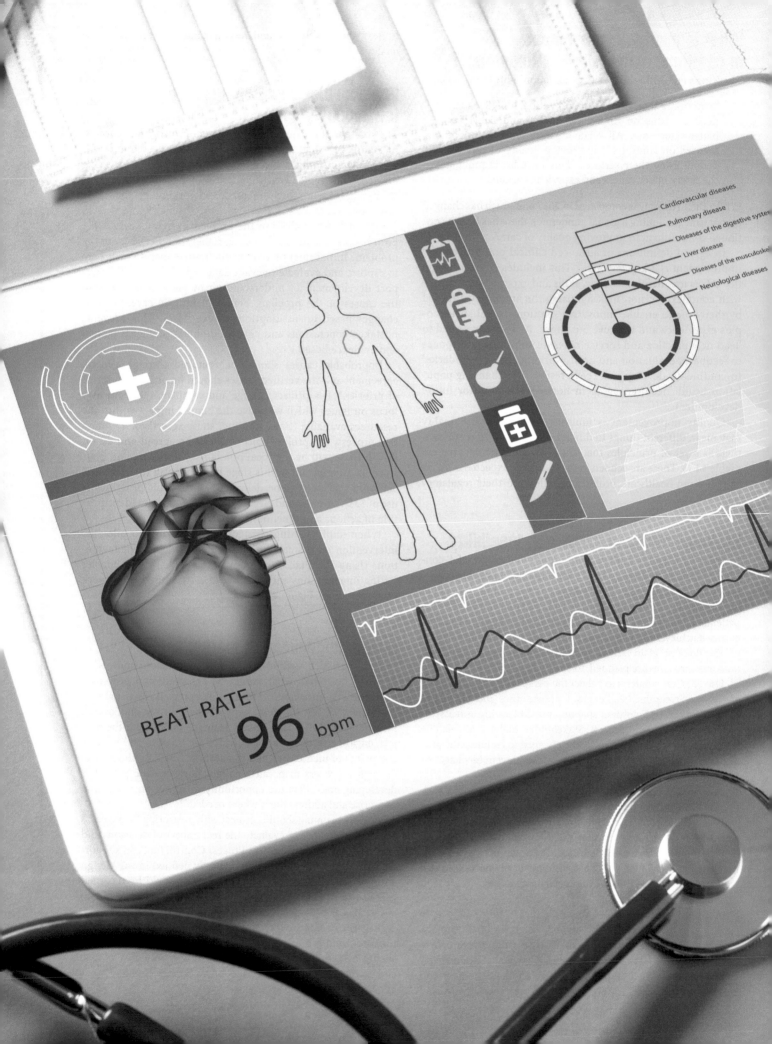

BEAT RATE
96 bpm

Cardiovascular diseases
Pulmonary disease
Diseases of the digestive system
Liver disease
Diseases of the musculoskel
Neurological diseases

Advanced clinical practice education

Part 6

Chapters

45 Exploring the challenges with advanced clinical practice education

Table 45.1 Challenges concerning ACP education and actions identified at system (macro) and regional (advanced practice faculties/employers/HEI) (meso) levels[1,2]

Challenges	Issues	Activities by/for: government agencies/HEIs/employers/tACPs
1. Ensuring that professionals working at ACP level have the knowledge, skills and behaviours relevant to their professional setting and job role	1a. Developing curricula to meet generic and specialist advanced practice content and capabilities aligned to four pillars of professional practice 1b. Defining and ensuring tACPs are able to meet area-specific/specialist capabilities in the ACP programme alongside generic knowledge and capabilities	1a. Developing curricula which meet HEI academic regulations, national ACP frameworks, generic and area-specific/specialist capabilities – with national accreditation or recognition for programmes where available 1b. Using national ACP frameworks and area-specific/specialist capabilities to inform curricula, programme structure, teaching, learning and assessment strategies to meet academic and clinical capabilities 1c. Collaboration between employers, HEIs and tACPs to confirm role requirements and ensure range of placements/experience available to meet role and area-specific/specialist capabilities and accreditation (see below) 1d. HEIs/employers identify relevant academic and workplace-based supervision, support and assessment (see below)
2. Promoting implementation and application that allow for local context but result in sufficient consistency to transform the workforce in line with national government priorities	2a. Informing the development and implementation of national ACP frameworks and area-specific capabilities to introduce greater consistency of role definition and capabilities between HEI programmes 2b. Working with Association of Advanced Practice Educators (AAPE), national ACP centres/boards and regional faculties for advanced practice, undertaking accreditation of ACP programmes, developing routes of equivalence, maintaining a directory of ACP practitioners	2a. HEIs/employers/tACPs: improving awareness of national ACP frameworks and developments, including impact of these frameworks on HEI programmes – level of award, learning outcomes, teaching, learning and assessment requirements 2b. HEIs/employers: engaging with developments in ACP credentials, roles, governance 2c. HEIs: incorporating recognition of prior learning and portfolio routes into programme approval and delivery
3. Encouraging collaboration between educators and employers to enable practitioners to develop their abilities, particularly clinical capabilities, and for supervisory and assessment purposes		3a. Employers/ACPs/tACPs: map core capabilities and area-specific/specialist capabilities to service opportunities to identify appropriate placements and where gaps may exist requiring reciprocal arrangements to be developed 3b. Health boards/regional HEE/employers: establish process for local reciprocal arrangements between organisations to enable tACPs access to services/supervision to achieve workplace-based supervision and achievement of clinical capabilities 3c. HEIs/employers: agree criteria for workplace-based co-ordinating education supervisors and associate supervisors; recruit and provide training and support 3d. HEIs/employers: consider a formal support network across regions for ACP practice co-ordinating education supervisors and associate supervisors 3e. HEIs/employers/ACPs: discuss continuing supervision and support needs of ACPs following successful completion of programme and transition to ACP role
4. Focus on an outcome-driven approach	4. Ensuring rigour across all four pillars of professional practice with associated standard of teaching, learning and assessment	4a. HEIs/employers: collaborative curriculum development meeting HEI regulations, national frameworks and area-specific/specialist credentials, apprenticeship standard 4b. HEIs/employers/ACPs/tACPs: improve understanding about ACP developments across the workforce and service users 4c. HEIs: incorporate four pillars of professional practice and associated capabilities in teaching, learning and assessment strategies

Table 45.1 (Continued)

Challenges	Issues	Activities by/for: government agencies/HEIs/employers/tACPs
5. Promote portfolio approaches and consistent, transparent processes for accreditation or recognition of prior learning		5a. HEE (or equivalent)/HEIs/AAPE: guidance for establishing an equivalence route for demonstrating advanced practice capabilities and Master's level thinking and practice – how to understand, measure, test and evidence these
6. Collaborating across an area or place if necessary to optimise cost-effective training with flexibility to develop generic capabilities and area-specific/specialist competence	6. Specialist module(s)/programmes may need to be delivered across each country, regionally to be educationally and financially viable	6a. HEIs/employers: co-ordinate recruitment to tACP roles, identifying range of programmes and modules required and available
7. ACP developments must be multiprofessional and encompass interprofessional learning and support		7a. Employers: reviewing service delivery and identifying opportunities for developing multiprofessional ACP services/roles 7b. Employers/HEIs: interprofessional learning and teaching strategies; range of clinical supervisors
8. Responding to apprenticeship requirements and royal colleges/faculties involvement in credentialling programmes	8. Concerns re erosion of professional identity if royal colleges drive credentialing of specialist skills in ACP education and if ACP roles regarded, or used, as doctor substitutes in service	8a. Employers/HEIs/ACPs/tACPs: develop understanding of apprenticeship requirements and structuring programmes to accommodate the end point assessment 8b. HEIs: contribute nationally (for example, via AAPE) to development of area-specific/specialty credentials
9. Enable ACP education to flourish	9a. Planning and long- term investment for HEIs to develop capacity and capability, investing in ACP programmes. 9b. Timely notification about commissions– funding and applications. Fees funding for learners	9a. Funding identified by UK nations for ACP workforce development 9b. HEIs/employers: working regionally to establish timely and co-ordinated processes for recruitment to ACP programmes, clinical educator criteria, opportunities for shared placements, sharing innovative practice

This chapter explores the challenges with ACP education for governmental bodies, higher education institutions (HEIs), employers and trainee ACPs (tACPs) resulting from historic and current system-wide changes, and the work being undertaken to achieve the clarity, consistency and standardisation required for the role and to facilitate wider service transformation.

Background/context

Globally, the integration of advanced practice roles into healthcare organisations and systems has evolved iteratively over time as roles have been introduced in an *ad hoc* manner and the formal policies and practices necessary to support optimal role implementation, legislation, regulation, competencies and education have lagged behind the informal introduction of the roles. These significant variations in ACP education, skills and experiences have led to a bespoke approach to role deployment, impeded system-wide innovation and created challenges to recruitment and ongoing professional development of role holders.

Calls for clarity, consistency and standardisation of the ACP role and education pathway led to the creation of national frameworks which aim to support UK healthcare providers to deliver sustainable ACP services. These frameworks make evident the changes required at system (macro), regional (meso) and individual employer/higher education institution (HEI)/tACP (micro) levels when introducing, developing and supporting ACP and embedding ACP roles in the workplace.

The introduction of these system-wide changes to ACP across the four UK nations has also required changes to ACP education and support to establish consistent education standards and credentialling systems, including work to define area-specific or specialty capabilities within the four pillars of professional practice, and secure sustainable funding to develop this workforce. This is a rapidly developing field, requiring co-ordination nationally, regionally and locally, and there also exists variation in academic and clinical support and supervision arrangements for tACPs associated with geography, pathway, practice context and roles.

System standard setting for, and co-ordination of, ACP education

In response to the rapidly evolving ACP policy developments, in 2018, the Council of Deans of Health together with Health Education England (HEE) and other stakeholders discussed the future of ACP education to optimise the outcomes required by health policy, employers and the workforce. The challenges and actions identified at system (macro) and regional (advanced practice faculties/employers/HEI) (meso) levels are summarised in Table 46.1 alongside those obtained from a region-wide survey of employers/HEIs/tACP (micro) levels.[1]

Broadly, challenges for ACP education relate to the following.

- *Curriculum development and programme delivery*: using national frameworks defining generic and area-specific/specialist capabilities in education programmes; HEI and external accreditation and quality assurance processes of programmes; co-ordination of ACP programme development, recruitment and delivery; recognition of prior learning.

- *Education routes to ACP roles and sustainable funding*: co-ordinating and aligning recruitment to tACP roles and education programmes; apprenticeship standard and levy (in England); portfolio equivalence route; development and inclusion of area-specific/specialist ACP curriculum, capabilities and accreditation.
- *Teaching, learning and assessment*: interprofessional learning/teaching; Master's level achievement of capabilities for four pillars of professional practice; academic and work-place support, supervision and assessment.
- *Workplace-based supervision and assessment*: securing access to range of experience to achieve generic/core and area-specific/specialist capabilities; supervisor/assessor criteria, role descriptors and preparation; assuring quality of supervision and assessment.

Whilst focused on HEIs in England, challenges similar to those identified in Table 45.1 may emerge for UK and international education providers. As is evident in Table 46.1, significant collaboration is required at all levels between employers, HEIs, ACPs and tACPs to ameliorate these challenges.

Development and delivery of ACP education – workplace-based and academic support and supervision

The challenges identified in Table 45.1 illustrate the workplace-based (clinical) supervision and support, alongside ongoing professional supervision, that tACPs require to ensure achievement of the generic and area-specific/specialist capabilities across the four pillars of practice, alongside meeting the academic requirements of the ACP programme.

In the workplace, tACPs are supported through clinical supervision from experienced practitioners. Clinical supervision provides an opportunity for practitioners to reflect on their clinical practice, discuss individual case studies and identify changes to practice required to maintain professional and public safety. It provides an opportunity to identify training and continuing development needs. For tACPs, clinical supervision also relates to developing and demonstrating achievement of the core generic capabilities of advanced practice, and national/local, area-specific/specialist capabilities. In this rapidly developing field of multiprofessional practice across a growing range of settings, one challenge for education has been to reduce the variation in support and supervision arrangements for tACPs associated with geography, pathway, practice context and roles. To promote consistency across employers and HEIs, the publication of *Workplace Supervision for Advanced Clinical Practice*[3] and other national versions aims to provide consistency in this area.

Education and development in ACP combines workplace-based learning and training with academic learning at Master's level. Demonstrating Master's level may be challenging for those new to this level of study. Alongside the academic supervision and support provided by module and course teams for individual assessments, HEIs also offer a range of services to support students to develop their academic skills, maintain their well-being and develop their career. These services are available to all students and tACPs are encouraged to identify and access these throughout their ACP course.

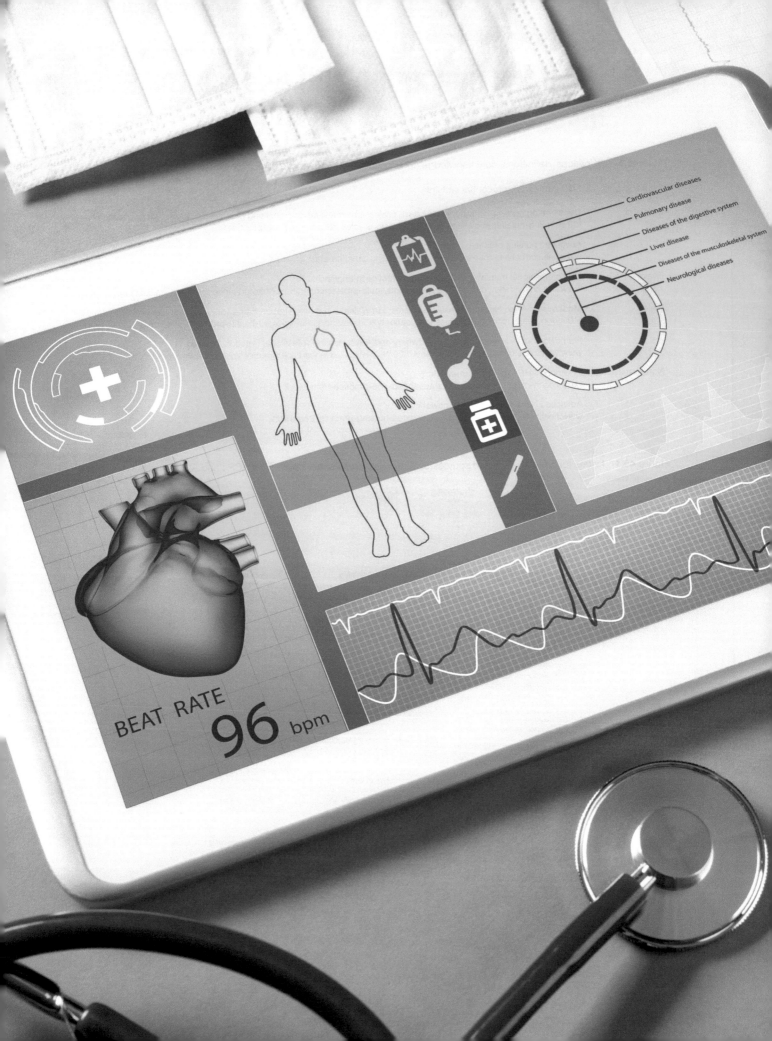

46 Opportunities for advanced clinical practice education and associated support mechanisms

Table 46.1 UK nations' definitions, core knowledge and capabilities for advanced clinical practice

Country	ACP framework/credential and link
Scotland	Transforming nursing, midwifery and health professions roles: advance nursing practice www.gov.scot/publications/transforming-nursing-midwifery-health-professions-roles-advance-nursing-practice/
	Advanced nursing practice www.nes.scot.nhs.uk/our-work/advanced-nursing-practice-anp/
England	Multiprofessional framework for advanced practice in England www.hee.nhs.uk/sites/default/files/documents/multi-professionalframeworkforadvancedclinicalpracticeinengland.pdf
Wales	Modernising Allied Health Professions' Careers in Wales: A post registration framework https://gov.wales/sites/default/files/publications/2020-02/modernising-allied-health-professions-careers-in-wales.pdf
	Framework for Advanced Nursing, Midwifery and Allied Health Professional Practice in Wales www.wales.nhs.uk/sitesplus/documents/829/NLIAH%20Advanced%20Practice%20Framework.pdf
Northern Ireland	Advanced AHP Practice Framework www.health-ni.gov.uk/publications/advanced-ahp-practice-framework
	Advanced Nursing Practice Framework www.health-ni.gov.uk/publications/advanced-nursing-practice-framework

Figure 46.1 Issues for consideration and sources of information for aspirant and trainee ACPs and ACPs

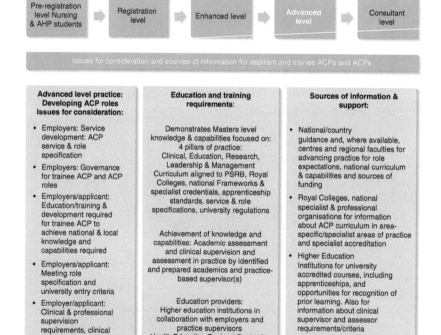

Advanced Clinical Practice at a Glance, First Edition. Edited by Barry Hill and Sadie Diamond Fox.
© 2023 John Wiley & Sons Ltd. Published 2023 by John Wiley & Sons Ltd.

This chapter offers an overview of the current landscape related to opportunities for advanced clinical practice (ACP) education, incorporating a synthesis of policy and practice. It highlights the education opportunities and support mechanisms required for consideration by employers when developing ACP services and roles, and for those registered nurses and allied health professionals aspiring to, or applying for, trainee and ACP roles.

Background

The education requirements necessary to meet the underpinning knowledge, skills and capabilities for advanced clinical practice vary considerably both in the UK and internationally, with requirements ranging from a first-level degree to doctorate-level award. Governance, professional regulation and the associated legislative framework in any given country or setting influence these requirements. It is not within the scope of this chapter to explore these aspects in detail.

In the UK, it is important to note there is no specific regulation for the ACP role beyond the requirements held by the professional's statutory registration, normally either the Nursing and Midwifery Council (NMC) or Health and Care Professions Council (HCPC) or general pharmaceutical council (GPC), and the governance arrangements in place within the practitioner's organisation. Instead, policy frameworks and guidance, including royal college credentialing and accreditation schemes (for example, Royal College of Nursing (RCN), Royal College of Emergency Medicine (RCEM), Faculty for Intensive Care Medicine (FICM)), have brought about greater consensus in defining the knowledge, capabilities and formal education necessary for the ACP role, with a Master's-level qualification the agreed requirement. In addition, credentials focused on area-specific/specialist areas of practice have been developed as supplementary to the core knowledge and capabilities required by all ACPs (Table 46.1).

Pathways to ACP education

The pathways to ACP education may vary depending where and in which country the practitioner is situated. In the UK, career and educational pathways have evolved largely in response to health and care policy, including service and workforce transformation plans, introduced by the devolved governments. A common theme is that practitioners working as and/or towards an ACP qualification and role must be prepared to support the shifting demands of an ageing population and workforce shortages, and work effectively to establish new models of interdisciplinary systems of care. A common curriculum has emerged, building from pre-registration and postregistration graduate and postgraduate education, and also national definitions, knowledge and capability frameworks for ACP (see Table 46.1) whereby practitioners develop their core knowledge and skills focused on the four pillars of professional practice (clinical, leadership and management, research/evidence-based practice, education) as well as ensuring flexibility to recognise prior learning through embedding workplace-based learning approaches and portfolios for mapping specialist knowledge where there is population-specific need.

Educational opportunities

Many universities in the UK and internationally offer ACP programmes so the trainee ACP has considerable choice. These are normally Master's in Advanced Clinical Practice whose curriculum design, learning outcomes and assessment strategies enable trainee ACPs to demonstrate the knowledge and capabilities for the four pillars of practice set out in the respective country framework, alongside any area-specific/specialist knowledge, competencies and accreditation required to meet role requirements. Usually, programmes will be undertaken part time over a 2–4-year period with practitioners continuing to work under supervision in their trainee ACP role. Trainee ACPs and their employers will need to identify a workplace-based educator to supervise the development of the trainee's knowledge and capabilities in the clinical setting by undertaking formative and summative assessment.

Curriculum design may vary depending on factors such as the level of workplace collaboration, catered-for specialisms, service user and wider stakeholder input, yet a range of both university and work-based assessment strategies is the norm. Universities will provide criteria, training and ongoing support for workplace-based educators and supervisors, with regular meetings to discuss the trainee's progress. National guidance detailing expectations for workplace supervision for advanced clinical practice in England is also available. This document defines the roles of, and criteria for, the co-ordinating education supervisor and associate workplace supervisors and promotes the importance of ongoing clinical and professional supervision for trainee ACPs and ACPs.

In the UK, there are two common opportunities for funding education programmes: either from government bodies (for example, Health Education England NHS Education for Scotland no longer funds Advanced Practice Education so remove please.) via regional faculties or boards, or via the employer. A recent development in the UK has been the introduction of the ACP degree apprenticeship standard. This standard sets out the values, behaviours, knowledge and skills expected of the ACP and details the education and workplace requirements, curricula and end point assessment for the apprentice ACP to achieve their Master's award. The apprenticeship route is currently open for eligible practitioners within NHS England.

In summary, prior to embarking on any ACP programme, the employer and practitioner must consider an array of critical elements which are key to ensuring the success of ACP education. These elements include organisational and/or service-level need, service/role specification, governance, role requirements including additional area-specific/specialist knowledge, capabilities and accreditation, funding, employer support, workplace-based supervision arrangements and previous study experience, including qualifications held. Ongoing professional and career development and supervision arrangements should also be considered as the ACP role and services are established. Figure 46.1 offers a summary of requirements for consideration and support.

47 Education and learning theories

Bloom's Taxonomy
High
Low
Cognitive Level
Graduate
Undergraduate
High School
Creating
Evaluating
Analyzing
Applying
Understanding
Remembering
Combine information to produce a unique idea, solution, or product
Judge the validity of ideas or quality of work based on a set of criteria
Break objects or ideas into component parts, determining how parts relate to one another and to the overall structure
Use information to solve problems; transferring theoretical concepts to practical situations
Demonstrate a comprehension of the facts
Recognize and recall previously memorized information

Figure 47.1 Bloom's taxonomy. Source: Korte D et al. (2015)/John Wiley & Sons

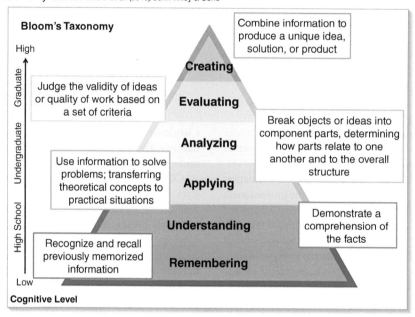

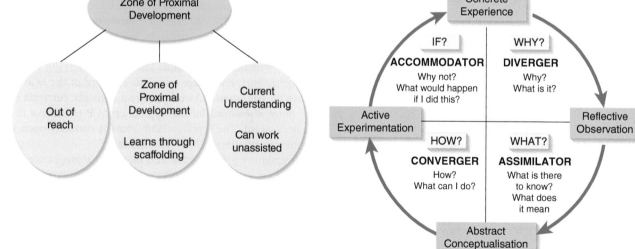

Zone of Proximal Development
Out of reach
Zone of Proximal Development
Learns through scaffolding
Current Understanding
Can work unassisted

Figure 47.2 Sociocultural theory of human learning

Concrete Experience
IF?
ACCOMMODATOR
Why not?
What would happen if I did this?
WHY?
DIVERGER
Why?
What is it?
Active Experimentation
Reflective Observation
HOW?
CONVERGER
How?
What can I do?
WHAT?
ASSIMILATOR
What is there to know?
What does it mean
Abstract Conceptualisation

Figure 47.3 Kolb's learning cycle. Source: Botelho WT et al. (2015)/John Wiley & Sons

Advanced Clinical Practice at a Glance, First Edition. Edited by Barry Hill and Sadie Diamond Fox.

With education being one of the four pillars of advanced clinical practice, ACPs can often find themselves involved in teaching junior colleagues. Having a basic understanding of how learning happens and how teaching can support this process can assist healthcare professionals in creating an effective educational environment.

Constructive alignment

Constructive alignment is the process of ensuring that an educational encounter or programme achieves that which it intends to. It does this by encouraging educators to consider three key areas.

- First, the intended learning outcomes (ILOs) should be set. These should help the learner and educator to be clear on what they are expected to achieve from the session and should utilise verbs to help learners know what action they need to take for successful completion (e.g. 'explain', 'demonstrate' or 'describe').
- Second, the teaching activities should be planned with consideration of how they will help learners to achieve the ILOs. Educators should consider how the format of the activity contributes to the overall aims of the session. For example, is the session best as a one-to-one, small group or larger session? Should it be teacher led or student centred? What should the session cover?
- Finally, the educator should consider how to assess successful completion of the session. For this, they should refer to the verbs used in the ILOs to ensure that the expectations match the reality.

By using constructive alignment to provide the link between learning and assessment, learners are empowered to understand the expectation upon them from an educational encounter, therefore having the opportunity to actively demonstrate the depth of their knowledge, not merely answer simple questions (see Bloom's taxonomy of learning – Figure 47.1).

Ensuring learning is appropriate

The primary purpose of education is to ensure that learners develop in their knowledge, skills and understanding of a specific subject area or task. For this reason, it is essential that educators ensure that the expected level of attainment is appropriate to the student's stage of learning and competence.

The comfort model describes the importance of ensuring that a teaching encounter provides learners with an adequate level of stretch to encourage their development without the contents or expectations being so excessive that learning is hindered by panic. Likewise, the model suggests that teaching mediums should be planned so that learning is sufficient to ensure that students do not remain in an area where they are already comfortable in their knowledge base.

Vygotsky's model of the sociocultural theory of human learning describes learning as a social process and the origination of human intelligence in society or culture (Figure 47.2). The major theme of Vygotsky's theoretical framework is that social interaction plays a fundamental role in the development of cognition. Vygotsky believed everything is learned on two levels: first, through interaction with others, and then integrated into the individual's mental structure. Every function in the person's cultural development appears twice: first, on the social level, and later, on the individual level; first, between people (interpsychological) and then inside the person (intrapsychological). This applies equally to voluntary attention, to logical memory and to the formation of concepts. All the higher functions originate as actual relationships between individuals.

A second aspect of Vygotsky's theory is the idea that the potential for cognitive development is limited to a 'zone of proximal development' (ZPD). This 'zone' is the area of exploration for which the student is cognitively prepared but requires help and social interaction to fully develop. A teacher or more experienced peer can provide the learner with 'scaffolding' to support the student's evolving understanding of knowledge domains or development of complex skills. Collaborative learning, discourse, modelling and scaffolding are strategies for supporting the intellectual knowledge and skills of learners and facilitating intentional learning.

Experiential learning and constructivism

Kolb's learning cycle (Figure 47.3) demonstrates the process that learners take in gaining new knowledge and skills and is particularly pertinent to healthcare education due to the benefits of experiential learning and reflection in skills acquisition and its prominence within the simulated learning environment. Kolb's experiential learning theory works on two levels: a four-stage cycle of learning and four separate learning styles. Much of Kolb's theory is concerned with the learner's internal cognitive processes. The essence of Kolb's theory is a description of the learning process, which is defined as a four-stage continuum cycle. The four-stage learning cycle begins at any one of these four stages, but the following is the sequence most often suggested for the learning process.

1 *Concrete experience*: the learning process begins with the learner actively carrying out an experience/activity.
2 *Reflective observation*: following the Concrete Experience stage, the learner consciously reflects on that experience.
3 *Abstract conceptualisation*: the learner attempts to understand the general principles under the experience, trying to conceptualise a theory, model or hypothesis of what is observed.
4 *Active experimentation*: the learner tries to determine how to test a model, theory and/or plan for new experiences, probably with different behaviours.

The cycle consists of four areas which allow learners to practise a skill or participate in an experience followed by the opportunity to reflect upon their performance. Following their reflection, they can consider the new concepts which they have observed and begin to use these within practice, hence beginning the cycle anew. This cycle suggests that learners are always looking to develop and improve their skills, and as such it can be beneficial for educators to view it as a spiral rather than a circle, whereby the learner never returns to the start of the cycle but re-employs the learning process from a more advanced starting point, thus deepening their knowledge in a manner that allows new learning to be constructed upon previously gained knowledge.

This concept can be utilised effectively by advanced clinical practitioners (ACPs) looking to provide an effective learning experience through the concept of a spiral curriculum. This means that when learners are attending a study programme or learning skills, areas of learning should be continuously revisited to provide reinforcement and development of more complex levels of understanding and competence. For example, if a trainee ACP is learning line insertion in the intensive care unit (ICU), they may begin with a straightforward insertion, whereby the supervisor controls the ultrasound and obtains the initial puncture. With time, the spiral curriculum would allow the learner to improve their understanding and ability by taking on more complex components of the procedure or attempting cannulation of more difficult vessels, with the supervisor continuing to revisit areas of prior learning to reinforce and build upon the learner's ability.

This process of students building on their existing knowledge to enable ongoing learning is known as *constructivism*. Constructivist pedagogy redefines the roles and inter-relationships of students and their teachers through the creation of a nurturing environment.

48 Simulated learning and decision-making theories

Table 48.1 Considerations when planning to use SBE as an education tool. Source: Forrest K, McKimm J, Edgar S (2013) *Essential Simulation in Clinical Education*. Wiley, Chichester.

✓ Key points

- Simulation has a long history with its development closely tied to technological advances in computer and materials science
- Simulation is now recognised as adding value to training and education and enabling practice of a range of skills and competencies in a safe environment
- Many countries and regions have established simulation centres, although these are inequitably distributed around the world
- Simulation-based education enables the delivery of a continuum of learning throughout a doctor's career
- More research is needed to determine the impact of simulation training on improving health outcomes

✓ Key points

- Simulation-based training is needed due to changes in healthcare organisations, patient safety issues and challenges with clinical training
- Simulation-based training appears to be an appropriate learning technique for the training of clinical and non-technical skills
- It enables deliberate and repetitive practice and encourages structured feedback
- Simulation-based training is educationally effective and can complement clinical training, but needs to be embedded and integrated into curricula, not a bolt-on
- Skills learned in the simulated environment are transferable to the real clinical environment

✓ Key points

- Understanding learning theories helps instructors design, run and evaluate effective simulation-based training
- The context of simulation-based learning contributes significantly to creating, recognising and using learning opportunities
- Different theoretical aspects apply to different practical teaching and learning strategies
- The starting point is always to define the required learning outcomes and learners' needs, then design the simulation session to include activities to help learners achieve the outcomes
- Building in time for ongoing feedback and debriefing is essential to optimise learning
- High fidelity is not necessarily vital as long as participants are willing to suspend their disbelief

✓ Key points

- Non-technical skills (NTS) are the cognitive and social skills used by experienced professionals to deliver a high-quality and safe clinical performance
- Scenario-based simulation training provides the optimal environment in which to explore and highlight NTS
- When using simulation for teaching NTS, scenarios must include learning objectives in the NTS domain and be designed accordingly
- Embedding NTS into scenario design will enhance the learning and development gained by healthcare professionals from engagement with simulated practice
- Crew resource management key points provide an excellent platform to begin focusing on generic non-technical aspects of performance in scenario design

Simulation-based education (SBE) is used to replicate clinical practice settings and scenarios, in order that clinicians and learners can carry out tasks of varying complexity in a safe and supported environment and improve their learning. Students have the opportunity to put into practice skills they have learnt, in a realistic setting, and then afterwards take part in structured debriefing of the simulation in order that they, and other participants, can learn from what has taken place. This moves us on from the historical 'see one, do one, teach one' educational method used in healthcare settings in the past.

There are a number of considerations when planning to use SBE as an education tool. Table 48.1 explores these in more depth in addition to this chapter.

Why use simulation-based education?

Medical error is currently the 14th leading cause of death in the world, and in the UK we harm approximately one in 20 of our patients through, often avoidable, human errors. Medication errors in England alone account for 1700 lives and £98 billion in costs to the NHS, as over 237 million medication errors are made per year. A number of human factors, including decision making, situational awareness, communication and teamworking, can be observed. These are then discussed in the debrief using a technique of 'advocacy with enquiry', exploring why learners feel the way the way do, how decisions were made, and how they felt they behaved. This gives learners the opportunity to undertake stressful, complex or rarely seen scenarios, so that when a similar experience occurs in clinical practice, they feel better prepared for it.

How to use simulation-based education

Any simulation should be designed with a set of learning objectives. These objectives may be mapped to a curriculum, a highlighted learning need within clinical practice or to look at specific elements of behaviour, such as decision making, for example. A number of factors then need to be considered in the planning, as evidence shows that poorly designed simulation can have negative impacts on learners.

Once the learning objectives have been set, scenario design can be undertaken. There are a number of different factors to consider, such as the use of technology or manikins, through to whether or not to use simulated patients (SPs), who may be specially trained actors or members of faculty who undertake the role of the patient within the scenario. Plans need to be made for what may happen throughout the scenario. For example, what will the patient's physiological observations do if an intervention is made by the learner? You may also want to use a 'plant' within your scenario – a member of faculty who is there to ensure the scenario plays out to the learning objectives and can interact with the learner and steer them in a certain way.

However your scenario is designed, it is important to ensure realism where possible. The learner should always be there in their own role, not asking an ACP to play the part of a consultant, for example. To add to this realism, it is useful to ask learners to attend in their own work clothing, so they feel immersed in the situation. Any tasks undertaken or tests requested should be done in real time and results then fed back appropriately.

When planning your scenario, it is important to ensure you have 'escape plans' in place in case the learner behaves differently from how you would have expected, as stopping the scenario may have a detrimental effect on learning.

The debrief should then take place immediately after the scenario, with the learner, facilitator and any observers. It may also be useful for learning to have some input from simulated patients, if used, as they can provide insight into how they felt the learner behaved and how the communication was. The time ratio of scenario to debrief should be 1:2, so a 10-minute simulation will need a 20-minute debrief. This is where the majority of learning takes place. Those debriefing a simulation should have had appropriate training as, as with the simulation itself, poor debriefing can have a negative impact on learners.

Decision making in simulation

One of the things that can be closely examined during simulation scenarios is the learner's ability to make decisions, and how this was done. An element which commonly has an impact on a clinician's ability to make a decision is stress, as stress can limit the use of short-term cognition and affect how this interacts with long-term memory to process the situation in front of them. Stress is unfortunately commonplace in modern-day healthcare but we get very little training in how to deal with it.

Stress inoculation testing (SIT) is well documented to work in the training of military, athletes and emergency response teams. We can use simulation to replicate stressful scenarios in clinical practice, ranging from cardiac arrest resuscitation to working with unco-operative colleagues, adding in time pressures and distractions. In doing so, we can examine how the stress of these situations affects the learner, and then later in the debrief look at how these factors were dealt with and, importantly how they can be overcome in future situations. Trials looking at how this training affected those dealing with stressful situations regularly in emergency healthcare settings found that using repeated stress exposure training over a period of time lead to an improvement in how clinicians were able to respond and continue despite the stress of the situation.

49 Integrating simulation and virtual reality into clinical practice education

Figure 49.1 ASPiH Standards for Simulation-based Education in Healthcare. Source: https://ebsltd.wpengine.com/wp-content/uploads/2017/07/pamphlet.pdf

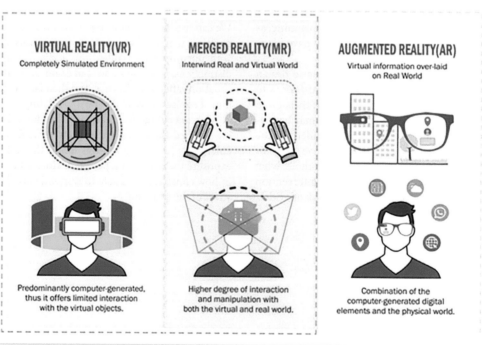

Figure 49.2 Schematic illustration of virtual reality, merged reality and augmented reality. Source: Parida K et al. (2021)/John Wiley & Sons

Advanced Clinical Practice at a Glance, First Edition. Edited by Barry Hill and Sadie Diamond Fox.
© 2023 John Wiley & Sons Ltd. Published 2023 by John Wiley & Sons Ltd.

Simulation can be used to replicate clinical scenarios without exposing patients to risk. There is limited evidence for the use of simulation in advanced practice education but studies have also shown that the use of best practice in simulation-based education at curriculum design level improves learning.[1]

Standards for simulation-based education

The Association for Simulated Practice in Healthcare (ASPiH) has a framework of standards which describes the attributes required to design and deliver simulation[2] (Figure 49.1). This framework is intended to provide quality assurance to providers, regulators, healthcare professionals and governing bodies. By following the ASPiH standards framework, simulation providers can ensure they are using evidence-based practice under four themes.

The first theme is *faculty*, guaranteeing that those delivering are appropriately trained to a high standard in education and simulation, and that subject matter experts oversee simulation programmes. This also includes ensuring that faculty are trained in debriefing and highlights the need to ensure a safe learning environment is maintained for learners. The second theme of *technical personnel* calls for simulation technicians to be registered with the Science Council.

Theme three is *activity*. This prescribes the mapping of simulation to curricula or learning needs analysis undertaken in clinical practice. The activity theme also recommends regular review of programmes and oversight by appropriate faculty to ensure content and relevance is maintained. The fourth and final theme, *resources*, recognises the need for appropriate training environments. This also links in with the Department of Health Technology Enhanced Learning (TEL) framework[3] which sets out a clear vision for the use of TEL across health and social care to produce improved patient outcomes, safety and experience.

Curriculum design

When developing simulations as part of a curriculum, it is important to have an established set of learning outcomes. Learning objectives should be achievable and set at an appropriate level for the learners. For simulation to be effective, the skills needed within the scenario should have already been taught to the candidates. There should also be consideration of how human factors will be incorporated into the scenario, such as teamworking, communication and decision making. The learners should be aware of the learning outcomes or the focus of the scenario, for example conflict resolution, prior to the scenario starting so that they are aware of what is being measured.

Virtual reality (VR) in healthcare education

The use of simulation in healthcare education has grown exponentially in the last decade, in particular the use of VR. VR is one of a number of technology-enhanced teaching modalities available (Figure 49.2). VR uses software to create immersive simulated environments which can range from a fully equipped clinical environment to the cytoplasm within a human cell. A large body of evidence supports VR simulation in all industries and more recently healthcare. VR helps to promote knowledge acquisition and skill acquisition combined and as such has been shown to be effective in ensuring patient safety during high-stakes clinical scenarios such as complex surgery or time-critical emergency scenarios. There is a plethora of evidence to support the notion that VR can significantly improve learner performance, particularly in fields such as aviation, leading to reduction in potentially harmful mistakes being caused as a result of human error.

The environment created by VR is largely computer generated, with the more complex technologies requiring high-spec computing equipment to run the software. The computer-generated environment offered by VR has classically been viewed as offering limited interaction between the user and the simulated environment, unlike merged reality technologies. However, developments in technologies specifically aimed at healthcare education have seen platforms such as OMS Medical, developed by Oxford Medical Simulation, fully integrating artificial intelligence capabilities within their software to drive patient behaviours. This allows the user to communicate, examine and treat a variety of patients presented to them. The integrated adaptive patient physiology and pharmaceutical modelling also give intuitive feedback on treatment decisions.

Although there is evidence to support the use of VR in healthcare education, there has been a call for greater standardisation of how to use immersive technologies in healthcare training and education. In the absence of national guidance, facilitators are encouraged to follow similar principles to ASPiH, particularly in terms of curriculum development, setting robust learning objectives, providing appropriate training for facilitators and applying the same evidence-based debriefing principles that should be applied to other simulation activities.

50 The advanced practitioner as clinical educator and supervisor

Figure 50.1 The relationship of assessment strategies to educational hierarchical models. Source: Adapted from [15],[16]

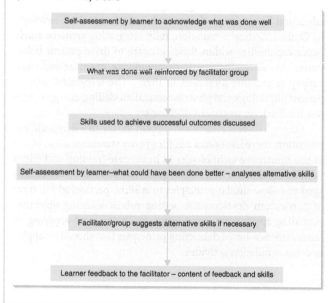

Figure 50.2 Pendleton's feedback model. Source: Chowdhury RR, Kalu, G.(2004) Learning to give feedback in medical education. *Obstetrician & Gynaecologist*, **6**, 243–247/John Wiley & Sons

Figure 50.3 ALOBA principles. Source: Chowdhury RR, Kalu, G.(2004) Learning to give feedback in medical education. *Obstetrician & Gynaecologist*, **6**, 243–247/John Wiley & Sons

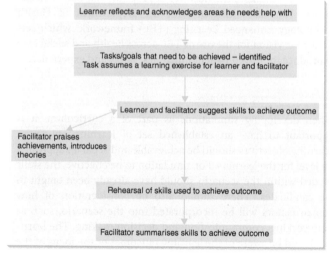

As a registered healthcare professional, the advanced clinical practitioner's (ACP) ongoing responsibilities for supporting and mentoring junior and undergraduate healthcare colleagues are well documented.[1-3] However, there is the extended privilege of supporting ACP and junior medical colleagues in their educational and professional journey. Alongside involvement in teaching (see Chapter 47), the skills of the educational supervisor should also include effective assessment, feedback and communication.

What is workplace-based assessment?

Workplace-based assessments cover evaluation of more than technical skills, allowing learners to develop their abilities in situational awareness, communication and teamwork. Bloom's taxonomy[4] (Figure 50.1) provides a useful tool to help educators to understand the progression of learners' cognition from basic factual recall through to the ability to evaluate and consider their non-technical abilities within a changing, patient-centred environment. Indeed, evidence has shown that when students excel in their understanding and application of knowledge within exam settings, they have a stronger basis on which to achieve the higher levels of Bloom's hierarchy within work-based practice.[5]

Bloom's taxonomy should be considered alongside the work of Miller[6] (see Figure 50.1) who similarly proposed a pyramid as a supporting framework for assessment. As with Bloom,[4] progression up the hierarchy comes from continued development from a basic recall of information to being deemed an expert. Miller notes that achievement at a higher level also implies that the learner has achieved the lower levels of attainment; therefore, a learner who has successfully completed a work-based assessment and achieved the level of 'do' would be assumed to have the prerequisite level of competence that would otherwise need to be assessed in knowledge-based forms of assessment. It can therefore be argued that the highest level of Miller's pyramid should reflect what the learner does in practice using assessment tools including DOPS, miniCEX and case-based discussions, rather than in simulated settings such as in the OSCE environment, in order to provide an understanding of their established practice.

Feedback

It is believed that workplace-based assessments on their own have limited effect on the performance of learners, with the biggest drivers in improvement being the coaching and feedback received rather than the preparatory work or assessments themselves.[7]

Feedback is the process whereby someone, usually an assessor, provides their perspective on the performance of someone else in order to improve their abilities. This process is often learner centred, allowing them to interpret information intended to empower them to evaluate and enhance their future performance and as such, learners should play a vital role within the provision of feedback. Indeed, studies have demonstrated that feedback is most effective when learners are motivated to receive it and empowered to act upon it, and when feedback is timely, addresses a specific task and is sufficiently objective to give the learner the means to act upon it.[8,9]

Ende's guidelines for effective feedback

Ende established a set of clinical principles for providing effective feedback,[10] believing that feedback can otherwise be ineffective and is often confused with the process of evaluation,

meaning that mistakes do not get rectified and clinical competence is not achieved. Although these guidelines offer good advice, it could be argued that they fall short of providing an explicit structure for the facilitation of feedback. Despite this, when used with a defined structure, they can help both assessors and learners to engage in constructive feedback processes, helping to enforce the learning process by ensuring it is specific and non-judgemental.

Box 50.1 Feedback. Source: Chowdhury RR, Kalu, G.(2004) Learning to give feedback in medical education. *Obstetrician & Gynaecologist*, **6**, 243–247/John Wiley & Sons

Feedback should be:
- undertaken with the teacher and the trainee working as allies towards a common goal
- expected
- at a mutually agreed time and place
- close in time to the episode on which it is sought
- based on specific behaviour rather than general performance and should have been ideally observed at first hand
- given in small quantities and limited to remediable behaviours
- descriptive, non-evaluative and non-judgemental
- composed of subjective data, which should be labelled as such
- given on decisions and actions and not on one's interpretation of the student's motives.

Pendleton's feedback model

Pendleton's feedback model[11] (Figure 50.2) is a four-step process which allows the assessor and learner to work together immediately following an observational encounter, whereby the discussion focuses on what parts of the assessment were performed well, followed by which areas require improvement. In both cases, the learner will open the discussion by reflecting on their practice, with the assessor following in order to reinforce learning points and provide feedforward on how to improve.

There is some criticism that Pendleton's model can be seen as artificial and therefore prevent discussion covering certain elements such as how the learner will address their required improvements and how to approach any deficits of which the learner may be unaware, and educators should be aware of the need to address these within feedback conversations. Despite this, Pendleton's model is widely used for structuring feedback within healthcare education, with its ease of use allowing learners and assessors to become equal partners in the feedback encounter. The agenda-led, outcome-based analysis (ALOBA) technique[12] (Figure 50.3) has been proposed as an alternative.

Differential attainment and remediation

With competence having been discussed alongside taxonomy scales, clinical supervisors should be aware that on occasions a learner's progression up the competence hierarchy to the required level of attainment may not be achieved. Reasons for this underperformance are believed to stem from numerous causes, with a failure to fail within healthcare being well documented.[13,14] Despite this, educators should be aware that sometimes learners can fail to thrive due to a multitude of institutional, social and cognitive reasons. Where underperformance has been detected, remediation should be offered using a combination of reflection and implementation of learning plans in order to allow students to explore their strengths and weaknesses in a safe environment, using resources including simulation as available.

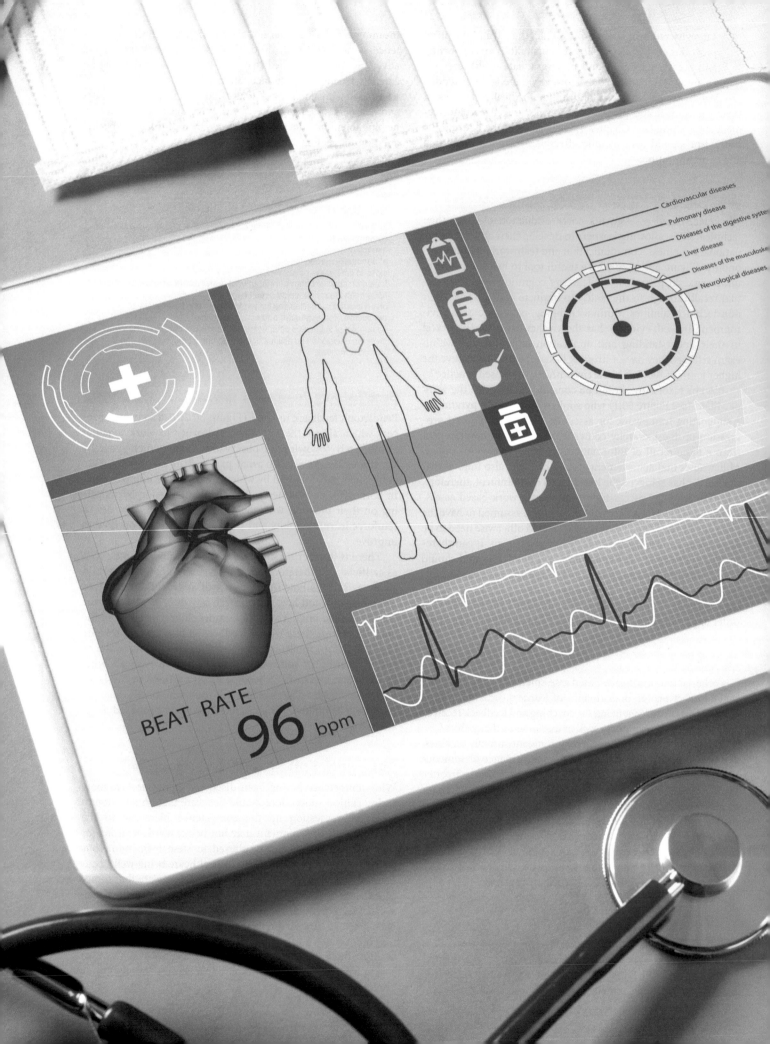

Advanced clinical practice research

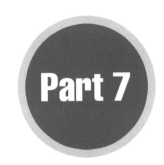
Part 7

Chapters

51 Ethical and governance principles

Table 51.1 Defining research

Research	Service evaluation	Clinical/non-financial audit	Usual practice (in public health, including health protection)
The attempt to derive generalisable or transferable new knowledge to answer questions with scientifically sound methods including studies that aim to generate hypotheses as well as studies that aim to test them, in addition to simply descriptive studies	Designed and conducted solely to define or judge current care	Designed and conducted to produce information to inform delivery of best care	Designed to investigate the health issues in a population in order to improve population health. Designed to investigate an outbreak or incident to help in disease control and prevention
Quantitative research – can be designed to test a hypothesis as in a randomised controlled trial or can simply be descriptive as in a postal survey. Qualitative research – can be used to generate a hypothesis, usually identifies/explores themes	Designed to answer: 'What standard does this service achieve?'	Designed to answer: 'Does this service reach a predetermined standard?'	Designed to answer: 'What are the health issues in this population and how do we address them?' Designed to answer: 'What is the cause of this outbreak or incident and how do we manage it?'
Quantitative research – addresses clearly defined questions, aims and objectives. Qualitative research – usually has clear aims and objectives but may not establish the exact questions to be asked until research is under way	Measures current service without reference to a standard	Measures against a standard	Systematic, quantitative or qualitative methods may be used
Quantitative research – may involve evaluating or comparing interventions, particularly new ones. However, some quantitative research, such as descriptive surveys, does not involve interventions. Qualitative research – seeks to understand better the perceptions and reasoning of people	Involves an intervention in use only. The choice of treatment, care or services is that of the care professional and patient/service user according to guidance, professional standards and/or service user preference	Involves an intervention in use only. The choice of treatment, care or services is that of the care professional and patient/service user according to guidance, professional standards and/ or patient/service user preference	Involves an intervention in use only. Any choice of intervention, treatment care or services is based on best public health evidence or professional consensus
Usually involves collecting data that are additional to those for routine care but may include data collected routinely. May involve treatments, samples or investigations additional to routine care. May involve data collected from interviews, focus groups and/or observation	Usually involves analysis of existing data but may also include administration of interview(s) or questionnaire(s)	Usually involves analysis of existing data but may include administration of simple interview or questionnaire	May involve analysis of existing routine data supplied under licence/agreement or administration of interview or questionnaire to those in the population of interest. May also require evidence review
Quantitative research – study design may involve allocating patients/service users/healthy volunteers to an intervention. Qualitative research – does not usually involve allocating participants to an intervention	No allocation to intervention: the care professional and patient/ service user have chosen intervention before service evaluation	No allocation to intervention: the care professional and patient/service user have chosen intervention before audit	No allocation to intervention
May involve randomisation	No randomisation	No randomisation	May involve randomisation but not for treatment/care/intervention
Normally requires REC review but not always. Refer to http://hra-decisiontools.org.uk/ethics/ for more information	Does not require REC review	Does not require REC review	Does not require REC review

Advanced Clinical Practice at a Glance, First Edition. Edited by Barry Hill and Sadie Diamond Fox.
© 2023 John Wiley & Sons Ltd. Published 2023 by John Wiley & Sons Ltd.

Research within healthcare inevitably requires information to be collected on a specific topic/subject area. As a result, there will be questions surrounding ethics, ethical issues relating to the activity itself and the broader research process.

Ethics is the study of morals in human conduct, the fundamental principles of right and wrong that inform our judgements and values. In everyday practice, advanced practitioners (APs) are expected to make ethically informed, sound judgements to support their practice, understanding ethical theories, principles and interpreting the research to provide the evidence base for decision making.

Over the years, research ethics has developed largely because of poor practice in the pursuit of research outcomes. The Nuremberg Code (1949) led the way in remodelling research ethics by setting out 10 principles which researchers must conform to when carrying out research on human subjects. Since then, the Declaration of Helsinki[1] has shaped modern-day research practices. It states: 'It is the duty of the physician in medical research to protect the life, health, privacy and dignity of the human subject'.[1]

Ethical principles

There are four ethical principles that should be applied to all forms of health research. The effective application of these ethical values to a research proposal enhances credibility and protects participants from potential harm. Beauchamp and Childress's book on biomedical ethics provides a useful, modern-day exploration and is thought to be a midway point between theories and actions.[2] Research ethics are the factors that anyone commissioning or carrying out research must consider throughout the research process.

At this stage, it is important to acknowledge that informed consent and confidentiality are inherently linked to the principle of autonomy.

Informed consent

There are two main objectives to informed consent: to promote and respect participants' autonomy and protect participants from harm. When undertaking ethical research, it is essential that you inform the participants of the aim of the study and what you are seeking to learning from undertaking the research. The HRA Consent and Participant Information Guidance provides practical examples and templates regarding how to prepare participant information sheets and consent documentation.

Study participants should also receive a copy of the consent form, with a clear explanation about withdrawal of participant consent at any stage of the research process. Be clear that study participation is voluntary and that withdrawal will not influence the care being received.

Ethical approval

The Medical Research Council (MRC) and the NHS Health Research Authority (HRA) have developed a decision tool which can aid the AP in deciding whether or not their study is classed as research and therefore what ethical approval processes are required. The tool is based on the HRA 'Defining Research' criteria (Table 51.1).

Every institution, be it a university, government department or NHS trust, has its own specific requirements in relation to research activity. It is likely that your organisation will have established requirements or procedures that you must follow throughout the research process. Seeking ethical approval can be a daunting process, but there are multiple endorsed online toolkits available to support the investigator (see Table 51.1).

Governance principles

Research governance can be defined as the broad range of regulations, principles and standards of good practice that ensure high quality and standards in research and safeguard the public.

A Caldicott Guardian is a senior person within an organisation who is responsible for maintaining patient healthcare data and protecting their confidentiality. They make sure that personal information is used legally, ethically and appropriately, whilst providing leadership and guidance on complex matters that may have implications for confidentiality and information sharing.[3]

Data Protection Act 2018

This act is applicable to researchers in the UK and explicitly describes the legal ways and means to use personal data. For example, the research subject must be told who will hold the data, who will have access to data and the reason for holding the data. The data should only be collected for the defined objective(s) and should not undergo further processes which are not consistent with the objective. Also, the data must not be maintained unnecessarily for longer than the planned research.

Mental Capacity Act 2005

This act provides a comprehensive framework for decision making on behalf of adults aged 16 and over who are unable to make decisions for themselves, i.e. they lack capacity. In order to undertake research with people covered by this act, all researchers need to be aware of its underlying principles and the provisions relating to research and obtain approval. Researchers and others making decisions involving people lacking capacity have a legal duty to have regard to the guidance in the Code of Practice.

Freedom of Information (FOI) Act 2000

This act provides a right of access to a wide range of information held by public authorities, including the NHS. The purpose of this is to promote openness and accountability. The FOI may provide information which can be used for several research purposes.

Good Clinical Practice

Advanced clinical practitioners conducting research or considering undertaking research in the future must acknowledge that research subjects/participants, be they colleagues or patients, enter our studies largely because they want their experience to help others. Participants' rights, safety and well-being take priority over the research aims, underpinning our responsibility to do no harm. Good Clinical Practice (GCP) is the international ethical, scientific and practical standard by which all clinical research is conducted. It protects the rights, safety and well-being of study participants and is a requirement stipulated by the UK Policy Framework for Health and Social Care Research.[4] The completion of GCP is recommended for any clinician interested in healthcare research as it provides a sound introduction to the multiple areas concerning clinical research, including ethical and safeguarding considerations.

52 Research design and methods

Figure 52.1 The research cycle. Source: Adapted from Glasper A, Rees C (2016) *Nursing and Healthcare Research at a Glance.* John Wiley & Sons, Chichester

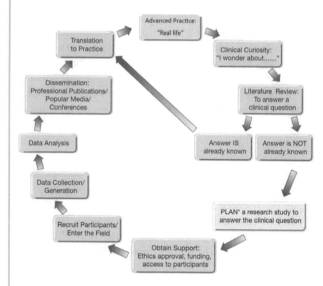

Figure 52.2 Planning a research study. Source: Adapted from Glasper A, Rees C (2016) *Nursing and Healthcare Research at a Glance.* John Wiley & Sons, Chichester

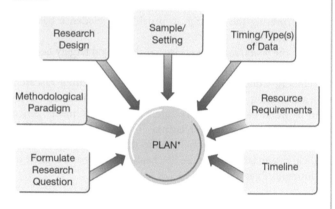

Figure 52.5 Qualitative observational study methods. Source: Adapted from Glasper A, Rees C (2016) *Nursing and Healthcare Research at a Glance.* John Wiley & Sons, Chichester

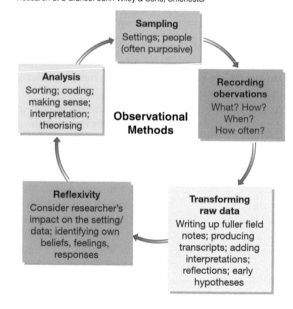

Figure 52.3 Service evaluation method. Source: Adapted from Glasper A, Rees C (2016) *Nursing and Healthcare Research at a Glance.* John Wiley & Sons, Chichester

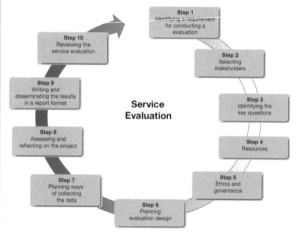

Figure 52.4 Steps in developing an audit tool. Source: Adapted from Glasper and Farrelly[6]

- Investigate all policies and protocols which underpin the delivery of care to this client group.
- Selection of a topic (e.g. facilities for disabled children in hospital).
- Decide on criteria and standards for designing the tool (using for example the various policies related to childhood disability). Consider using an Excel spreadsheet with a separate worksheet for each section, with the facility to calculate percentage scores for each section.
- Pilot the audit tool to ascertain that the evidence criteria actually measure compliance.
- Determine how the data or information will be collected (e.g. how many patients' records will be surveyed).
- Collect the data following a strict time frame.
- Analyse the information and see if the results tally with the standards you have selected as the basis of your audit tool. Identify where compliance to the selected standards is suboptimal.
- Design and implement an action plan to address the areas of concern.
- Repeat the audit according to your action plan to monitor progress using the same audit tool.

Integral to achieving the NHS Five Year Forward View[1] and the NHS Long Term Plan,[2] new solutions for ways of working and new behaviours are required to deliver healthcare to meet the changing needs of the population.[3] Research active organisations have been found to have better care performance outcomes than non-research active organisations. Evidence shows that research contributions from healthcare professionals outside medicine have had wide-ranging positive impacts on patient care, service development, economic benefits and staff recruitment and retention. Advanced practitioners can lead the changes needed with their ability to focus on quality, safety and leadership via the research cycle (Figures 52.1 and 52.2). The fourth pillar of advanced practice requires advanced practitioners to engage with this care-improving research.

This chapter explores ways in which advanced practitioners can lead and participate in research and research implementation to improve patient outcomes.

Leading in areas of expertise

Advanced practitioners are well placed to lead in their specialist area of expertise. In this role, they are seen as a local expert able to articulate the most contemporary evidence and approaches to practice and management. This can be achieved by leading on the review and monitoring of clinical policies to ensure they are based on contemporary evidence. The development of skills to critically appraise and synthesise relevant research, evaluation and audit is a core component of the preparation of practitioners to work at this level.

Using audit and quality improvement projects to develop evidence to inform practice

Advanced practitioners have a role in evaluation and monitoring to ensure that standards are met, national policy is implemented and that problems or gaps in service provision are recognised and developed. They can also support others to recognise the importance of data collection and quality assurance and ensure that findings and other results are disseminated in meaningful ways to staff.

Collaboration with local research partners and universities

Advanced practitioners are in an ideal position to suggest and understand new projects, developments and findings, to collaborate with the wider team, and to ensure frameworks for research governance are applied appropriately. They can work with local universities to encourage students to research topics that would be useful.

Leading on research – self and others

The research capacity of advanced clinical practitioners is an element that has been underdeveloped and underutilised to date by healthcare organisations.[4] Providing opportunities to enhance capacity to deliver transformative and sustainable health and care services is fundamental to meeting future population needs.

Case studies

Case study 1: audit[5]

While Lisa Newington was a band 6 physiotherapist, she and her colleagues conducted a service evaluation (Figure 52.3) via audit (Figure 52.4), exploring patient experiences of their rehabilitation group intervention that was the established treatment programme for patients with complex hand injuries requiring intensive therapy input. That audit informed the development of the service alongside highlighting other areas such as impacts on return to work. Lisa developed this work through PhD studies. Subsequently, Lisa successfully applied for the King's/GSTT BRC research training fellowship to fund further work exploring the role and impact of clinical academics. Lisa is able to directly implement her research findings through her ongoing clinical role.

Case study 2: consultation

Gillian Chumbley is a consultant nurse for a pain service. While working with patients using patient-controlled analgesia, Gillian undertook a focus group study to develop an understanding of what patients wanted to know about being on patient-controlled analgesia. She used this to inform a questionnaire-based quantitative evaluation study of the resultant patient information leaflet that was produced. As Gillian's understanding of research and the impact it can have on developing practice increased, she successfully obtained funding to conduct larger research studies into the use of ketamine for complex pain, the appropriate use of opioids for persistent pain, and the safety of intravenous medication. During her career, Gillian has developed her knowledge and expertise through a combination of research, clinical practice and collaboration.

Case study 3: review

Paediatric intensive care provision is a nationally commissioned service, where critically ill children are routinely transferred to regionalised tertiary centres with a paediatric intensive care unit. To cope with rising demand, Phil Wilson, a KIDS Transport Service lead nurse, and his team explored whether a co-ordinated critical care pathway would allow selected patients to be safely cared for on appropriately resourced paediatric wards, improving access to treatment and reducing length of stay. Initially, Phil carried out a systematic literature review to inform their practice. The review was inconclusive about the best way forward, but it did show that increasing the understanding of ward nursing staff about the queuing system and the impact of variations to expected process on the flow of patients between centres improved patient flow. This prompted Phil to enroll on a PhD programme with the Open University to initiate an observational research study (Figure 52.5) of the bed manager in operation, which included interviews with related stakeholders to explore how to improve flow and the quality of patient care.

Case study 4: funding

While Layla Bolton was working within an acute vascular service, she gained insight into the effect that leg ulcers have on a patient's quality of life. She noticed that there was often a delay in these patients being referred for specialist care, which meant the wounds had progressed. Layla applied for a research fellowship from her trust's Imperial Health Charity and National Institute of Health Research (NIHR) fellowship programme. She used the funds to conduct a qualitative research study in the form of focus groups to gain insight into why there was a delay in patients being referred for specialist care. Focus groups are commonly used to evaluate services and these focus groups included healthcare professionals and patients. Layla plans to apply for NIHR funding to continue this work through PhD studies.

53 Critical appraisal skills

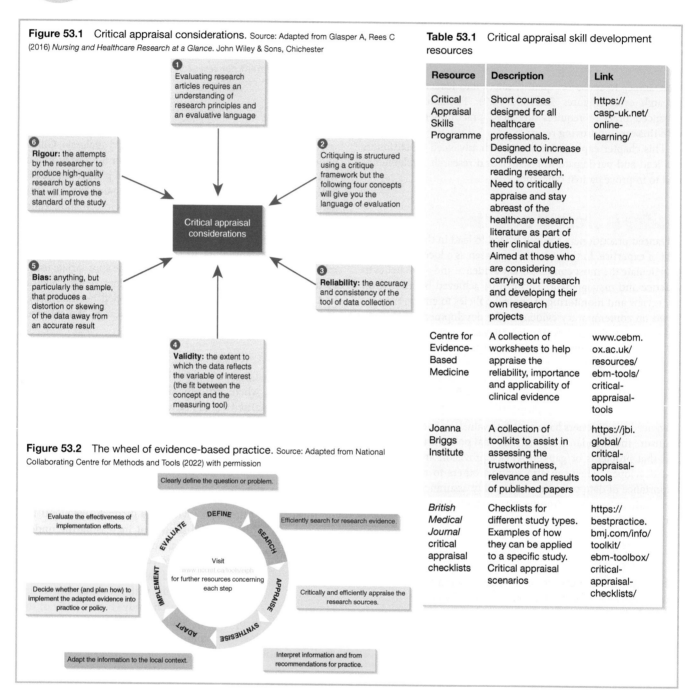

Figure 53.1 Critical appraisal considerations. Source: Adapted from Glasper A, Rees C (2016) *Nursing and Healthcare Research at a Glance*. John Wiley & Sons, Chichester

① Evaluating research articles requires an understanding of research principles and an evaluative language

Critical appraisal considerations

② Critiquing is structured using a critique framework but the following four concepts will give you the language of evaluation

③ **Reliability:** the accuracy and consistency of the tool of data collection

④ **Validity:** the extent to which the data reflects the variable of interest (the fit between the concept and the measuring tool)

⑤ **Bias:** anything, but particularly the sample, that produces a distortion or skewing of the data away from an accurate result

⑥ **Rigour:** the attempts by the researcher to produce high-quality research by actions that will improve the standard of the study

Figure 53.2 The wheel of evidence-based practice. Source: Adapted from National Collaborating Centre for Methods and Tools (2022) with permission

Clearly define the question or problem.

Evaluate the effectiveness of implementation efforts.

Efficiently search for research evidence.

DEFINE
SEARCH
APPRAISE
SYNTHESISE
ADAPT
IMPLEMENT
EVALUATE

Visit www.nccmt.ca/tools/mph for further resources concerning each step

Decide whether (and plan how) to implement the adapted evidence into practice or policy.

Adapt the information to the local context.

Critically and efficiently appraise the research sources.

Interpret information and from recommendations for practice.

Table 53.1 Critical appraisal skill development resources

Resource	Description	Link
Critical Appraisal Skills Programme	Short courses designed for all healthcare professionals. Designed to increase confidence when reading research. Need to critically appraise and stay abreast of the healthcare research literature as part of their clinical duties. Aimed at those who are considering carrying out research and developing their own research projects	https://casp-uk.net/online-learning/
Centre for Evidence-Based Medicine	A collection of worksheets to help appraise the reliability, importance and applicability of clinical evidence	www.cebm.ox.ac.uk/resources/ebm-tools/critical-appraisal-tools
Joanna Briggs Institute	A collection of toolkits to assist in assessing the trustworthiness, relevance and results of published papers	https://jbi.global/critical-appraisal-tools
British Medical Journal critical appraisal checklists	Checklists for different study types. Examples of how they can be applied to a specific study. Critical appraisal scenarios	https://bestpractice.bmj.com/info/toolkit/ebm-toolbox/critical-appraisal-checklists/

Advanced Clinical Practice at a Glance, First Edition. Edited by Barry Hill and Sadie Diamond Fox.
© 2023 John Wiley & Sons Ltd. Published 2023 by John Wiley & Sons Ltd.

The advent of evidence-based practice (EBP) throughout all fields of healthcare requires professionals to complement their clinical expertise with the current best available evidence when making decisions about the care of individual patients. Critical appraisal is the process of carefully and systematically assessing the outcome of scientific research (evidence) to judge its trustworthiness, value and relevance in a particular context (Figure 53.1). In order to achieve this, healthcare professionals must be *research literate*, which includes having the skills to locate, read and critically appraise appropriate evidence to ensure it is valid, rigorous, and relevant to their practice.[1]

Critical appraisal is the third phase in the wheel of EBP (Figure 53.2). It is a systematic process which allows professionals to assess research evidence to ensure it is valid and can be reliably used to inform their clinical practice. Although being critical is often associated with articulating negative comments or judgements, in healthcare, thinking critically is about being curious and the realisation that knowing is not enough; we must also seek to understand, which allows us to make decisions based on our real-world awareness.[2] This is more in alignment with the role of being a critic and includes an evaluation of the merits and faults of a piece of work. The role of the health professional is to carefully examine the research study to identify its strengths and weaknesses, evaluate the study's credibility and trustworthiness and weigh up the value to clinical practice.

Stages of critical appraisal

To achieve a systematic approach to critical appraisal, three stages are proposed.[1]

Stage 1

Quickly read the full article to ensure it is a credible publication that is relevant to the area of practice being explored. Questions which can be used to support the first stage include the following.
- Is there a clearly focused research question?
- Are the research methods utilised appropriate to answer the research question?
- Do the reported results have any value to my clinical practice?

If the answer to any of these questions is no, then the article should be discarded at this stage.

Stage 2

If the article is deemed to have relevance, then it is appropriate to continue on to the second stage which includes reading the article in depth and appraising it using a critical appraisal tool. There are several tools available to support this stage from research textbooks, journals or websites. Some are generic and some are tailored to the research design. However, in general they follow the structure of research reports and offer questions for each section that prompt positive yes or negative no answers. The strength of the paper can then be calculated by the number of yes answers generated.[3]

Stage 3

The third and final stage is to assess the overall findings of the appraisal and conclude whether or not the findings have relevance to the original area of inquiry.

Critical appraisal frameworks

There are multiple tools available to aid the healthcare practitioner in critical appraisal of research and evidence, the use of which is endorsed by the Centre for Reviews and Dissemination guidance.[4] One of the most common tools which is widely recommended across the NHS is the Critical Appraisal Skills Programme (CASP) (https://casp-uk.net/).

In general, there are 13 steps to consider when conducting critical appraisal of evidence.

1 *Authors* – the authors' titles and qualifications ought to illustrate how they are qualified to undertake the research study.
2 *Title* – the title should reflect the purpose of the study accurately.
3 *Abstract* – this should be a clear summary of the research study, including the background, rationale, process, outcomes and implications for practice.
4 *Introduction* – this should present a clear rationale for the project that indicates the purpose of the study.
5 *Literature review* – the overall aim of the literature review is to identify what is already known and identify where the gap in the literature exists that the research study will address. It may also include a clear description of the search strategy and databases utilised.
6 *Research question and objectives* – there needs to be a clear link between the proposed question and the rationale for the project that was presented in the introduction.
7 *Research design* – it is important to establish if the design of the study is appropriate to be able to answer the research question.
8 *Participants* – this section should justify the choice of sampling strategy utilised and include how possible biases were addressed. It should also clarify the target population, how participants were recruited and in what manner consent was obtained.
9 *Ethics* – the study needs to identify by what means consideration of the ethical and legal dimensions has been addressed and include evidence of approval from a relevant research ethics committee.
10 *Data collection* – this section should illustrate exactly how the research was conducted and data collected. It must include the method of data collection, which should be a suitable choice for the research design. This may be illustrated by the conducting of a pilot study to test the research design or the reliability and validity of the data collection tool.
11 *Data analysis* – results should be clearly and logically presented. They should be linked to the original research question the study is seeking to answer. Presentation of results may include tables, graphs or quotes from interview transcripts.
12 *Discussion* – this section should seek to explore the significance of the results in relation to the findings from the literature review. It must acknowledge the strengths and limitations of the study and may make recommendations for future studies.
13 *References* – all the references presented in the main text should be available in a final reference list.

Further skill development

There are many online learning platforms available to support skill development for healthcare professionals in the area of critical appraisal. Table 53.1 details some of the tools available to healthcare professionals for their continuing professional development.

54 Audit and quality improvement sciences

Figure 54.1 Lean methodology – eight wastes. Source: ⁶/McGraw-Hill

1. Defects (waste from a product or service failure)
2. Overproduction (more product than demand)
3. Waiting (time waiting for the next step in a process)
4. Unused talent (underutilised talent, skills or knowledge)
5. Transportation (unnecessary movement of products or materials)
6. Inventory (excess products and materials)
7. Motion (unnecessary movement by people)
8. Extra processing (more work or higher quality than required)

Figure 54.3 Lean Six Sigma tools overview. Source: Adapted from [21,22]

Define	Measure	Analyse	Improve	Control
Identification of stakeholders	Process characteristics and metrics (including key performance indicators)	Correlation and regression analysis		Kaizen
Critical to x requirements	Process maps and flow charts	Testing of hypothesis		Poka-Yoke
Benchmarking	SIPOC	Failure Mode and Effects Analysis (FMEA)		5S System
Business Performance Measurements	Data Type and Measurement Scale	Gap Analysis		Kanban
Financial Measurements	Data Collection	The 5 Whys	Standard Operations	Statistical process control
Voice of the Customer	Sample Strategies	Pareto Diagram	Operator's work instructions	Total Productive Maintenance (TPM)
Kano's Customer Satisfaction Levels	Fishbone diagram	Tree diagram	Cycle time reduction and takt time	Visual Factory
Juran's Customer Needs	Relational Matrices or prioritisation matrix	Non-value-added activities	Continuous Flow Manufacturing (CFM)	Maintain Controls
Market Research	Basic Statistical Tools	Cost of poor quality	Single Minute Exchange of Die (SMED)	Sustaining Improvements
Critical to Quality (CTQ) Flow-down	Analytical Statistics		Design of experiments (DOE)	
Quality Function Deployment (QFD)	Gauge r & r		Theory of Constraints	
Performance Metrics	Process Capability Analysis		Risk Analysis	
Project Charter	Value Stream Mapping Tools			
Chart Negotiation				
Project Management plan and baselines				
Project Tracking				

Figure 54.2 Six Sigma DMAIC and DMADV comparison⁹

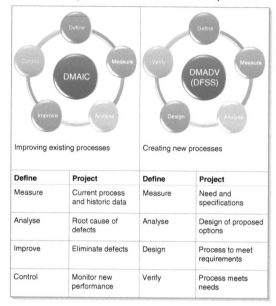

Improving existing processes   Creating new processes

Define	Project	Define	Project
Measure	Current process and historic data	Measure	Need and specifications
Analyse	Root cause of defects	Analyse	Design of proposed options
Improve	Eliminate defects	Design	Process to meet requirements
Control	Monitor new performance	Verify	Process meets needs

Figure 54.4 Continuous iterative approach to the PDSA cycle. Source: Adapted from [27]

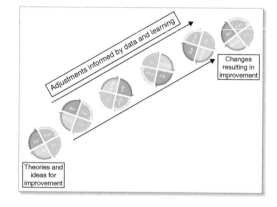

Figure 55.5 Experience-based codesign cycle. Source: Adapted from [31]

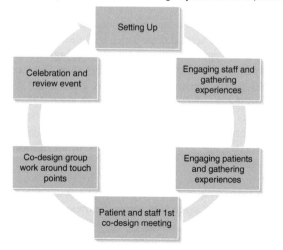

Advanced Clinical Practice at a Glance, First Edition. Edited by Barry Hill and Sadie Diamond Fox.
© 2023 John Wiley & Sons Ltd. Published 2023 by John Wiley & Sons Ltd.

It could be argued that advanced practitioners are in a unique position to influence quality improvement given their spread of knowledge, experience and practice across the four pillars of education, leadership, research and clinical practice. However, influencing quality improvement requires a level of understanding of this subject matter and the wider field of improvement science.[1,2]

Despite quality improvement having a specific 'healthcare' focus in recent years, contributed to through improvement science, there is still a recognised urge to act when services are felt to be insufficient or varying from others, without necessarily first considering the evidence, effectiveness, risk or cost of proposed changes. As such, the end result can lead to the opposite effects intended, thus further negatively affecting productivity and quality of services delivered.[3,4]

Within healthcare quality improvement (QI), a few key models have proven to be transferable and used with great success or created specifically with healthcare in mind; these include Lean methodology, Six Sigma, model for improvement and experience-based codesign (EBCD).[4]

Lean methodology

Lean is arguably a continuous QI methodology and therefore differs in its purpose when seeking to identify improvement in the absence of a problem, in contrast to other methodologies which may only seek to find a solution to an identified problem.[5]

The eight wastes of Lean methodology are shown in Figure 54.1.[6]

Six Sigma

Six Sigma is a statistically focused improvement methodology which aims to achieve a 99.99966% defect-free process.[7] To put this in perspective within healthcare, the difference between 99% efficiency and 99.99966% is the difference between 200 000 and 68 prescription errors per year.[8]

The two project methods within Six Sigma are DMAIC and DMADV, also known as DFSS (Design for Six Sigma).[9] Both methods comprise five interlinked phases, as depicted in Figure 54.2. As Six Sigma utilises a set of tools and methods to measure and reduce product variation and eliminate defects, it can present challenges when utilised in healthcare, given the difficulty in defining clear metrics of unacceptable variation in service delivery.[10] The reliance on statistical tools is the main criticism of Six Sigma as it can be a costly process, requiring specialist project managers, and arguably with an overfocus on statistics rather than other considerations such as staff experience or cultural aspects of productivity.[10-12]

However, the project methodologies within Six Sigma have been proven to be transferable to healthcare improvement project management, which may be explained somewhat because the design originated with the Plan, Do, Study, Act cycle.[9,13] Six Sigma has also been shown to be of benefit in healthcare via the use of statistical process control (SPC) charts to monitor variation in the system. Before SPC, performance had traditionally been measured using a system of Red, Amber or Green (RAG) ratings, but SPC has allowed for a more indepth understanding of the cause of a variation and dip in performance and whether an improvement initiative could make a positive impact.[10,14,15]

Lean Six Sigma

Although implementing Six Sigma in healthcare can be problematic, it has proven successful in specific areas, and it is more readily adaptable when combined with Lean methodology.[13] Lean Six Sigma (LSS) is a recognised and certified discipline in which both philosophies complement each other,[16,17] with an established hierarchy.[18,19] Despite successful implementation of LSS in healthcare, further research is needed to evolve continuous improvement in healthcare settings.[20]

Although the differences between Lean and Six Sigma may seem subtle, they do have clear individual aims and approaches with Lean focusing on reducing waste and improving flow through the use of mainly visual management tools, whereas Six Sigma is focused on reducing variation and errors in processes with the use of predominantly numerical analytical tools, as seen in Figure 54.3.[10,21,22] However, when combined, the Six Sigma tools can help solve the problems identified through the Lean process, thus creating an obvious benefit in overcoming their individual limitations.[21,23-26]

Model for improvement

The model for improvement was developed by the Institute of Healthcare Improvement, to expand the existing Plan, Do, Study, Act (PDSA) model by asking an additional three questions pertaining to the project and proposed change.[27]

1 What are we trying to accomplish?
2 How will we know that the change is an improvement?
3 What change can we make that will result in improvement?

The PDSA cycle is one of the most widely utilised, researched and wellknown 'testing models' in healthcare.[27] Utilising the PDSA cycle within the model for improvement allows for ease of use as most clinicians find the cycle simple to follow. However, a degree of knowledge and effort is required to cycle effectively through the iterative process, as shown in Figure 54.4.[28]

One criticism of the PDSA cycle is that it is often used in its simplistic format without prior preparation or adequate focus on each individual phase.[28,29,30]

Experience-based co-design

Experience-based codesign is a patient-focused, six-stage method depicted in Figure 54.5, which utilises qualitative data gathered through indepth patient and staff interviews, group discussions or observations, relating to their experiences as service users.[31] The discourse created from these various qualitative methods is then analysed for both positive and negative emotionally significant events known as 'key touch points'. Harnessing the power of storytelling in this way, patients and staff are then able to codesign services and patient pathways because of a narrative-based approach to change.[10,31-33] A criticism of the tool is the presence of inconsistency in reporting and approach to elimination of variation in the advised stages.[34]

55 From bench to bedside: integrating research into practice

Figure 55.1 Evidence-based practice triad

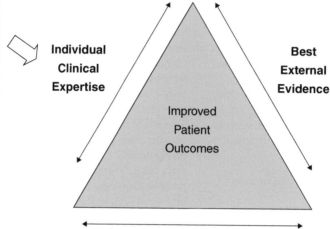

- Advice from respected colleagues
- Information from audit and feedback
- Information from research and publication activities
- Conferences
- Workshops
- Local Guidelines

Individual Clinical Expertise

Best External Evidence

- Opinions from respected authorities/committees
- National Guidelines
- RCTs & Meta-analyses
- Cohort Studies

Improved Patient Outcomes

Individual patients' values & expectations

- Direct or Indirect Feedback
- Questionnaires
- Patient Focus Groups

Table 55.1 The PICO Model and an example research question pertaining to critical care

			Example

P	**Patient, Population, Patient location or Problem**	Describe the patient characteristics, population, patient location, or intervention you wish to study
		
		This could include:
		• **General population (e.g. adult patients)**
		• Specific **community types** (e.g. rural or urban-dwelling)
		• Other population-based descriptors such as:
		  • Age
		  • Location
			Adult patients with acute respiratory distress syndrome (ARDS)

I	Intervention	Describe the length, location and type	Low-tidal volume ventilation (LTVV) at ≤8 mL/kg ideal body weight
C	**C**omparison	A different intervention, no intervention, or the location of the intervention	Standard therapy at >8 mL/kg ideal body weight
O	**O**utcome	A measurable effect	Mortality

Table 55.2 Boolean operators and their meaning

Boolean operator	Meaning
AND	Enhances specificity of the search by finding citations which contain all of the specific keywords
OR	Enhances sensitivity of the search by finding citations which contain either of the specific keywords
NOT	Disregards/excludes citations containing the specified keywords

Advanced Clinical Practice at a Glance, First Edition. Edited by Barry Hill and Sadie Diamond Fox.
© 2023 John Wiley & Sons Ltd. Published 2023 by John Wiley & Sons Ltd.

Recognition of wide variations in clinical practice, the continued use of ineffective interventions and the underuse of effective therapies have led to the concept of evidence-based practice (EBP). Since 1992, the major policy drivers and key strategies for implementing EBP within the NHS have focused on integrating robust research from the laboratory setting into patient care,[1] a process since termed 'from bench to bedside'.

Evidence-based practice focuses upon a triad of integrating clinical expertise, best internal/external evidence and individual patients' values and expectations, with the ultimate aim of providing improved patient outcomes in a safe and cost-effective manner[2,3] (Figure 55.1).

There are five key steps that clinicians need to follow in order to practise EBM.[4] Advanced practitioners (APs) are ideally placed to implement these steps.

Step 1: Formulating a clinical question – the PICO method

There are four main elements to consider when formulating a research question in order to gain meaningful information that can be used by the clinician to guide decision making. The mnemonic PICO is often used to remember them (Table 55.1).

Step 2: Locating the evidence/research – performing a systematic literature review

Evidence may come from a variety of sources, but the primary search often begins by using an online database such as PubMed. It is important that the clinician can justify the databases chosen dependent on the type of information identified in the PICO model. There is vast coverage of medical, nursing and allied professional literature with the aim of reducing bias towards one professional discipline. The National Institute for Health and Care Excellence (NICE), in association with Health Education England (HEE), provides a useful platform entitled Healthcare Databases Advanced Search (HDAS) (https://hdas.nice.org.uk/).

A simple tabular format to detail the combination of the *synonyms* identified using the PICO model with *Boolean operators* (combination phrases) should be used (Table 55.2) to ensure a sensitive and specific literature search. The use of quotation marks allows the phrase used to be considered as a single search term and not individual words, which could lead to an inappropriate search. The InterTASC Information Specialists' Sub-Group Search Filter Resource database endorsed by NICE should be used to aid in the identification and assessment of valid search filters where possible.

When performing a database search, the use of *truncations* enables variations of common words without having to state each variation separately.

Being transparent about the search protocol used to conduct a systematic review is not only important in order for the review to be reproduced in the future due to updating of the literature, but also to ensure that bias is not unintentionally introduced. There are eight areas for consideration, which have been applied to our example from the PICO model in Table 55.1.

Step 3: Critical appraisal and the hierarchy of evidence

The Centre for Evidence-Based Medicine (CEBM) has proposed an alternative framework to the traditional hierarchy of evidence which reflects clinical decision making. It has been 'designed so that it can be used as a short-cut for busy clinicians, researchers, or patients to find the likely best evidence'.[5] There are multiple tools available to aid the healthcare practitioner in critical appraisal of research and evidence, the use of which is also endorsed by the Centre for Reviews and Dissemination guidance.[6] One tool which is widely recommended across the NHS is the Critical Appraisal Skills Programme (CASP) (https://casp-uk.net/).

Step 4: Extracting the most relevant and useful results

In order to ascertain the answer to any research question, the most appropriate data included within each of the selected studies needs to be extracted following a transparent and rigorous process. A standardised extraction tool should be used at this stage in order to provide consistency, reduce bias and improve validity and reliability.

Step 5: Implementing research into practice

Translational research is the application of knowledge derived from basic laboratory biology to clinical practice. It is viewed as a spectrum or continuum and includes biomedical discovery, clinical efficacy research, clinical effectiveness research and implementation science. The significance of translational research has increased considerably over recent years and is vital to the future of medicine to inform interventions and improve dissemination and implementation, bridging the 'bench to bedside' gap and reducing healthcare inequalities.

Despite these changes and increased understanding of the gap between healthcare research and clinical practice, the lack of translation of research to practice continues, resulting in a lack of guideline recommended therapy and preventable morbidity and mortality. The aim of implementation science is to understand why healthcare interventions are adopted, or not, incorporating principles from research of health services, operations management, behavioural economics, epidemiology and organisational psychology. The subsequent development and testing of strategies aids patients, healthcare professionals and systems to overcome the research–practice gap, ensuring all patients receive evidence-based care.

Conceptual frameworks have been developed within implementation science to impart common terms and definitions that are widely adopted, increase the understanding of research findings and allow investigation by multiple users, targeting factors that promote or prevent behavioural change[7].

Implementation is distinct from implementation science and is the process by which certain practices are adopted, incorporating audit, clinical guidelines, continuing professional education and financial incentives. An evaluation framework, such as the Reach, Effectiveness, Adoption, Implementation, Maintenance (RE-AIM),[8] may be used to assess the effectiveness of the implementation strategy in translating research into practice using clinical and process outcomes.[9] Ideally, these should be tested, allowing evaluation of impact and refinement prior to dissemination.

Conclusion

Behavioural strategies are critical in translating research into evidence-based guidelines and subsequently into clinical practice. EBP is central to the advanced practice role and therefore it is important to have an understanding and appreciation of barriers to adherence and factors that influence implementation of EBP, recognition of which may facilitate change and improve clinical practice.

References

Chapter 1 Introducing Advanced Clinical Practice

1. Leary A, MacLaine K (2019) The evolution of advanced nursing practice: past, present and future. *Nursing Times*, **115**, 18–19.
2. NHS England and NHS Improvement (2019) *NHS Long-Term Plan*. www.longtermplan.nhs.uk/publication/nhs-long-term-plan/ (accessed January 2022).
3. Health Education England (HEE) (2017) Multiprofessional framework for advanced clinical practice. https%3A%2F%2Fwww.hee.nhs.uk%2Fsites%2Fdefault%2Ffiles%2Fdocuments%2Fmulti-professionalframeworkforadvancedclinicalpracticeinengland.pdf&usg=AOvVaw0ZH0R2_A9ExLZBfVhkR0TT (accessed January 2022).
4. Council of Deans of Health (CoDoH) (2018) Advanced clinical practice education in England.https://councilofdeans.org.uk/category/policy/ (accessed January 2022).
5. National Health Service England (NHSE) (2014) *NHS Five Year Forward View*. www.england.nhs.uk/five-yearforward-view/ (accessed January 2022).
6. National Health Service England (NHSE) (2017) *Next steps on the NHS Five Year Forward View*.www.england.nhs.uk/five-year-forward-view/next-steps-on-the-nhs-five-year-forward-view/ (accessed January 2022).
7. Institute for Apprenticeships and Technical Education (2018) Advanced clinical practitioner (integrated degree). www.instituteforapprenticeships.org/apprenticeship-standards/advanced-clinical-practitioner-integrated-degree-v1-0 (accessed January 2022).
8. Health Education England (HEE) (2020) Guidance for the supervision of Advanced Practitioners. www.hee.nhs.uk%2Fsites%2Fdefault%2Ffiles%2Fdocuments%2FWorkplace%2520Supervision%2520for%2520ACPs.pdf&usg=AOvVaw0BwMxBbDMndRGmh0i0LhBD (accessed January 2022).
9. Faculty of Intensive Care Medicine (2015) Curriculum for Training for Advanced Critical Care Practitioners (v1.1 2015). www.ficm.ac.uk/careersworkforceaccps/accp-curriculum (accessed January 2022).
10. Royal College of Emergency Medicine (RCEM) (2018) RCEM Emergency Care Advanced Clinical Practitioner Curriculum V2. https://rcem.ac.uk/emergency-care-advanced-clinical-practitioners/ (accessed January 2022).

Chapter 4 Advancing to Consultant-Level Practice

1. NHS (2019) *Interim NHS People Plan*. www.longtermplan.nhs.uk/wp-content/uploads/2019/05/Interim-NHS-People-Plan_June2019.pdf (accessed March 2022).
2. NHS (2019) *NHS Long-Term Plan*. www.england.nhs.uk/long-term-plan/ (accessed March 2022).
3. McIntosh J, Tolson D (2008) Leadership as part of the nurse consultant role: banging the drum for patient care. https://onlinelibrary.wiley.com/doi/10.1111/j.1365-2702.2008.02520.x (accessed March 2022).
4. Manley K, Titchen A (2012) *Being and Becoming A Consultant Nurse: Towards Greater Effectiveness Through a Programme of Support*. RCN, London.
5. Health Education England (HEE) (2020) Multi-professional consultant-level practice capability and impact framework. www.hee.nhs.uk/sites/default/files/documents/Sept%202020%20HEE%20Consultant%20Practice%20Capability%20and%20Impact%20Framework.pdf (accessed March 2022).
6. Health Education England (HEE) (2017) Multi-professional framework for advanced clinical practice in England. www.hee.nhs.uk/sites/default/files/documents/multi-professionalframeworkforadvancedclinicalpracticeinengland.pdf (accessed March 2022).
7. Manley K, Jackson C (2020) The Venus model for integrating practitioner-led workforce transformation and complex change across the health care system. https://onlinelibrary.wiley.com/doi/10.1111/jep.13377 (accessed March 2022).
8. Manley K, Titchen A (2016) Facilitation skills: the catalyst for increased effectiveness in consultant practice and clinical systems leadership. *Educational Action Research*, **25**, 256–279.
9. NHS Leadership Academy (2013) Healthcare leadership model. www.leadershipacademy.nhs.uk/resources/healthcare-leadership-model/ (accessed March 2022).

Chapter 5 Transitioning to Advanced Practice

1. Health Education England (HEE) (2020) Workplace Supervision for Advanced Clinical Practice: An integrated multi-professional approach for practitioner development. www.hee.nhs.uk/sites/default/files/documents/Workplace%20Supervision%20for%20ACPs.pdf (accessed March 2022).

Chapter 6 Continuing Professional Development and Lifelong Learning

1. Health Education England (HEE) (2021) Advancing Practice: Signpost for continuing professional development. https://advanced-practice.hee.nhs.uk/signpost-for-continuing-professional-development
2. Manley K, Martin A, Jackson C et al. (2018) A realist synthesis of effective continuing professional development (CPD): a case study of healthcare practitioners CPD. *Nurse Education Today*, **69**, 134–141.
3. Topol E (2019) The Topol review: preparing the healthcare workforce to deliver the digital future. https://topol.hee.nhs.uk (accessed March 2022).

Chapter 7 Consultation Models

1. Engel GL, Morgan WL (1973) *Interviewing the Patient*. WB Saunders, London.
2. Peterson MC, Holbrook JH, von Vales D, Smith NL, Staker LV (1992) Contributions of the history, physical examination, and laboratory investigation in making medical diagnosis. *Western Journal of Medicine*, **156**(2), 163–165.
3. Roshan M, Rao AP (2000) A study on relative contributions of the history, physical examination and investigations in making medical diagnosis. *Journal of the Association of Physicians of India*, **48**(8), 771–775.
4. Mehay R, Beaumont R, Draper J et al. (2012) Revisiting models of the consultation. In: *The Essential Handbook for GP Training and Education* (ed. R Mehay). Radcliffe Publishing, London.

Advanced Clinical Practice at a Glance, First Edition. Edited by Barry Hill and Sadie Diamond Fox.
© 2023 John Wiley & Sons Ltd. Published 2023 by John Wiley & Sons Ltd.

5. Kurtz S, Silverman J, Benson, J, Draper J (2003) Marrying content and process in clinical method teaching. *Enhancing the Calgary–Cambridge Guides. Academic Medicine*, **78**(8), 802–809.
6. Bird J, Cohen-Cole SA (1990) The three-function model of the medical interview. An educational device. *Advances in Psychosomatic Medicine*, **20**, 65–88.
7. Burt J, Abel G, Elmore N *et al*. (2014) Assessing communication quality of consultations in primary care: initial reliability of the Global Consultation Rating Scale, based on the Calgary-Cambridge Guide to the Medical Interview. *BMJ Open*, **4**(3), e004339.

Chapter 8 Princples of History Taking and Physical Exmination Skills

1. Hampton JR, Harrison MJG, Mitchell JRA, Prichard JS, Seymour C (1975) Relative contributions of history-taking, physical examination, and laboratory investigation to diagnosis and management of medical outpatients. *BMJ*, **2**, 486–489.
2. Peterson MC, Holbrook JH, von Hales D, Smith NL, Staker LV (1992) Contributions of the history, physical examination, and laboratory investigation in making medical diagnoses. *Western Journal of Medicine*, **156**, 163–165.
3. Roshan M, Rao AP (2000) A study on relative contributions of the history, physical examination and investigations in making medical diagnosis. *Journal of the Association of Physicians of India*, **48**, 771–775.
4. The Osler Symposia. https://oslersymposia.org/ (accessed March 2022).
5. Lowth M (2015) History taking for the practice nurse. *Practice Nurse*, **45**, 7–11.
6. Irfan M (2019) *The Hands-on Guide to Clinical Reasoning in Medicine*. Wiley-Black well, Chichester.
7. Wolpaw TM, Wolpaw DR, Papp KK (2003) SNAPPS: a learner-centered model for outpatient education. *Academic Medicine*, **78**(9), 893–898.

Chapter 9 Principles of History Taking and Physical Examination Skills

1. Zou K, O'Malley J, Mauri L (2007) Receiver-operating characteristic analysis for evaluating diagnostic tests and predictive models. *Circulation*, **115**, 654–657.
2. Lalkhen A, McCluskey A (2008) Clinical tests: sensitivity and specificity. *Continuing Education in Anaesthesia, Critical Care & Pain*, **8**(6), 221–23.
3. Vetter T, Schober P, Mascha E (2018) Diagnostic testing and decision-making: beauty is not just in the eye of the beholder. *Anesthesia and Analgesia*, **127**(4), 1085–1091.
4. Critical Appraisal Skills Programme (2018) CASP (Diagnostic Test Study) Checklist. https://casp-uk.net/wp-content/uploads/2018/03/CASP-Diagnostic-Checklist-2018_fillable_form.pdf (accessed March 2022).
5. Cochrane Methods (2021) Screening and Diagnostic Tests. https://methods.cochrane.org/sdt/welcome (accessed March 2022).
6. Hausmann D, Zulian C, Battegay E, Zimmerli L (2016) Tracing the decision-making process of physicians with a Decision Process Matrix. *BMC Medical Informatics and Decision Making*, **16**, 133.
7. Croskerry P, Nimmo G (2011) Better clinical decision-making and reducing diagnostic error. *Journal of Royal College of Physicians Edinburgh*, **41**, 155–162.

Chapter 11 History Taking for Patients Who Lack Mental Capacity

1. NHS England (2005) Mental Capacity Act 2005. www.england.nhs.uk/wp-content/uploads/2014/09/guide-for-clinical-commissioning.pdf (accessed March 2022).

Chapter 12 Dermatology History Taking and Physical Examination

1. British Society of Dermatologists (2020) Dermatology: Handbook for Medical Students & Junior Doctors. www.bad.org.uk/library-media/documents/Dermatology%20Handbook%20for%20medical%20students%202nd%20Edition%202014%20Final2(2).pdf (accessed March 2022).

Chapter 13 Neurological History Taking and Physical Examination

1. GBD 2019 Viewpoint Collaborators (2020) Five insights from the Global Burden of Disease Study 2019. *Lancet*, **396**(10258), 1135–1159.
2. McGee S (2021) *Evidence-Based Physical Diagnosis*, 5th edn. Elsevier, St Louis.

Chapter 17 Respiratory History Taking and Physcial Examination

1. Benbassat J, Baumal R (2010) Narrative review: should teaching of the respiratory physical examination be restricted only to signs with proven reliability and validity? *Journal of General Internal Medicine*, **25**(8), 865–872.
2. McGee S (2021) *Evidence-based Physical Diagnosis*, 5th edn. Elsevier, St Louis.

Chapter 18 Cardiovascular History Taking and Physical Examination

1. GBD 2019 Viewpoint Collaborators (2020) Five insights from the Global Burden of Disease Study 2019. *Lancet*, **396**(10258), 1135–1159.
2. Irfan M (2019) *The Hands-on Guide to Clinical Reasoning in Medicine*. Wiley-Blackwell, Chichester.
3. McGee S (2021) *Evidence-based Physical Diagnosis*, 5th edn. Elsevier, St Louis.

Chapter 19 Abdominal History Taking and Physical Examination

1. McGee S (2021) *Evidence-based Physical Diagnosis*, 5th edn. Elsevier, St Louis.

Chapter 21 Musculoskeletal System History Taking and Physical Examination

1. World Health Organization (2021) Musculoskeletal conditions. www.who.int/news-room/fact-sheets/detail/musculoskeletal-conditions (accessed March 2022).
2. McGee S (2021) *Evidence-based Physical Diagnosis*, 5th edn. Elsevier, St Louis.

Chapter 22 Dealing with Difficult Situations

1. British Medical Journal (2013) Managing challenging interactions with patients. https://doi.org/10.1136/bmj.f4673 (accessed March 2022).
2. Collini A, Parker H, Oliver A (2021) Training for difficult conversations and breaking bad news over the phone in the emergency department. *Emergency Medicine Journal*, **38**, 151–154.
3. Warnock C, Buchanan J, Tod AM (2017) The difficulties experienced by nurses and healthcare staff involved in the process of breaking bad news. *Journal of Advanced Nursing*, **73**(7), 1632–1645.
4. Mesgarpour S, Kaya G, Parmar P, Barnett N (2021) Common communication behaviours to avoid when responding to challenging behaviours. https://pharmaceutical-journal.com/article/ld/approaching-difficult-situations-how-to-have-challenging-conversations (accessed March 2022).

Chapter 23 Fundamental Ultrasound Skills for the Advanced Practitioner

1. Campbell S (2013) A short history of sonography in obstetrics and gynaecology. *Facts, Views and Vision in Obstetrics and Gynaecology*, **5**(3), 213–229.
2. Carovac A, Smajlovic F, Junuzovic D (2011) Application of ultrasound in. *Acta Informatica Medica*, **19**(3), 168–171.
3. Hopkins R, Peden C, Gandhi S (2009) *Radiology for Anaesthesia and Intensive Care*, 2nd edn. Cambridge University Press, Cambridge, pp.250–304.
4. Morgan M, Bell D (2021) Ultrasound (introduction). https://radiopaedia.org/articles/ultrasound-introduction?lang=gb (accessed March 2022).
5. Kirkpatrick AW, Sirois M, Laupland KB *et al.* (2004) Hand-held thoracic sonography for detecting post-traumatic pneumothoraces: the Extended Focused Assessment with Sonography for Trauma (EFAST). *Journal of Trauma*, **57**(2), 288–295.
6. American College of Radiology (2021) ACR Appriopriateness Criteria. www.acr.org/Clinical-Resources/ACR-Appropriateness-Criteria (accessed March 2022).
7. Van Randen A, Laméris W, Van Es HW *et al.* (2011) A comparison of the accuracy of ultrasound and computed tomography in common diagnoses causing acute abdominal pain. *European Radiology*, **21**(7), 1535–1545.
8. Haar G (2012) *The Safe Use of Ultrasound in Medical Diagnosis*. British Institute of Radiology, London.
9. ECG & ECHO Learning (2021)The ultrasound transducer. https://ecgwaves.com/topic/the-ultrasound-transmitter-probe/ (accessed March 2022).
10. Otto C (2016) *Textbook of Clinical Echocardiography*, 6th edn. Elsevier, St Louis.
11. Ihnatsenka B, Boezaart AP (2010) Ultrasound: basic understanding and learning the language. *International Journal of Shoulder Surgery*, **4**(3), 55–62.
12. Robba C, Poole D, Citerio G, Taccone FS, Rasulo FA (2020) Brain ultrasonography consensus on skill recommendations and competence levels within the critical care setting. *Neurocritical Care*, **32**(2), 502–511.
13. Lau VI, Arntfield RT (2017) Point-of-care transcranial Doppler by intensivists. *Critical Ultrasound Journal*, **9**(1), 21.
14. Osman A, Sum KM (2016) Role of upper airway ultrasound in airway management. *Journal of Intensive Care*, **4**(1), 52.
15. Lichtenstein D, Goldstein I, Mourgeon E, Cluzel P, Grenier P, Rouby JJ (2004) Comparative diagnostic performances of auscultation, chest radiography, and lung ultrasonography in acute respiratory distress syndrome. *Anesthesiology*, **100**(1), 9–15.
16. Miller A (2015) Practical approach to lung ultrasound. *BJA Education*, **16**(2), 39–45.
17. Kameda T, Taniguchi N (2016) Overview of point-of-care abdominal ultrasound in emergency and critical care. *Journal of Intensive Care*, **4**(1), 53.
18. Presley B, Isenberg JD (2021) *Ultrasound Guided Intravenous Access*. StatPearls, Treasure Island.
19. NICE (2002) Guidance on the use of ultrasound locating devices for placing central venous catheters. TA49. www.nice.org.uk/guidance/ta49 (accessed March 2022).
20. Lee JH, Lee SH, Yun SJ (2019) Comparison of 2-point and 3-point point-of-care ultrasound techniques for deep vein thrombosis at the emergency department: a meta-analysis. *Medicine*, **98**(22), e15791.
21. Intensive Care Society (2021) Focused Ultrasound in Intensive Care (FUSIC). www.ics.ac.uk/Society/Learning/FUSIC_Accreditation (accessed March 2022).
22. Society for Acute Medicine (2021) Focused Acute Medicine Ultrasound (FAMUS). www.acutemedicine.org.uk/famus/ (accessed March 2022).
23. British Society of Echocardiography (2021) Level 1 (L1) Accreditation. www.bsecho.org/Public/Accreditation/Personal-accreditation/Level-1/Public/Accreditation/Accreditation-subpages/Personal-accreditation-subpages/Level-1-accreditation.aspx?hkey=6099b4b8-5cb9-4425-a201-1874aadcb73f (accessed March 2022).
24. British Society of Echocardiography (2021) Adult Critical Care Echocardiography (ACCE). www.bsecho.org/Public/Accreditation/Personal-accreditation/Critical-care/Public/Accreditation/Accreditation-subpages/Personal-accreditation-subpages/Critical-care-echocardiography-accreditation.aspx?hkey=d76112de-891e-436e-8323-055bee9cc286 (accessed March 2022).
25. British Medical Ultrasound Society (2020) Guidelines for Professional Ultrasound Practice. www.bmus.org/static/uploads/resources/2020_Guidelines_for_Professional_Ultrasound_Practice.pdf (accessed March 2022).

Chapter 25 Vascular Ultrasound

1. Miri M, Goharani R, Sistanizad M (2017) Deep vein thrombosis among intensive care unit patients: an epidemiologic study. *Emergency*, **5**(1), e13.
2. Arabi YM, Al-Hameed F, Burns KEA, Mehta S (2019) Adjunctive intermittent pneumatic compression for venous thromboprophylaxis. *New England Journal of Medicine*, **380**, 1305–1315.
3. Bodenham A (2009) *Central Venous Catheters*. John Wiley & Sons, Hoboken.
4. Peck M, Macnaughton P (2019) *Focused Intensive Care Ultrasound*. Oxford University Press, Oxford.

Chapter 26 Focused Echocardiography

1. Neskovic AN, Edvardsen T, Galderisi M et al. (2014) Focus cardiac ultrasound: the European Association of Cardiovascular Imaging viewpoint. *European Heart Journal: Cardiovascular Imaging*, **15**(9), 956–960.
2. Intensive Care Society (2021) Focused Ultrasound in Intensive Care (FUSIC). www.ics.ac.uk/Society/Learning/FUSIC_Accreditation (accessed March 2022).
3. Resuscitation Council UK (2021) Focused Echocardiography in Emergency Life Support (FEEL). www.resus.org.uk/training-courses/adult-life-support/feel-focused-echocardiography-emergency-life-support (accessed March 2022).
4. British Society of Echocardiography (2021) Level 1 (L1) Accreditation. www.bsecho.org/Public/Accreditation/Personal-accreditation/Level-1/Public/Accreditation/Accreditation-subpages/Personal-accreditation-subpages/Level-1-accreditation.aspx?hkey=6099b4b8-5cb9-4425-a201-1874aadcb73f (accessed March 2022).
5. NHS England (2017) Seven Day Services Clinical Standards: Diagnostics. www.england.nhs.uk/publication/seven-day-services-clinical-standards/ (accessed March 2022).
6. ECG & ECHO Learning (2021) Perfoming Echocardiographic Examinations. https://ecgwaves.com/topic/performing-echocardiographic-studies/ (accessed March 2022).
7. Harkness A, Ring L, Augustine DX, Oxborough D, Robinson S, Sharma V (2020) Normal reference intervals for cardiac dimensions and function for use in echocardiographic practice: a guideline from the British Society of Echocardiography. *Echo Research and Practice*, **7**(1), G1–G18.
8. Ciampi Q, Villari B (2007) Role of echocardiography in diagnosis and risk stratification in heart failure with left ventricular systolic dysfunction. *Cardiovascular Ultrasound*, **5**(1), 34.
9. Cheesman MG, Leech G, Chambers J, Monaghan MJ, Nihoyannopoulos P (1998) Central role of echocardiography

in the diagnosis and assessment of heart failure. *Heart*, **80**(suppl 1), S1–S5.

10. Schneider M, Aschauer S, Mascherbauer J et al. (2019) Echocardiographic assessment of right ventricular function: current clinical practice. *International Journal of Cardiovascular Imaging*, **35**(1), 49–56.

11. Isgro G, Yusuff HO, Zochios V (2021) The right ventricle in COVID-19 lung injury: proposed mechanisms, management, and research gaps. *Journal of Cardiothoracic and Vascular Anesthesia*, **35**(6), 1568–1572.

12. Zochios V, Lau G, Conway H, Yusuff HO (2021) Protecting the injured right ventricle in COVID-19 acute respiratory distress syndrome: can clinicians personalize interventions and reduce mortality? *Journal of Cardiothoracic and Vascular Anesthesia*, **35**(11), 3325–3330.

13. Naeije R, Badagliacca R (2017) The overloaded right heart and ventricular interdependence. *Cardiovascular Research*, **113**(12), 1474–1485.

14. Miller A, Mandeville J (2016) Predicting and measuring fluid responsiveness with echocardiography. *Echo Research and Practice*, **3**(2), G1–G12.

15. Miller A, Peck M, Clark T et al. (2021) *FUSIC HD. Comprehensive haemodynamic assessment with ultrasound. Journal of the Intensive Care Society*, **2021**, 17511437211010032.

16. Libby P, Zipes D (2018) *Braunwald's Heart Disease: A Textbook of Cardiovascular Medicine*. Elsevier, St Louis.

17. Stashko E, Meer J (2021) *Cardiac Tamponade*. StatPearls Publishing, Treasure Island.

18. Evangelista A, Flachskampf FA, Erbel R et al. (2010) Echocardiography in aortic diseases: EAE recommendations for clinical practice. *European Journal of Echocardiography*, **11**(8), 645–658.

19. Fields JM, Davis J, Girson L et al. (2017) Transthoracic echocardiography for diagnosing pulmonary embolism: a systematic review and meta-analysis. *Journal of the American Society of Echocardiography*, **30**(7), 714–723.

20. Via G, Price S, Storti E (2011) Echocardiography in the sepsis syndromes. *Critical Ultrasound Journal*, **3**(2), 71–85.

Chapter 27 Central Venous Catheter and Arterial Catheter Insertion

1. Zisquit J, Velasquez J, Nedeff N. Allen Test. StatPearls, Treasure Island. www.ncbi.nlm.nih.gov/books/NBK507816/ (accessed March 2022).

Chapter 28 Pleural Procedures

1. BTS (2018) Statement on criteria for specialist referral, admission, discharge and follow-up for adults with respiratory disease. http://dx.doi.org/10.1136/thx.2007.087627 (accessed March 2022).

2. Hooper C, Lee YCG, Maskell N, BTS Pleural Guideline Group (2020) Investigation of a unilateral pleural effusion in adults: British Thoracic Society pleural disease guideline 2010. *Thorax*, **65**, ii4–ii17.

3. Evison M, Blyth KG, Bhatnagar R et al. (2018) Providing safe and effective pleural medicine services in the UK: an aspirational statement from UK pleural physicians. *BMJ Open Respiratory Research*, 5, e000307.

4. National Patient Safety Alert (2020) Deterioration due to rapid offload of pleural effusion fluid from chest drains. www.england.nhs.uk/wp-content/uploads/2020/12/NatPSA-Pleural-Effusion-FINAL-v3.pdf (accessed March 2022).

5. Bielsa S, Panades MJ, Egido R et al. (2008) [Accuracy of pleural fluid cytology in malignant effusions.] *Anales d Medicina Interna*, **25**, 173–177.

6. Rahman NM, Ali N, Brown G et al. (2010) Local anaesthetic thoracoscopy: British Thoracic Society pleural disease guideline 2010. *Thorax*, **65**, ii54–60.

Chapter 30 The Advanced Practitioner's Role in Organ Donation and Transplantation

1. NHS Blood and Transplant Services (2021) Organ Donation and Transplantation. Donation after circulatory death. www.odt.nhs.uk/deceased-donation/best-practice-guidance/donation-after-circulatory-death/ (accessed March 2022).

2. Faculty of Intensive Care Medicine (2021) Diagnosing Death for Donation after Circulatory Death (DCD) for Advanced Critical Care Practitioners. www.ficm.ac.uk/sites/default/files/accp_dcd_guidance.pdf (accessed March 2022).

3. Academy of Medical Royal Colleges (2008) A Code of Practice for the Diagnosis and Confirmation of Death. https://aomrc.org.uk/wp-content/uploads/2016/04/Code_Practice_Confirmation_Diagnosis_Death_1008-4.pdf (accessed March 2022).

4. Faculty of Intensive Care Medicines (2021) Diagnosing Death using Neurological Criteria. www.ficm.ac.uk/news-events-education/news/diagnosing-death-using-neurological-criteria (accessed March 2022).

5. National Institute for Health and Care Excellence (2016) Organ donation for transplantation: improving donor identification and consent rates for deceased organ donation. CG135. www.nice.org.uk/guidance/cg135/resources/organ-donation-for-transplantation-improving-donor-identification-and-consent-rates-for-deceased-organ-donation-pdf-35109512048581 (accessed March 2022).

6. Mental Capacity Act (2005) HMSO, London. www.legislation.gov.uk/ukpga/2005/9/contents (accessed March 2022).

Chapter 31 Verification of Death

1. Office for National Statistics (2020) Deaths registered in England and Wales: 2020. www.ons.gov.uk/peoplepopulationandcommunity/birthsdeathsandmarriages/deaths/bulletins/deathsregistrationsummarytables/2020 (accessed March 2022).

2. Academy of Medical Royal Colleges (2008) A Code of Practice for the Diagnosis and Confirmation of Death. www.aomrc.org.uk/aomrc/admin/reports/docs/DofD-final.pdf (accessed March 2022).

3. Hospice UK (2020) Care after Death. Guidance for staff responsible for care after death. www.hospiceuk.org/what-we-offer/publications?kwrd=care%20after%20death&cat=72e54312-4ccd-608d-ad24-ff0000fd3330 (accessed March 2022).

4. Ministry of Justice (2020) Revised guidance for registered medical practitioners on the Notification of Deaths Regulations. https://assets.publishing.service.gov.uk/government/uploads/system/uploads/attachment_data/file/878083/revised-guidance-for-registered-medical-practitioners-on-the-notification-of-deaths-regulations.pdf (accessed March 2022).

5. Public Health England (2021) Guidance. Notifiable diseases and causative organisms: how to report. www.gov.uk/guidance/notifiable-diseases-and-causative-organisms-how-to-report#list-of-notifiable-diseases (accessed March 2022).

6. Births and Deaths Registration Act (1953) www.legislation.gov.uk/ukpga/Eliz2/1-2/20/section/28/enacted (accessed March 2022).

7. Association of Ambulance Chief Executives (2019) *Joint Royal Colleges Ambulance Liason Committee (JRCALC) Clinical Guidelines 2019*. Class Professional Publishing, Somerset.

8. Department of Health (2009) End of life care strategy: Quality markers and measures for end of life care. https://dementiapartnerships.com/wp-content/uploads/sites/2/EndofLifeQualityMarkers.pdf (accessed March 2022).

9. National Institute for Health and Care Excellence (2011) End of life care for adults. Quality Standard 13 (QS13). www.nice.org.uk/guidance/qs13 (accessed March 2022).

10. British Medical Association (2020) Verification of Death (VoD), Completion of Medical Certificates of Cause of Death (MCCD) and Cremation Forms in the Community in England and Wales. www.bma.org.uk/media/2843/bma-verification-of-death-vod-july-2020.pdf (accessed March 2022).

11. Scottish Government (2017) Verification of death by a registered healthcare professional: Chief Nursing Officer Guidance. www.gov.scot/publications/verification-of-death-by-a-registered-healthcare-professional-chief-nursing-officer-guidance/ (accessed March 2022).

12. British Medical Association (2020) Guidance for Remote Verification of Expected Death (VoED) Out of Hospital. www.bma.org.uk/media/2323/bma-guidelines-for-remote-voed-april-2020.pdf (accessed March 2022).

13. Faculty of Intensive Care Medicine (2021) Diagnosing Death for Donation after Circulatory Death (DCD) for Advanced Critical Care Practitioners. www.ficm.ac.uk/sites/default/files/accp_dcd_guidance.pdf (accessed March 2022).

14. Organ Donation Taskforce (2008) Organs for Transplant. www.dh.gov.uk (accessed March 2022).

15. Intensive Care Society (2021) Form for the diagnosis of death using neurological criteria. Long version. www.ics.ac.uk/Society/Guidance/PDFs/Diagnosis_of_Death (accessed March 2022).

16. Intensive Care Society (2021) Form for the diagnosis of death using neurological criteria. Short version. www.ics.ac.uk/Society/Guidance/PDFs/Diagnosis_of_Death (accessed March 2022).

17. Intensive Care Society (2021) Supplementary ECMO guideline. www.ics.ac.uk/Society/Guidance/PDFs/Diagnosis_of_Death accessed March 2022).

18. General Medical Council (2010) Treatment and care towards the end of life. www.gmc-uk.org/-/media/documents/treatment-and-care-towards-the-end-of-life---english-1015_pdf-48902105.pdf?la=en&hash=41EF651C76FDBEC141FB674C08261661BDEFD004 (accessed March 2022).

19. National Institute for Health and Care Excellence (2011) Organ donation for transplantation. Improving donor identification and consent rates for decreased organ donation. Clinical Guideline 135. www.nice.org.uk/guidance/cg135/evidence/full-guideline-pdf-184994893 (accessed March 2022).

20. University of Warwick and Joint Royal Colleges Ambulance Liason Committee (2006) Recognition of Life Extinct by Ambulance Clinicians. https://warwick.ac.uk/fac/sci/med/research/hsri/emergencycare/prehospitalcare/jrcalcstakeholderwebsite/guidelines/recognition_of_life_extinct_by_ambulance_clinicians_2006.pdf (accessed March 2022).

Chapter 32 Home-based Care, Crisis Response and Rehabilitation

1. NICE (2013) Myocardial infarction: cardiac rehabilitation and prevention of further cardiovascular disease. CG172. www.nice.org.uk/guidance/cg172 (accessed March 2022).

2. NICE (2013) Stroke rehabilitation in adults. CG162. www.nice.org.uk/guidance/cg162 (accessed March 2022).

3. NICE (2020) myCOPD for self-management of chronic obstructive pulmonary disease. MIB214. www.nice.org.uk/advice/mib214 (accessed March 2022).

Chapter 33 Frailty

1. Fried LP, Tangen CM, Watson J et al. (2001) Frailty in older adults: evidence for a phenotype. *Journals of Gerontology: Series A*, 56(3),146–156.

2. Rockwood K, Theou O (2020) Using the Clinical Frailty Scale in allocating scarce health care resources. *Canadian Geriatrics Journal*, 23(3), 254–259.

3. Song X, Mitnitski A, Rockwood K (2010) Prevalence and 10-year outcomes of frailty in older adults in relation to deficit accumulation. *Journal of the American Geriatric Society*, **58**, 681–687.

4. British Geriatric Society (2018) *Fit for Frailty Part 1. Consensus best practice guidance*. www.bgs.org.uk/sites/default/files/content/resources/files/2018-05-23/fff_full.pdf (accessed March 2022).

5. British Geriatric Society (2021) *Silver Book II*. www.bgs.org.uk/resources/resource-series/silver-book-ii (accessed March 2022).

6. Ellis G, Gardner M, Tsiachristas A et al. (2017) Comprehensive geriatric assessment for older adults admitted to hospital. *Cochrane Database of Systematic Reviews*, 9, CD006211.

Chapter 34 Advanced Practitioner-Led Inter- and Intrahospital Transfer

1. Droogh JM, Smit M, Absalom AR, Ligtenberg JJ, Zijlstra JG (2015) Transferring the critically ill patient: are we there yet? *Critical Care*, **19**(62), 1–7.

2. Iwashyna TJ (2012) The incomplete infrastructure for interhospital patient transfer. *Critical Care Medicine*, **40**, 2470–2478.

3. Foex B, Van Zwanenberg G, Ball J et al. (2019) *Guidelines for the Transport of the Critically Ill Adult*. Intensive Care Society, London.

4. Grier S, Brant G, Gould TH, von Vopelius-Feldt J, Thompson J (2020) Critical care transfer in an English critical care network: analysis of 1124 transfers delivered by an ad-hoc system. *Journal of the Intensive Care Society*, **21**(1), 33–39.

5. Bourn S, Wijesingha S, Nordmann G (2018) Transfer of the critically ill adult patient. *British Journal of Anaesthesia Education*, **18**(3), 63–68.

6. Droogh JM, Smit M, Hut J, de Vos R, Ligtenberg JJ, Zijlstra JG (2012) Inter-hospital transport of critically ill patients: expect surprises. *Critical Care*, **16**(1), R26.

7. Flabouris A, Runciman WB, Levings B (2006) Incidents during out-of-hospital patient transportation. *Anaesthesia and Intensive Care*, **34**, 228–236.

8. Healthcare Safety Investigation branch (2019) *Transfer of critically ill adults*. Summary report, I2017/002A. Healthcare Safety Investigation Branch, London.

9. Association of Anaesthetists of Great Britain and Ireland (2009) *AAGBI Safety Guideline: Interhospital Transfer*. AAGBI, London.

10. Foëx B, Fortune PM, Lawn C (2019) *Neonatal, Adult and Paediatric Safe Transfer and Retrieval: A Practical Approach to Transfers*. Wiley-Blackwell, Oxford.

11. Ash A, Whitehead C, Hughes B, Williams D, Nayyar V (2015) Impact of a transport checklist on adverse events during intra-hospital transport of critically ill patients. *Australian Critical Care*, **28**(1), 49–50.

12. Choi H, Shin S, Ro Y, Kim D, Shin S, Kwak Y (2012) A before- and after-intervention trial for reducing unexpected events during the intrahospital transport of emergency patients. *American Journal of Emergency Medicine*, **30**(8), 1433–1440.

13. Mowplass HC, Enfield, KB, Verghese GM et al. (2012) Interhospital intensive care transfer checklist facilitates early implementation of critical therapies and is associated with improved outcomes. *American Journal of Respiratory and Critical Care Medicine*, **185**, A6575.

14. Parmentier-Decrucq E, Poissy J, Favory R et al. (2013) Adverse events during intrahospital transport of critically ill patients: incidence and risk factors. *Annals of Intensive Care*, **3**(1), 10.

15. Paediatric Intensive Care Society (2015) *Quality Standards for the Care of the Critically Ill*, 5th edn. Paediatric Intensive Care Society, London.

16. National Institute of Clinical Excellence (2018) Standardised systems of care for intra- and inter-hospital transfers. Emergency and acute medical care in over 16s: service delivery and organisation. NICE guideline 94. National Institute of Clinical Excellence, London.

17. Faculty of Intensive Care Medicine (2015) *Curriculum for Training for Advanced Critical Care Practitioners*. Faculty of Intensive Care Medicine, London.

18. Denton G, Green L, Palmer M et al. (2019) The provision of central venous access, transfer of critically ill patients and advanced airway management: are advanced critical care practitioners safe and effective? *Journal of the Intensive Care Society*, **20**(3), 248–254.

Chapter 36 Non-pharmacological and Pharmacological Interventions

1. NICE (n.d.) Making Every Contact Count. https://stpsupport.nice.org.uk/mecc/index.html#group-Shared-learning-case-studies-M5U2aiZwo4 (accessed March 2022).

Chapter 38 Prescribing Practice and Patient Education

1. Agency for Healthcare Research and Quality (2013) Patient Education Materials Assessment Tool (PEMAT) and User's Guide. www.ahrq.gov/health-literacy/patient-education/pemat.html (accessed March 2022).

Chapter 39 Non-medical Authorisation of Blood Components

1. Blood Safety and Quality Regulations (2005) www.legislation.gov.uk/uksi/2005/50/contents/made (accessed March 2022).
2. Medicines (Medicines Act 1968 Amendment) Regulations 1977. www.legislation.gov.uk/uksi/1977/1050/made (accessed March 2022).
3. Green J, Pirie L (2009) A Framework to Support Nurses and Midwives Making the Clinical Decision and Providing the Written Instruction for Blood Component Transfusion. www.transfusionguidelines.org/document-library/documents/bt-framework/download-file/BTFramework-final010909.pdf (accessed March 2022)
4. Robinson S, Harris A, Atkinson S *et al.* (2018) The administration of blood components: a British Society for Haematology Guideline. *Transfusion Medicine*, **28**, 3–21.
5. Medicines Act (1968) www.legislation.gov.uk/ukpga/1968/67 (accessed March 2022).
6. Human Medicines Regulations (2012) www.legislation.gov.uk/uksi/2012/1916/contents/made (accessed March 2022).
7. Royal Pharmaceutical Society (2021) A Competency Framework for all Prescribers. www.rpharms.com/resources/frameworks/prescribing-competency-framework/competency-framework#framework (accessed March 2022).
8. National Institute for Health and Care Excellence (2015) Blood transfusion guidelines [NG24]. www.nice.org.uk/guidance/ng24 (accessed March 2022).
9. Narayan S, Poles D, on behalf of the Serious Hazards of Transfusion (SHOT) Steering Group (2021) The 2020 Annual SHOT Report. www.shotuk.org/shot-reports/report-summary-and-supplement-2020/2020-annual-shot-report-individual-chapters/ (accessed March 2022).
10. Tinegate H, Birchall J, Gray A, *et al.* (2012) Guideline on the investigation and management of acute transfusion reactions. Prepared by the BCSH Blood Transfusion Task Force. *British Journal of Haematology*, **159**, 143–153.

Chapter 40 Leadership in Healthcare Settings

1. O'Neil K. (2013) *Patient-centred Leadership: Rediscovering Our Purpose*. King's Fund, London.
2. Care Quality Commission (2014) Working together to assess leadership. www.cqc.org.uk/news/stories/working-together-assess-leadership (accessed March 2022).
3. NHS Leadership Academy (2013) *Healthcare Leadership Model: The Nine Dimensions of Leadership Behaviour*. NHS Leadership Academy, London.

4. Jasper M, Jumaa M (2008) *Effective Healthcare Leadership*. John Wiley & Sons, Chichester.
5. West M, Armit K, Loewenthal L, Eckert R, West T, Lee A (2015) *Leadership and Leadership Development in Health Care: The Evidence Base*. King's Fund, London.
6. Ham C, Baker G, Docherty J et al. (2011) *The Future of Leadership and Management in the NHS: No More Heroes*. King's Fund, London.
7. King's Fund (2014) *Culture and Leadership in the NHS. The King's Fund 2014 survey*. King's Fund, London.
8. Alderwick H, Dixon J (2019) The NHS long term plan. *British Medical Journal*, **364**, 184.
9. Eckert R, West M, Altman D, Steward K, Pasmore WA (2014) *Delivering a Collective Leadership Strategy for Health Care*. King's Fund, London.
10. West M, Eckert R, Collins B, Chowla R (2017) *Caring to Change. How Compassionate Leadership can Stimulate Innovation in Health Care*. King's Fund, London.
11. West MA (2021) *Compassionate Leadership : Sustaining Wisdom, Humanity and Prescence in Health and Social Care*. Swirling Leaf Press.
12. Manley K, Sanders K, Cardiff S, Webster J (2011) Effective workplace culture: the attributes, enabling factors and consequences of a new concept. *International Practice Development Journal*, **1**(2), 1–29.
13. Vize R (2017) *Swimming Together or Sinking Alone: Health, CARE and the Art of Systems Leadership*. Institute of Healthcare Management, London.

Chapter 43 Educational Leadership

1. NHSE (2017) *Multi-professional Framework for Advanced Clinical Practice in England*. NHS England, London.
2. Lamb A, Martin-Misener R, Bryant-Lukosius D, Latimer M (2018) Describing the leadership capabilities of advanced practice nurses using a qualitative descriptive study. *Nursing Open*, **5**, 400–413.

Chapter 44 Research Leadership

1. Grimshaw JM, Patey AM, Kirkham KR et al. (2020) De-implementing wisely: developing the evidence base to reduce low-value care. *BMJ Quality & Safety*, **29**, 409417.
2. Westwood G, Fader M, Roberts L, Green SM, Prieto J, Bayliss-Pratt L (2013) How clinical academics are transforming patient care. *Health Service Journal*, **123**(6368), 28–29.

Chapter 45 Improving Quality of Care

1. King's Fund and Health Foundation (2017) Making the case for quality improvement: lessons for NHS boards and leaders. www.kingsfund.org.uk/publications/making-case-quality-improvement (accessed March 2022).
2. NHS (2019) Long Term Plan. www.longtermplan.nhs.uk/ (accessed March 2022).
3. Health Education England (2017) Multi-Professional Framework for Advanced Clinical Practice in England. https://advanced-practice.hee.nhs.uk/multi-professional-framework-for-advanced-clinical-practice-in-england/ (accessed March 2022).
4. International Council of Nurses (2020) *Guidelines on Advanced Practice Nursing*. International Council of Nurses, Geneva.
5. Skills for Health (2018) Advanced Clinical Practitioner (Degree) Standard. https://haso.skillsforhealth.org.uk/standards/#standard-355 (accessed March 2022).
6. Nursing and Midwifery Council (2015) *Code of Professional Conduct*. Nursing and Midwifery Council, London.
7. Health and Care Professions Council (2016) *Standards of Conduct, Performance and Ethics*. Health and Care Professions Council, London.

8. NHS England and NHS Improvement (2021) Quality, service improvement and redesign (QSIR) tools. www.england.nhs.uk/sustainableimprovement/qsir-programme/qsir-tools/ (accessed March 2022).
9. NHS Institute for Innovation and Improvement (2010) The Handbook of Quality and Service Improvement Tools. https://webarchive.nationalarchives.gov.uk/ukgwa/20160805122939/http://www.nhsiq.nhs.uk/media/2760650/the_handbook_of_quality_and_service_improvement_tools_2010.pdf (accessed March 2022).
10. Jones B (2019) How to get started in quality improvement. *British Medical Journal*, **364**, k5408.
11. Hughes RG (2008) Tools and strategies for quality improvement and patient safety. In: Hughes RG (ed.) *Patient Safety and Quality: An Evidence-Based Handbook for Nurses*. Agency for Healthcare Research and Quality, Rockville.
12. Ogbeiwi O (2017) Why written objectives need to be really SMART. *British Journal of Healthcare Management*, **23**(7), 324–336.
13. Armstrong N, Herbert G, Aveling EL, Dixon-Woods M, Martin G (2013) Optimizing patient involvement in quality improvement. *Health Expectations*, **16**(3), 36–47.
14. Wandersman A, Alia KA, Cook B, Ramaswamy R (2015) Integrating empowerment evaluation and quality improvement to achieve healthcare improvement outcomes. *BMJ Quality and Safety*, **24**(10), 645–652.
15. Crowl A, Sharma A, Sorge L, Sorensen T (2003) Accelerating quality improvement within your organization: applying the Model for Improvement. *Journal of the American Pharmacists' Association*, **55**(4), 364–376.

Chapter 46 Exploring the Challenges with Advanced Clinical Practice Education

1. Taylor V (2021) *Workplace Supervision and Support for Trainee Advanced Clinical Practitioners across West Yorkshire*. Report to HEE Yorkshire and the Humber.
2. Council of Deans of Health (2018) Advanced clinical practice education in England. https://councilofdeans.org.uk/wp-content/uploads/2018/11/081118-FINAL-ACP-REPORT.pdf (accessed March 2022).
3. Health Education England (2021) Workplace supervision for advanced clinical practice. https://advanced-practice.hee.nhs.uk/workplace-supervision-for-advanced-clinical-practice-2/ (accessed March 2022).

Chapter 50 Integrating Simulation and Virtual Reality into Clinical Practice Education

1. Astbury J, Ferguson J, Silverthorne J, Willis S, Schafheutle E (2021) High-fidelity simulation-based education in pre-registration healthcare programmes: a systematic review of reviews to inform collaborative and interprofessional best practice. *Journal of Interprofessional Care*, **35**(4), 622–632.
2. Association for Simulated Practice in Healthcare (2016) The ASPiH St*andards Framework and Guidance: Standards for Simulation-based Education*. ASPiH, Lichfield.
3. Department of Health (2011) *A Framework for Technology Enhanced Learning*. Department of Health, London.

Chapter 51 The Advanced Practitioner s Clinical Educator and Supervisor

1. General Pharmaceutical Council (2017) Standards for pharmacy professionals. www.pharmacyregulation.org/sites/default/files/standards_for_pharmacy_professionals_may_2017_0.pdf (accessed March 2022).
2. Health Care Professions Council (2018) Standards of conduct, performance and ethics. www.hcpc-uk.org/globalassets/resources/standards/standards-of-conduct-performance-and-ethics.pdf (accessed March 2022).
3. Nursing and Midwifery Council (2018) The Code. *Professional Standards of Practice and behaviour for nurses, midwives and nursing associates*. www.nmc.org.uk/globalassets/sitedocuments/nmc-publications/nmc-code.pdf (accessed March 2022).
4. Bloom B.S (1956) *Taxonomy of Educational Objectives, Handbook I: The Cognitive Domain*. David McKay Co. Inc., New York.
5. Verenna AA, Noble KA, Pearson HE, Miller SM (2018) Role of comprehension on performance at higher levels of Bloom's taxonomy: findings from assessments of healthcare professional students. *Anatomical Sciences Education*, **11**(5), 433–444.
6. Miller GE (1990) The assessment of clinical skills/competence/performance. *Academic Medicine*, **65**(9), S63–S67.
7. Miller A, Archer J (2010) Impact of workforce based assessment on doctors' education and performance: a systematic review. *British Medical Journal*, **341**, c5064.
8. Pelgrim EAM, Kramer AWM. Mokkink HGA, van der Vleuten CPM (2012) The process of feedback in workplace-based assessment: organisation, delivery, continuity. *Medical Education*, **46**(6), 604–612.
9. Shute V.J (2008) Focus on formative feedback. *Review of Educational Research*, **78**(1), 153–189.
10. Ende J (1983) Feedback in clinical medical education. *JAMA*, **250**(6), 777–781.
11. Pendleton D, Schofield T, Tate P, Havelock P (2008) *The New Consultation: Developing Doctor-Patient Communication*. Oxford University Press, Oxford.
12. Silverman JD, Kurtz SM, Draper J (12996) The Calgary-Cambridge approach to communication skills teaching 1: Agenda-led, outcome-based analysis of the consultation. *Education for General Practice*, **4**, 288–299.
13. Duffy K (2003) Failing students: a qualitative study of factors that influence the decisions regarding assessment of students' competence in practice. www.researchgate.net/publication/251693467_Failing_Students_A_Qualitative_Study_of_Factors_that_Influence_the_Decisions_Regarding_Assessment_of_Students%27_Competence_in_Practice (accessed March 2022).
14. Luhanga FL, Larocque S, MacEwan L, Gwekwerere YN, Danyluk P (2014) Exploring the issue of failure to fail in professional education programs: a multidisciplinary study. *Journal of University Teaching & Learning Practice*, **11**(2), article 3.
15. Sweet C, Blythe H, Carpenter R (2016) Why the revised Bloom's Taxonomy is essential to creative teaching. *National Teaching & Learning Forum*, **26**(1), 7–9.
16. Al-Eraky M, Marei H (2016) A fresh look at Miller's Pyramid: assessment at the 'is' and 'do' levels. *Medical Education*, **50**(12), 1253–1257.

Chapter 52 Ethical and Governance Principles

1. World Medical Association (2013) Declaration of Helsinki – ethical principles for medical research involving human subjects. www.wma.net/policies-post/wma-declaration-of-helsinki-ethical-principles-for-medical-research-involving-human-subjects/ (accessed March 2022).
2. Beauchamp TL, Childress JF (2001) *Principles of Biomedical Ethics*, 5th edn. Oxford University Press, New York.
3. UK Caldicott Guardian Council (2017) *A Manual for Caldicott Guardians*. www.ukcgc.ck/caldicott-guardians-manual (accessed March 2022).
4. NHS Health Research Authority (2020) UK Policy Framework for Health and Social Care Research. www.hra.nhs.uk/planning-and-improving-research/policies-standards-legislation/uk-policy-framework-health-social-care-research/uk-policy-framework-health-and-social-care-research/

Chapter 53 Research Design and Methods

1. National Health Service (2014) NHS Five Year Forward View. www.england.nhs.uk/publication/nhs-five-year-forward-view/ (accessed March 2022).
2. NHS England (2019) *The NHS Long Term Plan*. NHS England, London.
3. Health Education England (2017) *Multi-professional Framework for Advanced Clinical Practice in England*. Health Education England, London.
4. Castro-Sánchez E, Russell AM, Dolman L, Wells M (2021) What place does nurse-led research have in the COVID-19 pandemic? *International Nursing Review*, **68**, 214–218.
5. Glasper A, Farrelly R (2009) Health care governance. In: Glasper A, McEwing G, Richardson J (eds) *Foundation Studies for Caring*. Palgrave Macmillan, Basingstoke.

Chapter 54 Critical Appraisal Skills

1. Moule P (2020) *Making Sense of Research*. Sage, London.
2. Waterkemper R, Prado M, Medina J, Reibnitz K (2014) Development of critical attitude in fundamentals of professional care discipline: a case study. *Nurse Education Today*, **34**(4), 581–585.
3. Polit D, Beck C (2018) *Essentials of Nursing Research: Appraising Evidence for Nursing Practice*, 9th edn. Wolters Kluwer, Philadelphia.
4. Centre for Reviews and Dissemination (2009) Systematic Reviews: CRD's guidance for undertaking reviews in health care. www.york.ac.uk/media/crd/Systematic_Reviews.pdf (accessed March 2022).

Chapter 55 Audit and Quality Improvement Sciences

1. Health Foundation (2011) *Evidence Scan: Improvement Science*. Health Foundation, London.
2. Chatfield C (2020) Quality improvement. In: Swanwick T, Vaux E (eds) *ABC of Quality Improvement in Healthcare*. Wiley-Blackwell, Oxford, pp.5–9.
3. Marshall M, Pronovost P, Dixon-Woods M (2013) Promotion of improvement as a science. *Lancet*, **381**, 419–421.
4. Swanwick T, Vaux E (eds) (2020) *ABC of Quality Improvement in Healthcare*. Wiley-Blackwell, Oxford.
5. Clark DM, Silvester K, Knowles S (2013) Lean management systems: creating a culture of continous quality improvement. *Journal of Clinical Pathology*, **66**, 638–643.
6. Gupta S, Jain SJ (2013) A literature review of lean manufactoring. *International Journal of Science and Engineering Management*, **8**, 241–249.
7. Pepper MP, Spedding TA (2010) The ivolution of Lean Six Sigma. *International Journal of Quality & Reliability Management*, **27**, 138–155.
8. Goh TN (2011) Six Sigma in industry: some obervations after twenty-five years. *Quality and Reliability Engineering International*, **27**, 221–227.
9. De Feo JA, Barnard W (2005) *JURAN Institiute's Six Sigma Breakthrough and Beyond – Quality Performance Breakthrough Methods*. McGraw-Hill, New York.
10. Evans K (2020) Models of improvement. In: Swanwick T, Vaux E (eds) *ABC of Quality Improvement in Healthcare*. Wiley-Blackwell, Oxford, pp.14–20.
11. Senapati NR (2004) Six Sigma in health care. *Leadership in Health Services*, **16**, 1–5.
12. Nakhai B, Neves JS (2009) The challenges of six sigma in improving service quality. *International Journal of Quality & Reliability Management*, **26**, 663–684.
13. Sehwail L, DeYong C (2003) Six Sigma in health care. *Leadership in Health Services*, **16**, 1–5.
14. Public Health England (2017) *Technical Guide: RAG Rating Indicator Values*. Public Health England, London.
15. NHS England (2020) Statistical process control tool. www.england.nhs.uk/statistical-process-control-tool/ (accessed March 2022).
16. Walshe K, Harvey G, Jas P (2010) *Connecting Knowledge and Performance in Public Services: From Knowing to Doing*. Cambridge University Press, Cambridge.
17. IASSC (2021) IASSC Lean Six Sigma Certification. https://iassc.org/about/ (accessed March 2022).
18. Professional Development (2020) Understanding Lean Six Sigma Belts. www.professionaldevelopment.ie/lean-six-sigma-belts (accessed March 2022).
19. Antony J (2004) Some pros and cons of Six Sigma: an academic perspective. *TQM Magazine*, **16**, 303–306.
20. Henrique DB, Moacir GF (2018) A systematic litertaure review of empirical research in Lean and Six Sigma in healthcare. *Total Quality Management & Business Excellence*, **31**, 429–449.
21. Wheat B, Mills C, Carnell M (2003) *Leaning Into Six Sigma: A Parable of the Journey to Six Sigma and a Lean Enterprise*. McGraw-Hill, New York.
22. Salah S, Rahim A, Carretero J (2010) The integration of Six Sigma and lean management. *International Journal of Lean Six Sigma*, **1**, 249–274.
23. Salah S, Rahim A (2019) *An Integrated Company-Wide Management System: Combining Lean Six Sigma with Process Improvement*. Springer, Cham, pp.49–93.
24. Vorne (2019) Top 25 Lean Tools www.leanproduction.com/top-25-lean-tools.html (accessed March 2022).
25. Bicheno J, Holweg M (2016) *The Lean Toolbox: A Handbook for Lean Transformation*, 5th edn. PICSIE Books, Buckingham.
26. Voehl F, Harrington HJ, Mignosa C et al. (2013) *The Lean Six SIgma Black Belt Handbook: Tools and Methods for Process Acceleration*. CRC Press, Boca Raton.
27. Langley GL, Moen R, Nolan KM et al. (2009) *The Improvement Guide: A Practical Approach to Enhancing Organizational Performance*. Jossey-Bass, San Francisco.
28. Mountford J (2020) Development and testing solutions. In: Swanwick T, Vaux E (eds) *ABC of Quality Improvement in Healthcare*. Wiley-Blackwell, Oxford, pp.34–38.
29. Reed JE, Card AJ (2016) The problem with Plan-Do-Study-Act Cycles. *BMJ Quality & Safety*, **25**, 147–152.
30. Taylor MJ, McNicholas C, Nicolay C et al. (2014) Systematic review of the application of the plan-do-study-act method to improve quality in healthcare. *BMJ Quality & Safety*, **23**, 290–298.
31. Robert G (2013) Particpatory action research: using experience-based co-design (EBCG) to improve healthcare services. In: Ziebland S, Calabrese J, Coulter A et al. (eds) *Understanding and Using Experienes of Health and Illness*. Oxford University Press, Oxford.
32. King's Fund (2021) Experience-based co-design toolkit. www.kingsfund.org.uk/projects/ebcd (accessed March 2022).
33. Bate SP, Robert G (2007) *Bringing User Experience to Healthcare Improvement: The Concepts, Methods and Practices of Experience-Based Design*. Radcliffe Publishing, Oxford.
34. Green T, Bonner A, Teleni L et al. (2020) Use and reporting of experience-based codesign studeos in the healthcare setting: a systematic review. *BMJ Quality & Safety*, **29**, 64–76.

Chapter 56 From Bench to Bedside: Integrating Research into Practice

1. Department of Health (1992) *The Health of the Nation – A Strategy for health in England*. Her Majesty's Stationery Office, London.
2. Sacket DL, Rosenberg W, Muir Gray J et al. (1996) Evidence based medicine: what it is and what it isn't. *British Medical Journal*, **312**, 71–72.
3. Hamer S, Collinson G (2005) *Achieving Evidence-based Practice. A Handbook for Practitioners*, 2nd edn. Baillière Tindall, Edinburgh.

4. Petrie A, Sabin C (2020) *Medical Statistics at a Glance*, 4th edn. Wiley-Blackwell, Chichester.
5. Centre for Evidence-Based Medicine (2011) CEBM Levels of Evidence. www.cebm.ox.ac.uk/resources/levels-of-evidence/ocebm-levels-of-evidence (accessed March 2022).
6. Centre for Reviews and Dissemination (2009) Systematic Reviews: CRD's guidance for undertaking reviews in health care. https://www.york.ac.uk/media/crd/Systematic_Reviews.pdf (accessed March 2022).
7. Wiess CH, Krishnan JA, Au DH et al (2016) An official American Thoracic Society Research Statement: Implementation science in pulmonary, critical care and sleep medicine. www.atsjournals.org/doi/pdf/10.1164/rccm.201608-1690ST (accessed March 2022).
8. Glasgow RE, Vogt TM, Boles SM (1999) Evaluating the public health impact of health promotion interventions: the RE-AIM framework. www.ncbi.nlm.nih.gov/pmc/articles/PMC1508772/pdf/amjph00009-0018.pdf (accessed March 2022).
9. Cabana MD, Rand CS, Powe NR et al. (1999) Why don't physicians follow clinical practice guidelines? A framework for improvement. *Journal of the American Medical Association*, **282**, 1458–1465.
10. Greenhalgh T (2019) *How to Read a Paper: The Basics of Evidence-Based Medicine*, 6th edn. Wiley-Blackwell, Chichester.

Index